ELSEVIER

1600 John F. Kennedy Boulevard • Suite 1800 • Philadelphia, Pennsylvania, 19103-2899

http://www.theclinics.com

PHYSICAL MEDICINE AND REHABILITATION CLINICS OF NORTH AMERICA Volume 28, Number 2
May 2017 ISSN 1047-9651, ISBN 978-0-323-52856-6

Editor: Lauren Boyle
Developmental Editor: Donald Mumford

Reprints. For copies of 100 or more of articles in this publication, please contact the Commercial Reprints Department, Elsevier Inc., 360 Park Avenue South, New York, NY 10010-1710. Tel.: 212-633-3874; Fax: 212-633-3820; E-mail: reprints@elsevier.com.

Physical Medicine and Rehabilitation Clinics of North America (ISSN 1047-9651) is published quarterly by Elsevier Inc., 360 Park Avenue South, New York, NY 10010-1710. Months of issue are February, May, August, and November. Business and Editorial Offices: 1600 John F. Kennedy Blvd., Suite 1800, Philadelphia, PA 19103-2899. Customer Service Office: 3251 Riverport Lane, Maryland Heights, MO 63043. Periodicals postage paid at New York, NY and additional mailing offices. Subscription price per year is $288.00 (US individuals), $560.00 (US institutions), $100.00 (US students), $210.00 (Canadian individuals), $737.00 (Canadian institutions), $210.00 (Canadian students), $210.00 (foreign individuals), $737.00 (foreign institutions), and $210.00 (foreign students). Foreign air speed delivery is included in all *Clinics* subscription prices. All prices are subject to change without notice. **POSTMASTER:** Send address changes to *Physical Medicine and Rehabilitation Clinics of North America*, Customer Service Office: Elsevier Health Sciences Division, Subscription Customer Service, 3251 Riverport Lane, Maryland Heights, MO 63043. **Customer Service: 1-800-654-2452 (US). From outside of the United States, call 314-447-8871. Fax: 314-447-8029. E-mail: JournalsCustomer Service-usa@elsevier.com (for print support); JournalsOnlineSupport-usa@elsevier.com (for online support).**

Physical Medicine and Rehabilitation Clinics of North America is indexed in *Excerpta Medica, MEDLINE/PubMed (Index Medicus), Cinahl,* and *Cumulative Index to Nursing and Allied Health Literature.*

Printed in the United States of America.

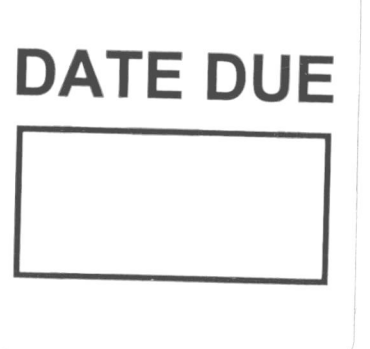

Traumatic Brain Injury Rehabilitation

Editors

BLESSEN C. EAPEN
DAVID X. CIFU

PHYSICAL MEDICINE AND REHABILITATION CLINICS OF NORTH AMERICA

www.pmr.theclinics.com

Consulting Editor
SANTOS F. MARTINEZ

May 2017 • Volume 28 • Number 2

Contributors

CONSULTING EDITOR

SANTOS F. MARTINEZ, MD, MS

Diplomate of the American Academy of Physical Medicine and Rehabilitation, Certificate of Added Qualification Sports Medicine, Assistant Professor, Department of Orthopaedics, Campbell Clinic Orthopaedics, University of Tennessee, Memphis, Tennessee

EDITORS

BLESSEN C. EAPEN, MD

Section Chief, Polytrauma Rehabilitation Center, Brain Injury Medicine/Polytrauma Fellowship Program Director, South Texas Veterans Healthcare System, Associate Professor, Department of Rehabilitation Medicine, UT Health, San Antonio, Texas

DAVID X. CIFU, MD

Associate Dean for Innovation and Herman J. Flax, MD Professor and Chairman, Department of Physical Medicine and Rehabilitation, Virginia Commonwealth University School of Medicine, Senior TBI Specialist, U.S. Department of Veteran Affairs; Director, Sports Science, NHL Florida Panthers, Principal Investigator, VA-DoD Chronic Effects of NeuroTrauma Consortium, Richmond, Virginia

AUTHORS

ELIZABETH V. ADAMOV, DO

Department of Physical Medicine and Rehabilitation, Spaulding Rehabilitation Hospital, Harvard Medical School, Boston, Massachusetts

PATRICK ARMISTEAD-JEHLE, PhD, ABPP-CN

Chief, Concussion Clinic, Munson Army Health Center, Fort Leavenworth, Kansas

LAUREN ELIZABETH AVELLONE, PhD

Research Associate, VCU-RRTC, Virginia Commonwealth University, Richmond, Virginia

SHEITAL BAVISHI, DO

Medical Director, Traumatic Brain Injury Rehabilitation Program, Department of Physical Medicine and Rehabilitation, Ohio State University Wexner Medical Center, Columbus, Ohio

HEATHER G. BELANGER, PhD, ABPP-CN

Staff Neuropsychologist and Training Director, Human Services Research and Development, Tampa VA TBI/Polytrauma Rehabilitation Center, Center of Innovation on Disability and Rehabilitation Research (CINDRR), James A. Haley Veterans' Hospital, Department of Mental Health and Behavioral Sciences, James A. Haley Veterans' Hospital, Associate Professor, Department of Psychiatry and Behavioral Neurosciences, University of South Florida, Tampa, Florida, Defense and Veterans Brain Injury Center, Tampa, Florida

ERICA BELLAMKONDA, MD
Assistant Professor, Department of Physical Medicine and Rehabilitation, Mayo Clinic, Rochester, Minnesota

ERIN BIGLER, PhD
Professor of Psychology and Neuroscience, Brigham Young University, Provo, Utah

DAVID X. CIFU, MD
Associate Dean for Innovation and Herman J. Flax, MD Professor and Chairman, Department of Physical Medicine and Rehabilitation, Virginia Commonwealth University School of Medicine, Senior TBI Specialist, U.S. Department of Veteran Affairs; Director, Sports Science, NHL Florida Panthers, Principal Investigator, VA-DoD Chronic Effects of NeuroTrauma Consortium, Richmond, Virginia

DOUGLAS B. COOPER, PhD, ABPP-CN
Research Director, Defense and Veterans Brain Injury Center, Department of Neurology, San Antonio Military Medical Center, Joint Base San Antonio, Fort Sam Houston, Texas; Adjunct Associate Professor, Department of Psychiatry, University of Texas Health Science Center, San Antonio, Texas

EDAN A. CRITCHFIELD, PsyD, ABPP
Staff Neuropsychologist, Psychology Service, South Texas Veterans Healthcare System, San Antonio, Texas

KIRSTY J. DIXON, PhD
Assistant Professor, Department of Physical Medicine and Rehabilitation, Virginia Commonwealth University, Richmond, Virginia

DAVID F. DRAKE, MD
Director, Department of Physical Medicine and Rehabilitation, Interventional Pain and Integrative Medicine, Richmond VAMC, Director, Interventional Pain Fellowship, Assistant Professor, Department of Physical Medicine and Rehabilitation, Virginia Commonwealth University, Richmond, Virginia

BLESSEN C. EAPEN, MD
Section Chief, Polytrauma Rehabilitation Center, Brain Injury Medicine/Polytrauma Fellowship Program Director, South Texas Veterans Healthcare System, Associate Professor, Department of Rehabilitation Medicine, UT Health, San Antonio, Texas

BRIAN L. EDLOW, MD
Department of Neurology, Massachusetts General Hospital, Boston, Massachusetts, Athinoula A. Martinos Center for Biomedical Imaging, Massachusetts General Hospital, Charlestown, Massachusetts

ANDREW J. GARDNER, PhD
Co-Director, Sports Concussion Program, Hunter New England Local Health District, Centre for Stroke and Brain Injury, School of Medicine and Public Health, University of Newcastle, Callaghan, New South Wales

JASON GEORGEKUTTY, DO
Staff Physiatrist, Kessler Institute for Rehabilitation, Chester, New Jersey

GARY GOLDBERG, BASc, MD
Professor, Department of Physical Medicine and Rehabilitation Service, Polytrauma Rehabilitation System of Care, Hunter Holmes McGuire VA Medical Center, Medical College of Virginia, Virginia Commonwealth University Healthcare System, Richmond, Virginia

KEVIN GUSKIEWICZ, PhD
Kenan Distinguished Professor, Department of Exercise and Sport Science, Dean, College of Arts and Sciences, University of North Carolina – Chapel Hill, Chapel Hill, North Carolina

ANNE M. HUDAK, MD
Director, Department of Physical Medicine and Rehabilitation, Polytrauma Network Site Clinic, Richmond VAMC, Associate Professor, Department of Physical Medicine and Rehabilitation, Virginia Commonwealth University, Richmond, Virginia

DIEGO IACONO, MD, PhD
Brain Tissue Repository and Neuropathology Core, Center for Neuroscience and Regenerative Medicine (CNRM), Uniformed Services University of the Health Sciences (USUHS), The Henry M. Jackson Foundation for the Advancement of Military Medicine (HJF), Bethesda, Maryland

MICHAEL A. McCREA, PhD
Professor and Eminent Scholar, Director of Brain Injury Research, Department of Neurosurgery, Medical College of Wisconsin, Milwaukee, Wisconsin

LINDSAY D. NELSON, PhD
Assistant Professor, Department of Neurosurgery, Medical College of Wisconsin, Milwaukee, Wisconsin

JUSTIN J.F. O'ROURKE, PhD, ABPP
Staff Neuropsychologist, Polytrauma Rehabilitation Center, South Texas Veterans Healthcare System, Clinical Neuropsychology of Texas, San Antonio, Texas

DANIEL P. PERL, MD
Brain Tissue Repository & Neuropathology Core, Center for Neuroscience and Regenerative Medicine (CNRM), Uniformed Services University of the Health Sciences (USUHS), Department of Pathology, F. Edward Hébert School of Medicine, Uniformed Services University of the Health Sciences (USUHS), Bethesda, Maryland

WILLIAM ROBBINS, MD
Assistant Professor, Department of Physical Medicine and Rehabilitation, Virginia Commonwealth University, Director, Polytrauma Transitional Rehabilitation Program, Richmond VAMC, Richmond, Virginia

BILLIE A. SCHULTZ, MD
Assistant Professor, Department of Physical Medicine and Rehabilitation, Mayo Clinic, Rochester, Minnesota

SHIRLEY L. SHIH, MD, MS
Department of Physical Medicine and Rehabilitation, Spaulding Rehabilitation Hospital, Harvard Medical School, Boston, Massachusetts

SHARON B. SHIVELY, MD, PhD
Brain Tissue Repository and Neuropathology Core, Center for Neuroscience and Regenerative Medicine (CNRM), Uniformed Services University of the Health Sciences (USUHS), The Henry M. Jackson Foundation for the Advancement of Military Medicine (HJF), Department of Pathology, F. Edward Hébert School of Medicine, Uniformed Services University of the Health Sciences (USUHS), Bethesda, Maryland

JASON R. SOBLE, PhD, ABPP-CN
Staff Neuropsychologist, Psychology Service, South Texas Veterans Healthcare System, San Antonio, Texas

BRUNO SUBBARAO, DO
Polytrauma/TBI Fellow, Polytrauma Rehabilitation Center, South Texas Veterans Healthcare System, San Antonio, Texas

REBECCA N. TAPIA, MD
Medical Director, Polytrauma Service, Polytrauma Network Site, South Texas Veterans Healthcare System, San Antonio, Texas

PAMELA SHERRON TARGETT, MEd
Research Associate, VCU-RRTC, Virginia Commonwealth University, Richmond, Virginia

ALEX B. VALADKA, MD
Professor and Chair, Department of Neurosurgery, Virginia Commonwealth University, Richmond, Virginia

PAUL HOWARD WEHMAN, PhD
Professor of Physical Medicine and Rehabilitation, Chairman, Division of Rehabilitation Research, Director of VCU-RRTC, Medical College of Virginia, Virginia Commonwealth University, Richmond, Virginia

WITTSTATT ALEXANDRA WHITAKER-LEA, MD
Resident, Department of Neurosurgery, Virginia Commonwealth University, Richmond, Virginia

ROSS D. ZAFONTE, DO
Director, Department of Physical Medicine and Rehabilitation, Spaulding Rehabilitation Hospital, Harvard Medical School, Massachusetts General Hospital Home Base Program, Brigham and Women's Hospital, Massachusetts General Hospital, Red Sox Foundation, Boston, Massachusetts

NATHAN D. ZASLER, MD, FAAPM&R, FACRM, BIM-C, FIAIME, DAIPM, CBIST
CEO & Medical Director, Concussion Care Centre of Virginia, Ltd, CEO and Medical Director, Tree of Life Services, Inc, Professor, Affiliate, Department of Physical Medicine and Rehabilitation, Virginia Commonwealth University, Richmond, Virginia; Associate Professor, Adjunct, Department of Physical Medicine and Rehabilitation, University of Virginia, Charlottesville, Virginia; Vice-Chairperson, International Brain Injury Association, Alexandria, Virginia

Contents

Traumatic brain injury (TBI) has become the signature injury of the military conflict in Iraq and Afghanistan and also has a high rate of occurrence in civilian populations in the United States. Although the effects of a moderate to severe brain injury have been investigated for decades, the chronic effects of single and repetitive mild TBI are just beginning to be investigated. Data suggest that the different types and severities of TBI have unique long-term outcomes and thus may represent different types of diseases. Therefore, this review outlines the causes, incidence, symptoms, and pathophysiology of mild, moderate, and severe TBI.

Traumatic brain injury (TBI) continues to be a major public health problem. Proposed treatments have not withstood testing in clinical trials because of failure to account for different types of TBI and other weaknesses in trial design. Management goals continue to be prevention and prompt treatment of secondary insults (hypotension, hypoxia, and other physiologic derangements). This goal is best accomplished by careful attention to airway, breathing, circulation, and basic principles of intensive care unit management. Attempts to intervene prophylactically to prevent intracranial hypertension or other complications have not been beneficial and may even have deleterious effects.

Disorder of consciousness (DOC) is a state of prolonged altered consciousness, which can be categorized into coma, vegetative state, or minimally conscious state based on neurobehavioral function. The pathophysiology of DOC is poorly understood but recent advances in neuroimaging and advanced electrophysiological techniques may provide an improved understanding for the neural network involved with consciousness. The primary aim of DOC rehabilitation programs is to promote arousal while preventing secondary medical complications while providing education and training to families. Treatment interventions include both pharmacologic and nonpharmacologic programs, but there are currently no consensus treatment guidelines for individuals with DOC.

> Brain injury specialists are experienced providers able to identify and treat the unique medical complications after moderate-severe traumatic brain injury, including posttraumatic seizures, paroxysmal sympathetic hyperactivity, spasticity, hydrocephalus, agitation, neuroendocrine dysfunction, heterotopic ossification, venous thromboembolism, and cranial nerve dysfunction. Owing to the potential negative impact on outcome if left untreated, identification and appropriate treatment is essential. An additional role of the brain injury specialist is to educate family about potential medical complications and anticipated outcomes after brain injury. The provider, patient, and family work together to identify and treat any potential sequelae of the moderate-severe brain injury.

> Over the past 2 decades, there have been major advances in the basic and clinical science of concussion and mild traumatic brain injury. These advances now provide a more evidence-informed approach to the definition, diagnosis, assessment, and management of acute concussion. Standardized clinical tools have been developed and validated for assessment of acute concussion across injury settings (eg, civilian, sport, military). Consensus guidelines now provide guidance regarding injury management and approaches to ensure safe return to activity after acute concussion. This article provides a brief, high-level overview of approaches to best practice in diagnosis, assessment, and management of acute concussion.

> One of the more challenging aspects beyond acute concussion management occurs when symptoms do not resolve as anticipated over time. The term postconcussion syndrome generally refers to a presentation of multiple ongoing symptoms months to years from injury, typically comprised of physical, cognitive, and emotional complaints such as headaches, poor sleep, poor concentration, dizziness, and irritability. Although individual factors vary, the condition is often regarded as multifactorial. Persistent issues can pose a threat to full community reintegration following concussion and reduce overall quality of life; thus early recognition and treatment are essential to optimize long-term outcomes.

> Chronic traumatic encephalopathy (CTE) is a neuropathologic diagnosis typically made in human brains with a history of repetitive traumatic brain injury (rTBI). It remains unknown whether CTE occurs exclusively after rTBI, or whether a single TBI (sTBI) can cause CTE. Similarly, it is unclear whether impact (eg, motor vehicle accidents) and non-impact (eg, blasts) types of energy transfer trigger divergent or common pathologies. While it

is established that a history of rTBI increases the risk of multiple neurode-generative diseases (eg, dementia, parkinsonism, and CTE), the possible pathophysiologic and molecular mechanisms underlying these risks have yet to be elucidated.

Patrick Armistead-Jehle, Jason R. Soble, Douglas B. Cooper, and Heather G. Belanger

Traumatic brain injury (TBI), in particular mild TBI (mTBI), is a relatively common injury experienced by service members across both deployed and nondeployed environments. Although many of the principles and practices used by civilian health care providers for identifying and treating this injury apply to military settings, there are unique factors that impact mTBI-related care in service members and Veterans. This article reviews several of these factors, including the epidemiology of TBI in the military/Veteran population, the influence of military culture on this condition, and identification and treatment of mTBI in the war zone.

Jason R. Soble, Edan A. Critchfield, and Justin J.F. O'Rourke

Clinical neuropsychology is a subspecialty of professional psychology that is concerned with the scientific study and clinical application of brain-behavior relationships. Broadly defined, a neuropsychological evaluation is a flexible clinical tool that involves integration of objective, psychometric test data along with various other sources of clinical information to comprehensively elucidate the cognitive, behavioral, and emotional sequelae after traumatic brain injury (TBI). In addition to characterizing TBI sequelae, evidenced-based neuropsychological assessment can contribute to TBI patient care by aiding with prognostic assessment, measuring interval change/recovery over time (eg, resolution of posttraumatic amnesia), informing and implementing rehabilitation strategies, and evaluating the effectiveness of interventions.

Paul Howard Wehman, Pamela Sherron Targett, and Lauren Elizabeth Avellone

This article describes some of the current issues related to return to school and employment for individuals with traumatic brain injury. A strong, collaborative partnership between an individual's health care providers and key stake holders is essential to a smooth transition back to school or work. Ways to improve current practices and ensure more timely and appropriate educational and employment services and supports for individuals with traumatic brain injury are described. Some recommendations on areas for future research are also offered.

David F. Drake, Anne M. Hudak, and William Robbins

Complementary and alternative medicine (CAM) is a group of diverse medical and health care systems, practices, and products that are not presently considered to be a part of conventional medicine. Integrative medicine combines treatment with conventional medical practices and elements of CAM in which there is strong evidence in efficacy and safety. Although there is growing interest in the integrative medical approach in treating the patient population with traumatic brain injury, there is a paucity in high-quality clinical trials supporting its use. This article reviews the background and current clinical data concerning some of the more common CAM interventions.

The role of the physiatrist in provision of medicolegal expert testimony in cases involving traumatic brain injury is challenging and complex. This article provides an overview of how such work should be conducted from a practical perspective including discussion of ethical, legal, medical, and business aspects of such activities. Additionally, pointers are provided with regards to how information including preinjury, injury, and postinjury (including neuroimaging and neuropsychological data) should be considered and integrated into medicolegal opinions and testimony.

A postmodern framework is proposed for conceptualizing the impact of brain injury on the subjective being of the injured person. Semiosis, the 'action of signs,' is argued as necessary for this recovery of subjectivity that escapes the mechanistic materialism and mind–matter dualism of modern science. Ethical dilemmas in brain injury care are best approached through an empirical 'semioethics' implemented as a dialogical practice among a group of selected stakeholders seeking a logical solution that best addresses the criterion of maximizing reasonableness as a tempering of rationality with relational concerns in the face of the constraints imposed by the injury.

With the continued advancement in technology, such as increasingly sophisticated neuroimaging parameters, and the ongoing development of various scientific fields, like serum and blood biomarkers, genetics, and physiology, traumatic brain injury (TBI) research is a dynamic field of study. TBI remains a significant public health concern and research has continued to grow exponentially over the past decade. This review provides an overview of the frontiers of TBI research, from sports concussion to severe TBI, from acute and subacute injury to long-term/chronic outcomes, from assessment and management to prognosis, specifically examining recent neuroimaging, biomarkers, genetics, and physiologic studies.

PHYSICAL MEDICINE AND REHABILITATION CLINICS OF NORTH AMERICA

VISIT THE CLINICS ONLINE!
Access your subscription at:
www.theclinics.com

Foreword

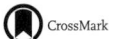 CrossMark

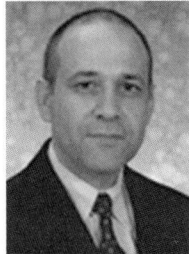

Santos F. Martinez, MD, MS
Consulting Editor

I would like to thank Dr Eapen and Dr Cifu for their hard work and enthusiasm in lining up a stellar team. Although the Physiatrist certainly is faced with a spectrum of pathology, the challenge in one's perception of self and family becomes ever more evident in those who have suffered traumatic brain injury. These patients force us to take an internal inventory as we observe one's place in society take a swift and drastic change.

This issue provides the reader with a comprehensive view of traumatic brain injury. The tools and conceptual format presented will certainly provide the clinician as well as the neuro-researcher with an enhanced appreciation and base of knowledge. I would be remiss if I did not acknowledge and thank Dr Nathaniel Mayer from The Drucker Brain Injury Center at MossRehab, who has dedicated his life to this population. Over the decades, he has been very influential in cultivating scores of future clinicians to take up the challenge of treating this population.

Santos F. Martinez, MD, MS
American Academy of Physical Medicine
and Rehabilitation
Campbell Clinic Orthopaedics
Department of Orthopaedics
University of Tennessee
Memphis, TN 38104, USA

E-mail address:
smartinez@campbellclinic.com

Phys Med Rehabil Clin N Am 28 (2017) xiii
http://dx.doi.org/10.1016/j.pmr.2017.03.001
1047-9651/17/© 2017 Published by Elsevier Inc.

Preface

Traumatic Brain Injury Rehabilitation

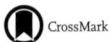

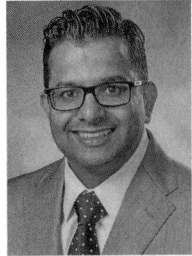 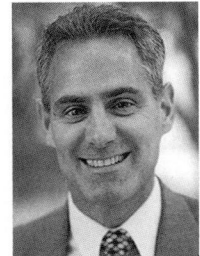

Blessen C. Eapen, MD   David X. Cifu, MD
Editors

Dear colleagues,

It is with great pleasure that we present this special issue of *Physical Medicine and Rehabilitation Clinics of North America* dedicated to traumatic brain injury (TBI) rehabilitation. This issue comes at a very timely juncture in light of the pervasive national headlines from the sport, civilian, military, and Veteran sectors and the increasing awareness of the short- and long-term effects of TBI seen in a wide range of federally funded longitudinal research networks, including the Department of Defense/Veterans Affairs Chronic Effects of Neurotrauma Consortium. We have assembled the foremost experts in the field of TBI rehabilitation medicine to develop this special issue.

The goal of this special issue is to provide readers with a glimpse of the current state of science and provide an overview of the advances in the field of brain injury rehabilitation. We describe the assessment, management, and rehabilitation of patients with TBI from coma to community reintegration. We also describe medicolegal issues and semioethics of brain injury care. Last, we discuss future frontiers in TBI research and describe the advancement in technology and ongoing developments across the field.

We would like to thank our contributing authors for their hard work and dedication to this special issue and the patients they treat. Also, we would like to thank Don Mumford and his team at Elsevier for their invaluable assistance in bringing this issue to publication. Lastly and most importantly, we would like to dedicate this special issue to the

Phys Med Rehabil Clin N Am 28 (2017) xv–xvi
http://dx.doi.org/10.1016/j.pmr.2017.02.001
1047-9651/17/© 2017 Published by Elsevier Inc.

courageous brain injury survivors and their caregivers for their continued journey toward recovery.

Blessen C. Eapen, MD
Physical Medicine and Rehabilitation Services PM&RS (MC 117)
South Texas Veterans Health Care System
7400 Merton Minter, Boulevard
San Antonio, TX 78255, USA

David X. Cifu, MD
Department of Physical Medicine and Rehabilitation
Virginia Commonwealth University
US Department of Veterans Affairs
Chronic Effects of NeuroTrauma Consortium
1223 E. Marshall Street, PO Box 980677
Richmond, VA 23284-0667, USA

E-mail addresses:
Blessen.Eapen2@va.gov (B.C. Eapen)
david.cifu@vcuhealth.org (D.X. Cifu)

Pathophysiology of Traumatic Brain Injury

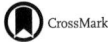

Kirsty J. Dixon, PhD

KEYWORDS

- Traumatic brain injury • TBI • Pathophysiology • Symptoms • Mild TBI
- Concussion • Blast TBI

KEY POINTS

- Traumatic brain injury (TBI) has become the signature injury of the military conflict in Iraq and Afghanistan and also has a high rate of occurrence in civilian populations in the United States.
- Although the effects of a moderate to severe brain injury have been investigated for decades, the chronic effects of single and repetitive mild TBI are just becoming investigated.
- Data suggest that the different types and severities of TBI have unique long-term outcomes and thus may represent different types of diseases.
- Therefore, this review outlines the causes, incidence, symptoms, and pathophysiology of mild, moderate, and severe TBI.

TRAUMATIC BRAIN INJURY: CAUSES, PREVALENCE, AND DEVELOPMENT OF THE NATIONAL RESEARCH ACTION PLAN

Traumatic brain injury (TBI) may have many different causes, including a blow to the head, penetration of the skull, fast acceleration or deceleration of the head, or exposure to a blast. In the United States, there are more than 5.3 million people living with a disability as a result of a TBI, and each year an additional 1.7 million Americans sustain a TBI.[1,2] These injuries have both short- and long-term effects on health, ranging from symptoms that have a minimal interference on lifestyle, through to physical, emotional, and psychosocial changes that may interfere with daily activities. As well as the burden to the individual, brain injuries also have an annual economic burden of more than US$60 billion, due to both direct and indirect costs, such as loss of productivity.[2] The reasons for the injuries depend on the age of the individual; for example, more than one-third of brain injuries in the United States are due to people falling, which is the leading cause of TBI among the elderly, whereas transportation-related brain injuries are the leading cause for individuals aged 15 to 24 years.[2]

Disclosures: There are no commercial or financial conflicts of interest to disclose.
Department of Physical Medicine and Rehabilitation, Virginia Commonwealth University, 1223 East Marshall Street, Richmond, VA 23298, USA
E-mail address: Kirsty.dixon@vcuhealth.org

Phys Med Rehabil Clin N Am 28 (2017) 215–225
http://dx.doi.org/10.1016/j.pmr.2016.12.001
1047-9651/17/© 2017 Elsevier Inc. All rights reserved.

In recent years, the media have had a strong focus on the long-term outcomes of mild TBI (mTBI) or concussions, such as that which may occur to American football players and military personnel. Pathophysiologic investigations on the brains of these individuals have revealed Alzheimer-like symptoms, termed chronic traumatic encephalopathy (CTE).[3,4] Although this disease has been known to occur in boxers since the 1960s (with numerous names, including dementia pugilistica and punch-drunk syndrome), the recent media attention has highlighted the high prevalence of this disease in other athletic arenas. This attention was followed by the Obama Administration releasing an Executive Order in 2012 to direct the Departments of Defense, Veterans Affairs, Health and Human Services, and Education to develop a National Research Action Plan (NRAP) on TBI, posttraumatic stress disorder (PTSD), and other common comorbidities. The NRAP was released in August 2013 and aims to (1) accelerate the understanding of the causes and mechanisms of TBI, PTSD, and other common comorbidities; (2) develop clinical innovations to detect disorders early and accurately; and (3) develop proven means to prevent and treat the devastating conditions caused by the injuries. To this end, understanding the acute and chronic pathophysiology of TBI is critical to determining the risk factors for individuals to develop symptoms as well as develop therapeutic innovations and interventions.

Given that current clinical imaging techniques do not detect minor changes in the human brain following injury, much of the knowledge on the cellular sequelae in the injured brain is based on rodent studies. To confirm these findings in the injured human brain, on arrival at the emergency department, an individual can be assessed for physical and cognitive functions, have a computed tomographic (CT)/MRI scan performed, have their intracranial pressure and cerebral blood flow measured, and possibly have bio-specimens collected for analysis of protein and messenger RNA expression. Subsequently, on autopsy, brain samples can be collected and analyzed.

MILD TRAUMATIC BRAIN INJURY
Causes, Diagnosis, and Symptoms

A mild brain injury is often caused by a blunt head trauma, and/or acceleration or deceleration forces to the head, and refers to the initial impact of the injury. The diagnosis of an mTBI is the subject of constant debate because no single test is available to definitively confirm the diagnosis. Currently, a combination of tools is used, including history of the injury, patient symptoms, and CT scans. Although most patients with an mTBI recover within weeks to months of the injury without specific intervention, 30% to 53% of affected individuals may still have disabling symptoms at least 1 year after the injury,[5,6] and this is often referred to as postconcussive syndrome. Because by definition mTBI is nonfatal and does not alter life expectancy (0.1% mortality[7]), prolonged symptoms can lead to life-long disabilities. Thus, the term mild brain injury can be misleading, because it does not refer to the severity or time course of injury symptoms.

In the acute period following an mTBI, an individual may experience a brief loss of consciousness (or altered consciousness), transient confusion, disorientation, loss of memory at the time of the injury (amnesia), and other neurologic and neuropsychological dysfunctions, including seizures, headaches, dizziness, irritability, fatigue, and poor concentration. More specifically, diagnosis is based on the Glasgow Coma Scale (GCS) that ranks functional ability from 1 (worst outcome) to 15 (best outcome), with a mild injury defined between 13 and 15.[8,9] Subsequently, these symptoms may evolve into persistent low-grade headaches, pain, poor attention and concentration, fatigue, anxiety, and depression, all or some of which may continue for months to years following the injury.[10–13]

Pathophysiology

After a violent hit to the head, the soft brain inside hits the intracranial surface of the skull, which may damage the area of the brain that comes in contact with the skull. This damage may occur in both the forward and the reverse locations as the brain "bounces" within the skull. In American football, which has a high incidence of mild repetitive TBIs, most of these impacts are on the side of the helmet, or from ground contact to the back of the head,[14] whereas the location of impact from concussions not related to football are difficult to document.

In addition to the brain hitting against the cranium, any rotational movement to the brain following the impact may stretch, and sometimes tear, axons within white matter tracts of the brain, which is known as "diffuse axonal injury."[15–18] Although traditional CT scans are unable to detect these injuries, modern imaging techniques such as altered fractional anisotropy using diffusion tensor imaging and MRI show promise to detect these changes.[18–21] Using rodent models, there is recent evidence to suggest this type of injury may impair neuronal function,[22] although the causes of this dysfunction are currently unclear. Some research suggests diffuse axonal injury may induce neuronal degeneration as evidenced by increased Fluoro-Jade staining,[23] whereas other research suggests it may only induce neuronal atrophy due to axotomy of the axon initial segment.[22,24] For the latter, 2 types of axonal abnormality have been observed. The first is progressive swellings along the axon termed "bulbs" that eventually lead to axonal disconnection and loss of function.[17,25] The second is a production of axonal varicosities and is thought to be due to microtubule breakage, thus slowing axonal transport to cause the varicosities.[17,26] It has been proposed these abnormalities may lead to delayed secondary disconnection and/or prolonged neuronal dysfunction.

In addition to these neuronal morphologic and functional alterations, a mild injury may also induce other pathophysiologic responses. Following mild injury, there is frequently a sustained proinflammatory cytokine upregulation, a reduction in oligodendrocyte cell numbers, and glial reactivity.[27–29] Furthermore, a mild injury may also disrupt the function of the cerebral vasculature. In a healthy brain, cerebral blood flow is tightly controlled to provide an adequate supply of oxygen and nutrients through a dense network of arteries and capillaries.[30–32] Following a traumatic injury, there is an initial reduction in cerebral blood flow (within hours of the injury), which can remain low for days, depending on injury severity.[33–36] This reduced blood flow could be attributed to increased nitric oxide expression after injury, causing vasodilation instead of a pressure-induced increase in vasoconstriction.[37] These changes are also associated with a reduction in blood vessel density in the perilesional region during the first few days after injury.[38,39] Over the next few days to weeks, there is usually a return of normal cerebral blood flow, which coincides with an increase in blood vessel density in the affected region.[36,38,39] Similar to the uninjured brain, the constant supply of blood then needs to be maintained, and this occurs by cerebral vessels undergoing vasodilation in response to dilatory stimuli, termed cerebrovascular reactivity. Unfortunately, following a brain injury, the cerebral blood vessels may be less able to respond to dilatory stimuli,[40–44] and this can lead to a poor prognosis, including a terminal event.[45]

In addition to the immediate effects of axonal injury and cerebral vascular dysregulation, in recent years there has been much attention paid to the discovery of CTE in athletes and some Veterans, whom have undergone repetitive mild brain injuries throughout their careers.[3,4,46] This disease is a form of tauopathy and is characterized by unusually high levels of tau deposition occurring as neurofibrillary tangles.[3,4,47] CTE has been classified into 4 clinical stages ranging from perivascular tangles in the initial stages of the disease, through to widespread tau deposition decades later.[48] Because only individuals with repetitive mild injuries appear to develop CTE, it is thought that this type of injury does not simply represent a milder form of moderate to severe TBI, but rather it represents a separate type of injury that can manifest to a different disease endpoint. However, unlike other neurodegenerative diseases such as Alzheimer, the development of CTE symptoms often occurs earlier in life and leads to an altered neuropathology.[46] Unfortunately, at this moment, definitive diagnosis of the disease can only be performed on postmortem analysis, although current technological advances with PET imaging may soon be used to detect tau accumulation in living individuals.[49] At present, the risk factors for developing CTE are under investigation.

MODERATE AND SEVERE TRAUMATIC BRAIN INJURY
Causes, Diagnosis, and Symptoms

According to the Centers for Disease Control and Prevention, the most common causes of a moderate or severe TBI are falls (40.5%), motor vehicle accidents (14.3%), assaults (10.7%), or being struck by or against (15.5%).[2] Moderate TBIs are diagnosed by a possible loss of consciousness lasting up to a few hours, confusion lasting from days to weeks, and physical, cognitive, and/or behavioral impairments lasting for months, or are sustained permanently, with a GCS score between 9 and 12.[9] In comparison, a severe brain injury is determined by a prolonged unconscious or vegetative state that can last for days to months, with a GSC score of less than 9.[9] Following a severe injury, patients may experience physical limitations (eg, headaches, nausea/vomiting, pupil dilation, slurred speech, aphasia, sensory deficits), along with cognitive (eg, memory, attention, concentration) and emotional (eg, motivation, irritability, aggression) dysfunctions. Although a patient with a moderate brain injury has the potential to make a good recovery through treatment, and/or learning to modify their behavior to compensate for any acquired deficits, a patient with a severe injury has the possibility of remaining permanently unresponsive.[2] Therefore, a risk factor for subsequent symptoms is injury severity, but also includes the location of the brain injury as well as the individual's age and gender.

Pathophysiology

Similar to a mild injury, a moderate or severe brain injury may cause the brain to hit against the intracranial portion of the skull, with or without penetration (from either skull fragments or foreign objects). As indicated above, the location and severity of the impact, as well as the depth and amount of brain penetration, likely have a significant impact on the patient's outcome. Any penetration of the brain's fragile structure can mechanically tear apart neurons and shear their axons to disrupt neuronal circuitry as well as damage the vasculature, allowing movement of blood and leukocytes into the normally immune privileged brain.[50–53] These effects have an immediate impact on the brain by inducing necrotic cell loss as well as inducing apoptosis of the surrounding cells.[50,54,55] Within minutes of these changes, a local inflammatory response occurs whereby astrocytes and microglia secrete proinflammatory cytokines, such as tumor necrosis factor, interleukin-6, and interleukin-1β, into the perilesional region.[56–60] These proinflammatory cytokines mobilize immune and glial cells to the injury site, causing edema and further inflammation.[59,61] This phase is associated with gliosis, demyelination, and continued apoptosis. Simultaneously, the cerebral vasculature is also undergoing further changes. Although there is some discrepancy within the literature, hypoperfusion may occur acutely after injury, likely caused by reduced blood pressure, impaired vasodilation (vascular reactivity), and elevated intracranial pressure.[62–65] Over the next few days, this may be followed by hyperemia, after which hypoperfusion may return and be accompanied by vasospasms.[33,66,67] At the same time, there may also be a reduction in the cerebral metabolic rate for oxygen,[33,66] suggesting impairments in energy metabolism; however, there are discrepancies in the literature on this matter, and it is unclear how much this may play a role in each patient's injury pathophysiology.

BLAST-INDUCED TRAUMATIC BRAIN INJURY
Causes, Diagnosis, and Symptoms

A blast TBI (bTBI) is a unique subtype of traumatic injury that occurs due to direct or indirect exposure to an explosion, primarily in combat situations. A "blast wave" generated from an explosion consists of a front of high pressure that quickly compresses the surrounding air, giving rise to negative pressure, but which rapidly expands and displaces an equal volume of air. This displacement of air then generates a "blast wind."[68] The Centers for Disease Control and Prevention have identified 4 types of injuries caused by exposure to a blast based on how the injury occurred. These injuries include injuries from the initial blast pressure wave (primary blast), penetrating or blunt injuries from flying debris and fragments, and injuries from individuals being thrown by the blast wind.[69] Although blast injuries are typically polytraumatic, here the focus is entirely on the effects of the pressure wave, because other aspects of the injury, such as penetration of the brain from flying debris, are covered in other sections of this review.

In recent years, retrospective studies have identified that approximately half of combat-related injuries sustained during the conflicts in Iraq and Afghanistan are due to explosions, of which up to 15% of the affected service members experienced a primary blast injury, although most are likely polytraumatic in nature.[69,70] The Centers for Disease Control and Prevention have identified that the severity of symptoms depends on factors such as the type of explosive used, the surrounding environment, the distance between the individual and the blast, and the presence of any protective or hazardous items between the individual and the blast. A retrospective study on service members shows an increased severity of the blast injury is associated with an increase in disability upon discharge.[71] In support of this, rodent data have revealed a dose-response relationship between blast intensity and behavioral deficits.[72] Diagnosis of whether the blast injury has caused a mild, moderate, or severe brain injury may include evaluation of the length of unconsciousness and GCS outcome, along with identifying any loss of memory at the time of the event, as well as any alteration in mental state. Similar to a nonblast civilian mTBI, a blast injury may commonly cause a concussion, with the individual experiencing physical, emotional, and/or cognitive difficulties. However, individuals with a blast-related concussion are likely to also experience other comorbid conditions, such as depression or PTSD.[73]

Pathophysiology

The blast wave caused by an explosion may interact with the brain in several ways. First, as the kinetic energy passes through the skull, it may directly induce acceleration or rotation of the brain, causing diffuse axonal injury and subsequent secondary injury mechanisms. Although these types of injuries may at first appear similar to nonblast civilian TBI, recent data suggest the type of axonal injury caused by a blast is unique to bTBI. Diffusion tensor imaging of military service members following brain injury indicates the axonal damage from bTBI is more widespread and spatially variable compared with non-blast civilian TBI[74] and includes brain regions such as the superior corona radiata of the frontal cortex, the cerebellum, and optic tracts.[75–77] In support of this, recent data from rodent models of bTBI, which induce similar behavioral outcomes to patients, also show that rotational brain injury produces a different set of behaviors compared with blast-induced neurotrauma.[78,79] Therefore, bTBI-induced axonal damage may need to be considered a separate type of diffuse axonal injury. Comparatively, the secondary mechanisms of injury produced from a bTBI appear to be similar to non-blast TBI, whereby a robust inflammatory response occurs that includes increased proinflammatory cytokines expression and glial reactivity.[80–83] In addition to these effects, edema and vasospasms are also far more prevalent following bTBI, compared with nonblast civilian mTBI,[80,84,85] which has been proposed to be due to narrowing of primary arteries,[75] and are supported by reduced vascular integrity following a blast injury in rodents,[72] thus providing support for a vascular-related mechanism of tissue damage.

In addition to the direct effects of a blast wave on the brain tissue, the blast wave may also act indirectly through 2 possible mechanisms. First, the blast may cause gas-containing compartments in the brain to compress, and subsequently expand, leading to damage of surrounding tissues.[86] Second, the blast wave may also cause shock waves in the blood or cerebrospinal fluid to be delivered to the brain within seconds of the impact.[86–89] This shock wave can lead to an acceleration of the elements of the tissue from their resting state to a rate dependent on the density of the medium, which may subsequently cause deformation and/or rupture of the affected brain tissue.[90]

SUMMARY

This review has outlined the causes, incidence, symptoms, diagnoses, and pathophysiology of mild, moderate, and severe TBI, including bTBI. Although many studies have attempted to link the brain's pathophysiology following injury to acute and subacute symptoms, individuals with a brain injury may suffer debilitating symptoms for months, if not years, following the incident or incidents. Unfortunately, at present, there is a dearth of knowledge regarding the long-term (chronic) effects of brain injury; specifically, the risk factors for long-term symptoms are unknown, as are many of the underlying pathophysiologic mechanisms. With the development of improved imaging techniques, and the expansion of longitudinal research studies, such as the Departments of Defense and Veterans Affairs–funded Chronic Effects of Neurotrauma Consortium, it is hoped these knowledge gaps can be filled.

REFERENCES

1. Centers for Disease Control and Prevention National Center for Injury Prevention and Control. Traumatic brain injury in the United States: a report to Congress. 1999. Available at: https://www.cdc.gov/traumaticbraininjury/pdf/tbi_in_the_us. pdf. Accessed January 28, 2017.
2. Faul M, Xu L, Wald MM, et al. Traumatic brain injury in the United States: emergency department visits, hospitalizations and deaths 2002-2006. Atlanta (GA): Centers for Disease Control and Prevention, National Center for Injury Prevention and Control; 2010.
3. McKee AC, Cantu RC, Nowinski CJ, et al. Chronic traumatic encephalopathy in athletes: progressive tauopathy after repetitive head injury. J Neuropathol Exp Neurol 2009;68(7):709–35.

4. McKee AC, Stein TD, Kiernan PT, et al. The neuropathology of chronic traumatic encephalopathy. Brain Pathol 2015;25(3):350–64.

5. Dikmen S, Machamer J, Fann JR, et al. Rates of symptom reporting following traumatic brain injury. J Int Neuropsychol Soc 2010;16(3):401–11.

6. Sterr A, Herron KA, Hayward C, et al. Are mild head injuries as mild as we think? Neurobehavioral concomitants of chronic post-concussion syndrome. BMC Neurol 2006;6:7.

7. af Geijerstam JL, Britton M. Mild head injury—mortality and complication rate: meta-analysis of findings in a systematic literature review. Acta Neurochir (Wien) 2003;145(10):843–50 [discussion: 850].

8. Department of Veterans Affairs and Department of Defense. VA/DoD clinical practice guideline for the management of concussion-mild traumatic brain injury. Version 2.0 ed2015. Available at: http://www.healthquality.va.gov/guidelines/Rehab/mtbi/mTBICPGFullCPG50821816.pdf. Accessed January 28, 2017.

9. Centers for Disease Control and Prevention. Report to Congress on traumatic brain injury in the United States: epidemiology and rehabilitation. Atlanta (GA): National Center for Injury Prevention and Control; Division of Unintentional Injury Prevention; 2015.

10. Nampiaparampil DE. Prevalence of chronic pain after traumatic brain injury: a systematic review. JAMA 2008;300(6):711–9.

11. Konrad C, Geburek AJ, Rist F, et al. Long-term cognitive and emotional consequences of mild traumatic brain injury. Psychol Med 2011;41(6):1197–211.

12. Smits M, Dippel DW, Houston GC, et al. Postconcussion syndrome after minor head injury: brain activation of working memory and attention. Hum Brain Mapp 2009;30(9):2789–803.

13. Lucas S, Smith BM, Temkin N, et al. Comorbidity of headache and depression after mild traumatic brain injury. Headache 2016;56(2):323–30.

14. Pellman EJ, Viano DC, Tucker AM, et al, Committee on Mild Traumatic Brain Injury NFL. Concussion in professional football: location and direction of helmet impacts—Part 2. Neurosurgery 2003;53(6):1328–40 [discussion: 1340–1].

15. Hill CS, Coleman MP, Menon DK. Traumatic axonal injury: mechanisms and translational opportunities. Trends Neurosci 2016;39(5):311–24.

16. Lafrenaye AD, Todani M, Walker SA, et al. Microglia processes associate with diffusely injured axons following mild traumatic brain injury in the micro pig. J Neuroinflammation 2015;12:186.

17. Browne KD, Chen XH, Meaney DF, et al. Mild traumatic brain injury and diffuse axonal injury in swine. J Neurotrauma 2011;28(9):1747–55.

18. Topal NB, Hakyemez B, Erdogan C, et al. MR imaging in the detection of diffuse axonal injury with mild traumatic brain injury. Neurol Res 2008;30(9):974–8.

19. Lipton ML, Gulko E, Zimmerman ME, et al. Diffusion-tensor imaging implicates prefrontal axonal injury in executive function impairment following very mild traumatic brain injury. Radiology 2009;252(3):816–24.

20. Rutgers DR, Fillard P, Paradot G, et al. Diffusion tensor imaging characteristics of the corpus callosum in mild, moderate, and severe traumatic brain injury. AJNR Am J Neuroradiol 2008;29(9):1730–5.

21. Inglese M, Makani S, Johnson G, et al. Diffuse axonal injury in mild traumatic brain injury: a diffusion tensor imaging study. J Neurosurg 2005;103(2):298–303.

22. Greer JE, Povlishock JT, Jacobs KM. Electrophysiological abnormalities in both axotomized and nonaxotomized pyramidal neurons following mild traumatic brain injury. J Neurosci 2012;32(19):6682–7.

23. Rachmany L, Tweedie D, Rubovitch V, et al. Cognitive impairments accompanying rodent mild traumatic brain injury involve p53-dependent neuronal cell death and are ameliorated by the tetrahydrobenzothiazole PFT-alpha. PLoS One 2013;8(11):e79837.

24. Greer JE, McGinn MJ, Povlishock JT. Diffuse traumatic axonal injury in the mouse induces atrophy, c-Jun activation, and axonal outgrowth in the axotomized neuronal population. J Neurosci 2011;31(13):5089–105.

25. Greer JE, Hanell A, McGinn MJ, et al. Mild traumatic brain injury in the mouse induces axotomy primarily within the axon initial segment. Acta Neuropathol 2013; 126(1):59–74.

26. Tang-Schomer MD, Johnson VE, Baas PW, et al. Partial interruption of axonal transport due to microtubule breakage accounts for the formation of periodic varicosities after traumatic axonal injury. Exp Neurol 2012;233(1):364–72.

27. Lotocki G, de Rivero Vaccari JP, Alonso O, et al. Oligodendrocyte vulnerability following traumatic brain injury in rats. Neurosci Lett 2011;499(3):143–8.

28. Yang SH, Gangidine M, Pritts TA, et al. Interleukin 6 mediates neuroinflammation and motor coordination deficits after mild traumatic brain injury and brief hypoxia in mice. Shock 2013;40(6):471–5.

29. Mouzon BC, Bachmeier C, Ferro A, et al. Chronic neuropathological and neurobehavioral changes in a repetitive mild traumatic brain injury model. Ann Neurol 2014;75(2):241–54.

30. Hoiland RL, Bain AR, Rieger MG, et al. Hypoxemia, oxygen content, and the regulation of cerebral blood flow. Am J Physiol Regul Integr Comp Physiol 2016;310(5):R398–413.

31. Rickards CA. Cerebral blood-flow regulation during hemorrhage. Compr Physiol 2015;5(4):1585–621.

32. Hotta H. Neurogenic control of parenchymal arterioles in the cerebral cortex. Prog Brain Res 2016;225:3–39.

33. DeWitt DS, Prough DS. Traumatic cerebral vascular injury: the effects of concussive brain injury on the cerebral vasculature. J Neurotrauma 2003;20(9):795–825.

34. McQuire JC, Sutcliffe JC, Coats TJ. Early changes in middle cerebral artery blood flow velocity after head injury. J Neurosurg 1998;89(4):526–32.

35. Golding EM, Robertson CS, Bryan RM Jr. The consequences of traumatic brain injury on cerebral blood flow and autoregulation: a review. Clin Exp Hypertens 1999;21(4):299–332.

36. Pasco A, Lemaire L, Franconi F, et al. Perfusional deficit and the dynamics of cerebral edemas in experimental traumatic brain injury using perfusion and diffusion-weighted magnetic resonance imaging. J Neurotrauma 2007;24(8):1321–30.

37. Villalba N, Sonkusare SK, Longden TA, et al. Traumatic brain injury disrupts cerebrovascular tone through endothelial inducible nitric oxide synthase expression and nitric oxide gain of function. J Am Heart Assoc 2014;3(6):e001474.

38. Hayward NM, Tuunanen PI, Immonen R, et al. Magnetic resonance imaging of regional hemodynamic and cerebrovascular recovery after lateral fluid-percussion brain injury in rats. J Cereb Blood Flow Metab 2011;31(1):166–77.

39. Park E, Bell JD, Siddiq IP, et al. An analysis of regional microvascular loss and recovery following two grades of fluid percussion trauma: a role for hypoxia-inducible factors in traumatic brain injury. J Cereb Blood Flow Metab 2009; 29(3):575–84.

40. Wei EP, Hamm RJ, Baranova AI, et al. The long-term microvascular and behavioral consequences of experimental traumatic brain injury after hypothermic intervention. J Neurotrauma 2009;26(4):527–37.

41. Gao G, Oda Y, Wei EP, et al. The adverse pial arteriolar and axonal consequences of traumatic brain injury complicated by hypoxia and their therapeutic
modulation with hypothermia in rat. J Cereb Blood Flow Metab 2010;30(3):
628–37.

42. Suehiro E, Ueda Y, Wei EP, et al. Posttraumatic hypothermia followed by slow re-
warming protects the cerebral microcirculation. J Neurotrauma 2003;20(4):
381–90.

43. Ueda Y, Wei EP, Kontos HA, et al. Effects of delayed, prolonged hypothermia on
the pial vascular response after traumatic brain injury in rats. J Neurosurg 2003;
99(5):899–906.

44. Baranova AI, Wei EP, Ueda Y, et al. Cerebral vascular responsiveness after experimental traumatic brain injury: the beneficial effects of delayed hypothermia combined with superoxide dismutase administration. J Neurosurg 2008;109(3):
502–9.

45. Petkus V, Krakauskaite S, Preiksaitis A, et al. Association between the outcome of
traumatic brain injury patients and cerebrovascular autoregulation, cerebral
perfusion pressure, age, and injury grades. Medicina (Kaunas) 2016;52(1):
46–53.

46. Stein TD, Alvarez VE, McKee AC. Concussion in chronic traumatic encephalopathy. Curr Pain Headache Rep 2015;19(10):47.

47. Kanaan NM, Cox K, Alvarez VE, et al. Characterization of early pathological tau
conformations and phosphorylation in chronic traumatic encephalopathy.
J Neuropathol Exp Neurol 2016;75(1):19–34.

48. McKee AC, Stern RA, Nowinski CJ, et al. The spectrum of disease in chronic traumatic encephalopathy. Brain 2013;136(Pt 1):43–64.

49. Barrio JR, Small GW, Wong KP, et al. In vivo characterization of chronic traumatic
encephalopathy using [F-18]FDDNP PET brain imaging. Proc Natl Acad Sci
U S A 2015;112(16):E2039–47.

50. Raghupathi R. Cell death mechanisms following traumatic brain injury. Brain
Pathol 2004;14(2):215–22.

51. Lotocki G, de Rivero Vaccari JP, Perez ER, et al. Alterations in blood-brain barrier
permeability to large and small molecules and leukocyte accumulation after traumatic brain injury: effects of post-traumatic hypothermia. J Neurotrauma 2009;
26(7):1123–34.

52. Johnson VE, Stewart W, Smith DH. Axonal pathology in traumatic brain injury. Exp
Neurol 2013;246:35–43.

53. O'Connor CA, Cernak I, Vink R. The temporal profile of edema formation differs
between male and female rats following diffuse traumatic brain injury. Acta Neurochir Suppl 2006;96:121–4.

54. Wang JY, Huang YN, Chiu CC, et al. Pomalidomide mitigates neuronal loss, neuroinflammation, and behavioral impairments induced by traumatic brain injury in
rat. J Neuroinflammation 2016;13(1):168.

55. Moro N, Ghavim SS, Harris NG, et al. Pyruvate treatment attenuates cerebral
metabolic depression and neuronal loss after experimental traumatic brain injury.
Brain Res 2016;1642:270–7.

56. Ekmark-Lewen S, Lewen A, Israelsson C, et al. Vimentin and GFAP responses in
astrocytes after contusion trauma to the murine brain. Restor Neurol Neurosci
2010;28(3):311–21.

57. Homsi S, Piaggio T, Croci N, et al. Blockade of acute microglial activation by min-
ocycline promotes neuroprotection and reduces locomotor hyperactivity after

closed head injury in mice: a twelve-week follow-up study. J Neurotrauma 2010; 27(5):911–21.

58. Morganti-Kossman MC, Lenzlinger PM, Hans V, et al. Production of cytokines following brain injury: beneficial and deleterious for the damaged tissue. Mol Psychiatry 1997;2(2):133–6.

59. Ghirnikar RS, Lee YL, Eng LF. Inflammation in traumatic brain injury: role of cytokines and chemokines. Neurochem Res 1998;23(3):329–40.

60. Taupin P. Adult neurogenesis, neuroinflammation and therapeutic potential of adult neural stem cells. Int J Med Sci 2008;5(3):127–32.

61. Lossinsky AS, Shivers RR. Structural pathways for macromolecular and cellular transport across the blood-brain barrier during inflammatory conditions. Review. Histol Histopathol 2004;19(2):535–64.

62. Scalfani MT, Dhar R, Zazulia AR, et al. Effect of osmotic agents on regional cerebral blood flow in traumatic brain injury. J Crit Care 2012;27(5):526.e7-12.

63. Stein DM, Hu PF, Brenner M, et al. Brief episodes of intracranial hypertension and cerebral hypoperfusion are associated with poor functional outcome after severe traumatic brain injury. J Trauma 2011;71(2):364–73 [discussion: 373–4].

64. Dore-Duffy P, Wang S, Mehedi A, et al. Pericyte-mediated vasoconstriction underlies TBI-induced hypoperfusion. Neurol Res 2011;33(2):176–86.

65. Bouma GJ, Muizelaar JP. Cerebral blood flow, cerebral blood volume, and cerebrovascular reactivity after severe head injury. J Neurotrauma 1992;9(Suppl 1): S333–48.

66. Jullienne A, Obenaus A, Ichkova A, et al. Chronic cerebrovascular dysfunction after traumatic brain injury. J Neurosci Res 2016;94(7):609–22.

67. Kenney K, Amyot F, Haber M, et al. Cerebral vascular injury in traumatic brain injury. Exp Neurol 2016;275(Pt 3):353–66.

68. Rossle R. German aviation medicine, world war II. Vol. 2. Washington, DC: Department of the Air Force. Pathology of Blast Effects; 1950.

69. Centers for Disease Control and Prevention National Center for Injury Prevention and Control. Explosions and blast injuries: a primer for clinicians. 2016. Available at: http://www.cdc.gov/masstrauma/preparedness/primer.pdf. Accessed June 29, 2016.

70. Ritenour AE, Blackbourne LH, Kelly JF, et al. Incidence of primary blast injury in US military overseas contingency operations: a retrospective study. Ann Surg 2010;251(6):1140–4.

71. Eskridge SL, Macera CA, Galarneau MR, et al. Combat blast injuries: injury severity and posttraumatic stress disorder interaction on career outcomes in male servicemembers. J Rehabil Res Dev 2013;50(1):7–16.

72. Mishra V, Skotak M, Schuetz H, et al. Primary blast causes mild, moderate, severe and lethal TBI with increasing blast overpressures: Experimental rat injury model. Sci Rep 2016;6:26992.

73. Centers for Disease Control and Prevention National Center for Injury Prevention and Control. Blast injuries: Fact Sheets for professionals. 2016. Available at: https://stacks.cdc.gov/view/cdc/21571/Print. Accessed January 28, 2017.

74. Davenport ND, Lim KO, Armstrong MT, et al. Diffuse and spatially variable white matter disruptions are associated with blast-related mild traumatic brain injury. Neuroimage 2012;59(3):2017–24.

75. Bauman RA, Ling G, Tong L, et al. An introductory characterization of a combat-casualty-care relevant swine model of closed head injury resulting from exposure to explosive blast. J Neurotrauma 2009;26(6):841–60.

76. Gilmore CS, Camchong J, Davenport ND, et al. Deficits in visual system functional connectivity after blast-related mild TBI are associated with injury severity and executive dysfunction. Brain Behav 2016;6(5):e00454.
77. Meabon JS, Huber BR, Cross DJ, et al. Repetitive blast exposure in mice and combat veterans causes persistent cerebellar dysfunction. Sci Transl Med 2016;8(321):321ra6.
78. Stemper BD, Shah AS, Budde MD, et al. Behavioral outcomes differ between rotational acceleration and blast mechanisms of mild traumatic brain injury. Front Neurol 2016;7:31.
79. Zuckerman A, Ram O, Ifergane G, et al. Controlled low-pressure blast-wave exposure causes distinct behavioral and morphological responses modelling mild traumatic brain injury, post-traumatic stress disorder, and comorbid mild traumatic brain injury-post-traumatic stress disorder. J Neurotrauma 2017;34(1): 145–64.
80. Zhang Y, Yang Y, Tang H, et al. Hyperbaric oxygen therapy ameliorates local brain metabolism, brain edema and inflammatory response in a blast-induced traumatic brain injury model in rabbits. Neurochem Res 2014;39(5):950–60.
81. Dalle Lucca JJ, Chavko M, Dubick MA, et al. Blast-induced moderate neurotrauma (BINT) elicits early complement activation and tumor necrosis factor alpha (TNFalpha) release in a rat brain. J Neurol Sci 2012;318(1–2):146–54.
82. Cho HJ, Sajja VS, Vandevord PJ, et al. Blast induces oxidative stress, inflammation, neuronal loss and subsequent short-term memory impairment in rats. Neuroscience 2013;253:9–20.
83. Ahmed F, Gyorgy A, Kamnaksh A, et al. Time-dependent changes of protein biomarker levels in the cerebrospinal fluid after blast traumatic brain injury. Electrophoresis 2012;33(24):3705–11.
84. Armonda RA, Bell RS, Vo AH, et al. Wartime traumatic cerebral vasospasm: recent review of combat casualties. Neurosurgery 2006;59(6):1215–25 [discussion: 1225].
85. Divani AA, Murphy AJ, Meints J, et al. A novel preclinical model of moderate primary blast-induced traumatic brain injury. J Neurotrauma 2015;32(14):1109–16.
86. Wolf SJ, Bebarta VS, Bonnett CJ, et al. Blast injuries. Lancet 2009;374(9687): 405–15.
87. Courtney A, Courtney M. The complexity of biomechanics causing primary blast-induced traumatic brain injury: a review of potential mechanisms. Front Neurol 2015;6:221.
88. Tumer N, Svetlov S, Whidden M, et al. Overpressure blast-wave induced brain injury elevates oxidative stress in the hypothalamus and catecholamine biosynthesis in the rat adrenal medulla. Neurosci Lett 2013;544:62–7.
89. Celander H, Clemedson CJ, Ericsson UA, et al. A study on the relation between the duration of a shock wave and the severity of the blast injury produced by it. Acta Physiol Scand 1955;33(1):14–8.
90. Chu SJ, Lee TY, Yan HC, et al. L-Arginine prevents air embolism-induced acute lung injury in rats. Crit Care Med 2005;33(9):2056–60.

Acute Management of Moderate-Severe Traumatic Brain Injury

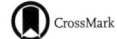 CrossMark

Wittstatt Alexandra Whitaker-Lea, MD, Alex B. Valadka, MD*

KEYWORDS

- Intracranial pressure • Management • Outcome • Traumatic brain injury

KEY POINTS

- Neurocritical care management of traumatic brain injury (TBI) patients focuses on prevention and prompt treatment of secondary insults.
- The acutely injured brain is highly vulnerable to brief deviations from normal physiologic values that would normally be well-tolerated.
- Treatments administered prophylactically against intracranial hypertension or other harmful sequelae have not been shown to be beneficial in clinical trials and have sometimes produced undesirable effects.
- Future advances in the management of TBI require treatments tailored to specific subtypes of patients, such as those with diffuse injury or with surgically evacuated traumatic hematomas.

INTRODUCTION

Traumatic brain injury (TBI) has long been a major public health problem. Commonly cited statistics indicate that 1,365,000 Americans visit emergency departments every year because of TBI.[1] It is likely that many more suffer TBI but receive other types of medical care (such as from their primary care physicians) or no care at all. In the United States, TBI causes 275,000 hospitalizations and 52,000 deaths every year, and it is a contributing factor in more than 30% of all injury-related deaths. The number of Americans living with the sequelae of TBI is as high as 5.3 million.[2]

TBI represents a leading cause of death and disability not just in the United States, but across the globe. Many low- and middle-income countries are burdened by a sharp increase in the numbers of motor vehicle-related injuries, a situation often aggravated by poor roads, inadequate enforcement of traffic laws, and underdeveloped prehospital emergency care systems.

Disclosure Statement: The authors have nothing to disclose.
Department of Neurosurgery, Virginia Commonwealth University, 417 North 11th Street, 6th Floor, PO Box 980631, Richmond, VA 23298-0631, USA
* Corresponding author.
E-mail address: avaladka@gmail.com

Phys Med Rehabil Clin N Am 28 (2017) 227–243
http://dx.doi.org/10.1016/j.pmr.2016.12.002

TBI is often classified as mild, moderate, or severe based on the Glasgow Coma Scale (GCS; **Tables 1** and **2**).[3,4] It has frequently been stated that 80% of TBI cases are mild, 10% moderate, and 10% severe. More recently, the proportion of mild cases seems to have increased, possibly because of greater awareness and recognition of concussion and other forms of mild TBI, which are discussed elsewhere in this volume.

Classically, the stereotypical TBI patient is a male in his late teens or early twenties. Fortunately, the incidence of interpersonal violence and motor vehicle crashes, which disproportionately affect males in this age group, has decreased in recent years. However, the number of falls among the elderly has increased dramatically as that segment of the population has grown in number. Many of these patients also take newer antiplatelet or anticoagulant medications, which can increase the likelihood and severity of intracranial hemorrhage after a fall.

Research and clinical care in TBI have been held back by persistent use of categorization based on physical examination instead of on underlying pathophysiology. No one would base a huge infrastructure of research, acute care, and rehabilitation on something as nebulous as "abdominal pain" because that term is so broad as to be almost meaningless. Abdominal pain can be caused by gastric ulcer, appendicitis, ischemic bowel, diverticulitis, pancreatitis, and a host of other diseases, which all have their own causes and treatments. A single medication or other treatment cannot be expected to be effective against such a variety of conditions. But the term "TBI" is used to describe any mechanically induced alteration of neurologic function, regardless of the underlying pathophysiologic cause, such as enlarging extraaxial hematoma, diffuse swelling, ischemia, blossoming contusion, and so on. Applying the same uniform approach to these different conditions makes as little sense as applying a single intervention to all patients with abdominal pain. It is no surprise that clinical trials in TBI, which have adopted this approach to patient enrollment, have failed to demonstrate improved outcome from any proposed intervention.

Both the public health burden of this severe and common disease and the exasperating stubbornness with which it has resisted attempts to develop effective treatments illustrate the magnitude of the challenges posed by TBI. This article focuses on the management of adults with moderate and severe closed brain injuries sustained in a civilian setting. The basic principles of management of severe TBI apply to children as much as to adults, but specific goals and parameters may differ. Also, pediatric TBI is characterized by a lower incidence of traumatic mass lesions than seen in adults. Of course, the possibility of intentionally inflicted injury must always be considered in children, just as it is in elderly and other vulnerable patients. Penetrating brain injuries may present interesting challenges in terms of surgical approaches and techniques, but

Table 1 Glasgow Coma Scale			
Score	Eye Opening (E)	Verbal (V)	Motor (M)
6	—	—	Obeys commands
5	—	Oriented	Localizes stimulus
4	Spontaneous	Confused	Withdraws from noxious stimulus
3	To voice	Inappropriate words	Abnormal flexion
2	To pain	Incomprehensible sounds	Extension
1	No eye opening	No sounds	No response

Table 2	
Classification of traumatic brain injury severity based on Glasgow Coma Scale	
Severity	Glasgow Coma Scale Score
Mild	13–15
Moderate	9–12
Severe	3–8

nonsurgical management has much in common with that of closed TBI patients. Similarly, military TBI is often caused by blast injury, which may produce massive brain swelling and cerebral vasospasm. However, other tenets of management are the same as those for nonblast injuries.

PATIENT EVALUATION AND MANAGEMENT OVERVIEW

The acute management of moderate and severe TBI is similar and varies primarily in degree of intervention, with the sickest patients requiring and receiving the most aggressive care.

History

Patient evaluation begins with a brief determination of the events surrounding the injury. Although such information is often incomplete and contradictory in the first minutes and hours after injury, it may prove useful for guiding initial management.

Physical Examination

The core of the evaluation is the physical examination. For TBI, as well as other neurologic emergencies, the initial assessment is usually based on the GCS (see **Table 1**).[3]

- The 3 components of the GCS are eye opening, verbal function, and motor examination. The score for each component should be listed separately and not lumped into a single overall score.
- For the eye opening and motor assessments, the right and left sides should be listed separately.
- If a patient's responses vary during a particular assessment, the highest level of function (best score) should be recorded.

Pupil size and reactivity are also important and should be noted for each eye.

- Dilatation and loss of reactivity may indicate that the pupil-constricting nerve fibers on the periphery of the third cranial nerve are significantly compressed by edematous or displaced brain tissue.
- Ischemia of the midbrain (where the third nerve arises from the Edinger-Westphal nucleus) may also be a cause.
- In a significant percentage of cases, local ocular trauma may be responsible.
- Pupillary dilatation and loss of reactivity resulting from extensive intracranial metabolic derangement is an ominous sign.

Completion of even this straightforward neurologic assessment may be impossible if patients have received sedation or paralytics, if one or both eyes are swollen shut, if the arms have sustained orthopedic or vascular injury, or for other reasons. The only recourse in such situations may be to document those parts of the examination that can be performed and to rely on others' reports (if available) of what the patient was doing initially. A more detailed neurologic assessment can be conducted after more pressing assessments and interventions have been carried out.

Careful initial assessment serves as the baseline against which subsequent improvement or deterioration in neurologic examination will be gauged.

Along with the neurologic assessment, a careful systematic examination is necessary to optimize treatment of non–nervous system injuries and, if necessary, to help balance different treatment priorities.

Prevention of Secondary Insults

Management of TBI patients, especially those at the severe end of the spectrum, is focused on preventing secondary cerebral injury.[5] This fundamental concept is based on the preclinical and clinical observation that the acutely traumatized brain is exquisitely sensitive to even mild deviations from normal homeostasis that would be well-tolerated in the absence of acute injury.[6]

The clinical outcome can be adversely affected by secondary insults. Among the most common are hypotension and hypoxia.[7] Because management of blood pressure and oxygenation is often performed by other specialists besides neurosurgeons, many different types of providers can intervene to prevent and treat these potentially devastating secondary insults.

Another common secondary insult is increased intracranial pressure (ICP). Potential interventions are discussed below. Etiologies can include the following:

- Impaired autoregulation with elevated cerebral blood volume (CBV)
- Presence or expansion of a large hematoma or contusion
- Edema around a cerebral contusion
- Hydrocephalus
- Diffuse brain swelling with reduced cerebral compliance
- Combinations of these and other causes

ABCs

As in any medical emergency, the first priority is assessment and stabilization of the ABCs (airway, breathing, and circulation; **Fig. 1**). Counterintuitively, endotracheal intubation has been reported to worsen the outcome in many published series. Many first responders do not perform endotracheal intubation sufficiently often to maintain their skill level in this technique, especially in prehospital environments that often pose a challenge to successful endotracheal intubation. Patients may become hypoxic during prolonged attempts at securing endotracheal access.

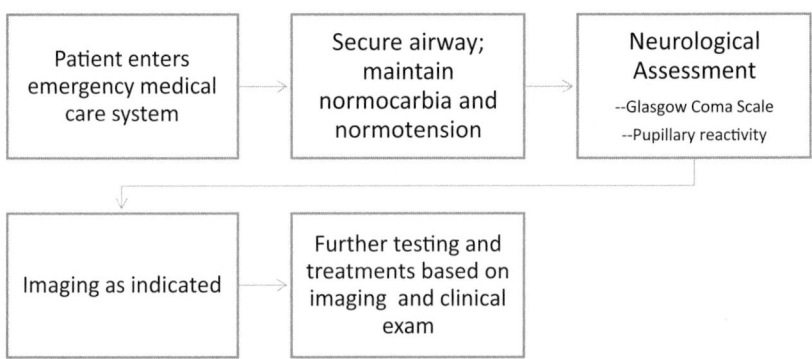

Fig. 1. Initial management of traumatic brain injury patients.

For breathing, the goals are simple: provide adequate oxygen to the injured brain and ensure sufficient ventilation to keep arterial carbon dioxide levels within a normal range because an increase in $Paco_2$ can lead to dilatation of cerebral arteries, with the consequent increase in CBV leading to an increased ICP. Regardless of whether an endotracheal tube is in place, care must be taken to avoid hyperventilation because hypocarbia can promote cerebral vasoconstriction and subsequent decrease in blood flow to an injured brain, potentially contributing to neuronal death from ischemia.[8]

Deliberate elevation of cerebral perfusion pressure (CPP, derived by subtracting the ICP from the mean arterial pressure) to supranormal levels has been demonstrated not to improve outcomes in severe TBI patients.[9] However, widespread recognition of the deleterious effects of hypotension in TBI patients has caused considerable attention to be placed on maintenance of normal blood pressure and avoidance of hypotension, the goal being not to worsen cerebral hypoperfusion and ischemia. Simply put, there is a floor below which the CPP is generally not allowed to fall, but deliberate elevation of CPP above this level is not beneficial. The Brain Trauma Foundation's *Guidelines for the Management of Severe Traumatic Brain Injury, 3rd edition*, specifies that this floor for CPP is 50 mm Hg for most patients, with a target of 50 to 70 mm Hg.[10] In North America, this recommendation is frequently simplified to target a minimum CPP of 60 mm Hg.

Monitoring

All intensive care unit (ICU) patients undergo detailed metabolic monitoring. Unique to neurocritical care is monitoring of parameters reflecting neurologic function. This is most commonly manifest as monitoring of ICP. For several decades, it was recommended widely that certain TBI patients undergo ICP monitoring, including most of those with severe TBI and some with less severe injuries. However, it was widely perceived that ICP monitoring was not being practiced as widely as one might expect. A review of the National Trauma Data Bank found that ICP monitoring was performed in fewer than one-half of patients who met Brain Trauma Foundation guidelines for such monitoring.[11] Moreover, ICP monitoring was associated with a 45% reduction in survival.

A prospective trial to investigate the effect of ICP monitoring on outcome was carried out in several South American countries.[12] The presence of intracranial hypertension in 2 groups of patients was determined either by invasive monitoring or by inference from findings on imaging and clinical examination. The 2 groups did not differ in outcome. This study has been criticized for several reasons, including the less-advanced prehospital emergency medical systems in the locations of the study hospitals when compared with those in high-income countries. Nevertheless, this study has been helpful for questioning a long-held dogma and for opening a discussion about the optimal use of ICP monitoring in TBI patients.

Many other neurologic monitoring technologies are available commercially, both invasive and noninvasive. Although adverse values for the specific parameters measured by these devices have been linked to worse outcomes, it has not been shown that intervention to treat those parameters can improve outcomes. One technology that is further along than most on the pathway toward demonstration of clinical efficacy is brain tissue oxygen monitoring. A phase II trial has suggested some benefit from intervening to correct low brain tissue oxygen levels,[13] and a phase III trial is in the planning stages.

Initial Imaging

After the ABCs have been addressed and an initial evaluation for associated injuries has been completed, patients are usually taken for immediate computed tomography

(CT) scanning. Typically, CT scans are obtained of the head, cervical spine, and chest, abdomen, and pelvis, including the thoracic and lumbar spines. Although MRI scanning may provide more detail about the brain parenchyma, it requires much more time than a CT scan. Also, CT scanning is highly sensitive for detecting acute blood, skull fractures, mass effect, and other traumatic pathologies that may require immediate intervention. CT scanning also puts few restrictions on access to an acutely injured patient, unlike MRI scanning. Finally, MRI scanning is not compatible with the ferromagnetic monitoring and therapeutic equipment that often accompanies trauma patients from the emergency department to the CT scanner.

Of note, CT scanning has become so rapid that, even if the head CT demonstrates a large hematoma requiring immediate evacuation, the remainder of the scan (cervical spine and chest, abdomen, and pelvis) can be completed while the operating room makes hurried preparations for an emergency craniotomy. This is time well-spent because the identification of other injuries may affect positioning or other preparations for the craniotomy, or may even require concurrent treatment while the intracranial hematoma is being evacuated.

Although many neurosurgeons have long favored clinically based classification systems like the GCS, it is also possible to classify TBI according to imaging features. Marshall and colleagues[14] used the Traumatic Coma Data Bank to develop a CT-based scheme (**Table 3**). Maas and colleagues[15] used a large clinical trial database to construct a prognostic scheme in which selected CT features are used to calculate a CT score (**Table 4**). The trauma surgery community often uses the Abbreviated Injury Scale to classify the severity of TBI, and it is possible to translate Abbreviated Injury Scale data into the appropriate Marshall classification.[16]

Follow-up Imaging

The need for routine follow-up CT scans in TBI patients has been a subject of several recent reports. Specific questions include whether, when, and how often to obtain follow-up brain imaging. Certainly, when patients exhibit unexplained or unanticipated neurologic deterioration or fail to improve as expected after surgery and other resuscitative interventions, prompt CT scanning should be considered. Otherwise, if patients with mild TBI and minimal findings on initial head CT remain neurologically stable for several hours after injury, follow-up scanning is not necessary.[17]

Avoiding repeat CT scanning saves the patient from additional radiation exposure, which has become a growing concern, especially in pediatric patients. Because mild

Table 3	
Marshall CT classification of traumatic brain injury	
Classification	**Definition**
Diffuse injury I	No intracranial pathology on CT scan
Diffuse injury II	Midline shift <5 mm. Cisterns present. High- or mixed-density lesions <25 mL.
Diffuse injury III	Midline shift <5 mm. Cisterns compressed or absent. High- or mixed-density lesions <25 mL.
Diffuse injury IV	Midline shift >5 mm. Absent cisterns. High- or mixed-density lesions <25 mL.
Evacuated mass lesion	Any surgically evacuated mass lesion.
Nonevacuated mass lesion	High- or mixed-density lesion >25 mL, not surgically evacuated.

Abbreviation: CT, computed tomography.

| Table 4 | | |
| Rotterdam CT scoring system | | |
Component	Description	Score
Basal cisterns	Normal	0
	Compressed	1
	Absent	2
Midline shift	≤5 mm	0
	>5 mm	1
Intraventricular blood or subarachnoid hemorrhage	Absent	0
	Present	1
Sum score		+1

TBI is such a common problem, eliminating low-yield or unnecessary scans in even a few of these patients can have a significant impact on reducing costs and administrative burdens to the health care system.

For moderate or severe TBI, however, planned repeat CT scanning is often wise. Recommended intervals vary from a few hours after injury to 24 hours or longer. Patients who remain stable and who demonstrate low ICP may be scanned at longer intervals, whereas those who have especially worrisome CT scans or those taking antiplatelet or anticoagulant medications may be scanned earlier.

Molecular Biomarkers

In the not-too-distant future, point-of-care serial monitoring of biochemical markers to detect new or worsening neurologic injury may become a routine part of the care of TBI patients.[18] Bedside testing using minimal volumes of blood may eliminate the potential risks of transport and excessive phlebotomy if biomarkers indicate that the cerebral response to injury is appropriate. However, adverse trends in levels of biochemical markers may indicate that prompt transport to the CT scanner is warranted. Some markers may even increase several hours before the ICP increases, thereby acting as a type of early warning system that might allow clinicians to intervene early to treat increases in ICP or even obviate them altogether. Future technologies will also permit analyses of body fluids and biospecimens other than blood.

PHARMACOLOGIC TREATMENT OPTIONS

Although potential pharmacologic treatments have been evaluated in many clinical trials, none has been shown to directly improve outcome after TBI. Nevertheless, several medications are used commonly to manage various aspects of the ICU course of moderate and severe TBI patients.

Osmotic Diuretics

Osmotic diuretics like mannitol and hypertonic saline are often effective at lowering ICP by decreasing blood viscosity (thereby triggering reflex constriction of the cerebral arteries, with resultant decrease in CBV and thus a decrease in ICP)[19] and drawing fluid across the blood–brain barrier from the brain to the vasculature. However, this ICP-lowering effect has not been demonstrated to lead directly to improved outcomes. Similarly, the recently popularized practice of continuously infusing hypertonic agents in hopes of creating a beneficial osmotic gradient between brain and blood remains unproven.[20]

Analgesics and Sedatives

Analgesics and sedatives like morphine, fentanyl, propofol, lorazepam, and others are administered to TBI patients frequently. Controlling pain from injuries is an important part of all medical care. Sedation may help to minimize coughing, fighting against an endotracheal tube or mechanical ventilator, and so on. However, the direct neuroprotective effect of specific medications has not been demonstrated. In patients with increased muscle tone from sympathetic hyperactivity, muscle spasms, and so on, pharmacologic neuromuscular blockade is sometimes used. Concerns have been expressed about myopathy from prolonged use of neuromuscular blocking agents. More important, a retrospective analysis of Traumatic Coma Data Bank patients found that prophylactic use of neuromuscular blocking agents did not improve outcome but did result in longer ICU duration of stay and a trend toward a greater mortality rate.[21]

Anticonvulsants

Anticonvulsants are often administered to TBI patients to prevent seizures. Phenytoin and valproate have been studied in the highest-quality clinical trials,[22,23] which suggested that prophylactic anticonvulsants lower the incidence of seizures in TBI patients for the first week or so after injury but not thereafter. Thus, a 1-week course of anticonvulsant prophylaxis is ordered commonly. The results of those trials are often extrapolated to other anticonvulsants. Levetiracetam is popular because of a perceived lower incidence of side effects and because it is not necessary to check serum drug levels as a guide to dosing. Of interest, the decreased incidence of seizures during the first week has not been shown to translate into improved long-term outcome.

Steroids

In prior decades, steroids were used routinely in TBI patients in attempts to mitigate cerebral edema. However, this practice was not supported by high-quality clinical trials. More recent studies found an association between steroid administration and increased mortality rates in TBI patients.[24] For these reasons, the routine administration of steroids to these patients is not recommended generally.

Pressors

Pressors may be required to achieve the goal of avoiding or treating hypotension and potentially inadequate CPP. However, the choice of specific pressor does not seem to affect outcome from TBI.

NONPHARMACOLOGIC TREATMENT OPTIONS

Because of the lack of pharmacologic treatments to stimulate neural repair or to minimize inflammation and other potentially harmful processes, the goals of management of moderate and severe TBI patients continue to be the prevention of secondary insults and the maintenance of physiologic processes as close to normal as possible so that the brain has an optimal environment in which to heal. So far, every treatment that has been initiated on a prophylactic basis—in other words, in an attempt to prevent deleterious cerebral metabolic events from occurring—has failed to demonstrate benefit in clinical trials. In fact, many such preventive treatments have actually worsened outcomes. Thus, the best practice continues to be close monitoring of patients so that appropriate interventions can instituted as soon as harmful deviations from normal physiologic homeostasis are detected.

Goals

Commonly recommended goals for various physiologic parameters are summarized in **Table 5**.[25] The pattern underlying those goals is that recommended values fall into normal ranges. These include Pao_2, $Paco_2$, and blood pressure. Normal values are also recommended for serum sodium levels, despite the widespread practice of deliberately increasing serum sodium concentration and osmolality in an attempt to prevent cerebral edema. Such a practice is often not needed because ICP does not increase in many patients, and in others, it will increase even after prophylactic hypernatremia has been achieved. In many such cases, the clinician must then manage elevated ICP without being able to use mannitol or hypertonic saline because stopping limits for those treatments have already been exceeded.

Temperature

Another controversial practice is aggressive prevention of fever. Although induced hypothermia has so far failed to show benefit in the treatment of TBI patients, the association of increased temperature with worse outcomes has led many ICUs to institute measures for aggressive maintenance of normothermia. However, high-quality clinical data to support this practice are lacking.

Hyperbaric Oxygen

Even more controversial is the use of hyperbaric oxygen in the treatment of TBI. At the moderate/severe end of the spectrum, transport of critically ill patients to a hyperbaric chamber for multiple treatments may pose significant logistical difficulties. Trials reported to date have varied in postinjury time of initiation of this treatment, extent of pressure increase in each session, frequency and total number of treatments, and other parameters. Standardization of these and other details of treatment would be

Table 5
Physiologic targets in traumatic brain injury patients

Physiologic Parameter	Goal
CPP	$\geq$60 mm Hg
Glucose	80–180 mg/dL
Hemoglobin	$\geq$7 g/dL
ICP	20–25 mm Hg
INR	$\leq$1.4
$Paco_2$	35–45 mm Hg
Pao_2	$\geq$100 mm Hg
$PbtO_2$	$\geq$15 mm Hg
pH	7.35–7.45
Platelets	$\geq$75,000/μL
Pulse oximetry	$\geq$95%
SBP	$\geq$100 mm Hg
Serum sodium	135–145 mEq/L
Temperature	36–38°C

Abbreviations: CPP, cerebral perfusion pressure; ICP, intracranial pressure; INR, international normalized ratio; $Paco_2$, arterial partial pressure of carbon dioxide; Pao_2, arterial partial pressure of oxygen; $PbtO_2$, brain tissue oxygen tension; SBP, systolic blood pressure.

necessary before conducting a definitive trial of hyperbaric oxygen in the moderate/severe TBI population.

Increased Intracranial Pressure

Secondary insults can be neurologic as well as systemic in origin. The most common of these is an increased ICP. Ideally, management would be tailored to the component(s) of intracranial volume that is contributing most to the intracranial hypertension: intravascular blood (increased CBV), hematoma/contusion (large mass lesion), cerebrospinal fluid (hydrocephalus), or cerebral parenchyma (edema).

- Increased CBV can be treated with careful hyperventilation to constrict the cerebral vasculature and lower the ICP, but care must be taken not to provoke cerebral ischemia from excessive vasoconstriction and lowered cerebral blood flow in the metabolically challenged brain tissue.
- Mannitol can also reduce CBV because its reduction of blood viscosity causes a reflex reduction in vascular diameter.
- Maintenance of normal or, in some cases, slightly increased CPP may induce reflex cerebral vasoconstriction.
- Large mass lesions are usually evacuated surgically.
- Accumulation of cerebrospinal fluid is managed by external drainage via a ventriculostomy catheter.
- Cerebral edema may require aggressive use of mannitol or hypertonic saline, or even decompressive craniectomy (DC) in select cases.

In the clinical setting, however, it is often difficult to make such distinctions. As a result, a common practice is to apply a standard ICP management algorithm in a one-size-fits-all approach, with the sequence of interventions ordered such that minimally invasive or least-risk maneuvers are implemented before progression to more worrisome treatments (**Fig. 2**). It has become common to place different treatments into "tiers" based on their perceived potential risk, but variability exists among

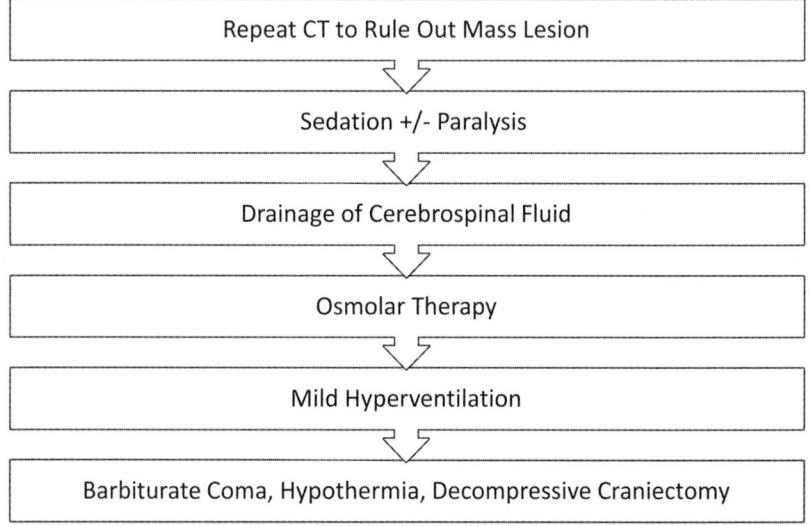

Fig. 2. Management algorithm for increased intracranial pressure. CT, computed tomography.

different authors concerning which treatments belong in which tiers, and the relationship of this classification scheme to outcome is not clear.

Last-ditch measures to control an increased ICP are frequently effective at treating intracranial hypertension, but in clinical trials this effect has failed to translate into demonstrably improved clinical outcomes. Treatments that fall into this category include barbiturate coma, hypothermia, and DC.

Pentobarbital has long been known to lower the ICP in many TBI patients in whom other ICP-lowering treatments had been ineffective. However, despite the ICP-lowering effects of pentobarbital, prospective, randomized, controlled trials have failed to demonstrate improved overall outcome when barbiturates were used in the management of intracranial hypertension.[26–28] Barbiturate administration often led to hypotension, which may have negated any neuroprotective effect. As with many trials of potential TBI treatments, it is unclear if benefit may have been shown in a trial that had been designed differently.

Therapeutic hypothermia has a powerful protective effect in experimental TBI. However, when tested as a prophylactic intervention in the clinical setting of severe TBI, therapeutic hypothermia has not been associated with an improved outcome.[29,30] A retrospective analysis of the databases from the National Acute Brain Injury Study: Hypothermia trials suggested that patients with surgically evacuated traumatic mass lesions benefited if hypothermia was initiated within 1.5 hours of the start of surgery.[31] This beneficial effect was not seen in nonsurgical patients. The Eurotherm3235 trial investigated therapeutic hypothermia not as a prophylactic measure, but as a therapeutic intervention initiated when preliminary efforts failed to lower intracranial hypertension.[32] This study also found no benefit to induced hypothermia.

At the time of this writing, the results of the RESCUEICP trial (Randomised Evaluation of Surgery with Craniectomy for Uncontrollable Elevation of Intracranial Pressure) are due to be released soon. This study investigates the value of DC to treat elevated ICP in TBI patients after less aggressive measures have failed,[33] and the results are awaited eagerly.

SURGICAL TREATMENT OPTIONS

The goal of surgery for most patients with moderate/severe TBI is to evacuate intracranial hematomas or contusions. The most frequently encountered lesions are epidural hematomas, subdural hematomas, cerebral contusions, and intraparenchymal hematomas (**Fig. 3**). The first 2 may often be lumped together as "extraaxial hematomas" in reference to their location outside the neuraxis. An intraparenchymal hematoma consists of extravasated blood, whereas a contusion is characterized by extravasated blood mixed with brain tissue, leading to a more heterogeneous CT scan appearance than seen in pure hematomas.

Mass Lesions

The key to planning the surgical approach to an acute subdural hematoma (ASDH) is the creation of as large a scalp incision as possible. This is necessary for 3 reasons.

- The source of the bleeding can arise anywhere from the midline to the skull base, and it is quite difficult to control bleeding without direct visualization of the source, especially when the brain is injured and swollen.
- ASDHs often extend over most of the hemisphere, requiring generous exposure to ensure evacuation of as much of the clot as possible.

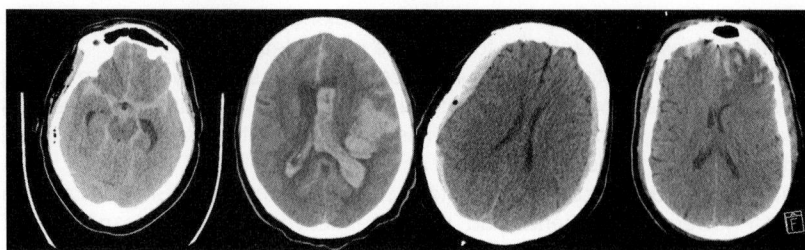

Fig. 3. Examples of different hemorrhagic lesions after traumatic brain injury. From left to right: subarachnoid hemorrhage, intraparenchymal hemorrhage with intraventricular extension, subdural (right side of picture) and epidural (left side of picture) hematomas, and cerebral contusion.

- In the event that significant intraoperative brain swelling makes it impossible to replace the bone flap, a wide craniectomy is necessary to allow sufficient room for the swollen brain to expand without strangulation of cerebral tissue and vasculature on the edges of the bony opening.

After opening of the scalp and removal of bone, the dura is incised and care is taken to ensure that the underlying cortex is not injured. The hematoma is evacuated, followed by either bipolar cauterization of sites of active bleeding or verification that active bleeding has ceased. This portion of the operation must proceed quickly because injured brain often expands once the physical constraints imposed by the dura have been removed. After hemostasis has been verified, it is the authors' preference to close the dura and replace the bone flap. Reconstruction of the normal dural and bony structures seems to result in less cerebral edema than duraplasty and craniectomy, and this clinical observation is supported by experimental data.[34] Furthermore, leaving the bone flap off has not been shown to improve outcomes, but it does expose the patient to a high rate of complications both from the craniectomy itself and from subsequent cranioplasty.[35]

These same basic principles apply to surgical evacuation of acute epidural hematomas and parenchymal lesions, except that it may be possible to evacuate these lesions through exposures smaller than those used for ASDHs.

Decompressive Craniectomy

As mentioned, DC must be performed via a large bony opening if it is to be successful. Some surgeons leave bone flaps off in most of their operations for ASDH, with the assumption that the underlying brain is likely to swell in the days after surgery. The ongoing RESCUE-ASDH trial (Randomised Evaluation of Surgery with Craniectomy for patients Undergoing Evacuation of Acute Subdural Haematoma) is intended to evaluate the effect of this practice on patient outcome.[33] Another common indication for DC is intracranial hypertension refractory to less aggressive interventions in potentially salvageable patients. In general, performance of DC in patients with diffuse brain swelling and no large mass lesion has become less popular in recent years, largely because of the results of the DECRA trial (Early Decompressive Craniectomy in Patients With Severe Traumatic Brain Injury).[36]

Cranioplasty

The preferred timing of the subsequent cranioplasty has evolved over the years. Earlier reports had advocated delays of 6 months or longer. More recently, it has become generally recognized that, in the absence of prior infection or gross contamination of wounds, patients fare better with earlier cranioplasty, which is often performed as soon as brain swelling has decreased sufficiently. Restoration of a normal calvarium seems to normalize cerebral pressure dynamics and may help to prevent the extraaxial fluid collections and enlarged ventricles that often occur after craniectomy. Case series describe improvements in such cerebral metabolic parameters as cerebral blood flow and glucose metabolism, and some patients seem to undergo mild neurologic improvement after cranioplasty.

TREATMENT RESISTANCE AND COMPLICATIONS

As emphasized, the monitoring of ICP and the prevention and treatment of its elevations are major areas of emphasis in the management of moderate and severe TBI patients. At the same time, these patients are also susceptible to the same systemic complications that can affect any critically ill patient. Basic ICU protocols for infection prevention, nutrition, decubitus ulcer prevention, and other generic measures should be implemented, with modification as necessary for individual patients and/or for the presence of TBI.

Prophylaxis against deep venous thrombosis can be problematic in TBI patients. Mechanical measures, such as compressive stockings and pneumatic compressive devices, are safe in both operated and nonsurgical TBI patients. Pharmacologic prophylaxis with unfractionated or low-molecular-weight heparin has been more controversial. Historically, neurosurgeons have been highly averse to any interventions that may cause or worsen intracranial bleeding. Waiting times of 1 or 2 weeks postinjury or even longer were often recommended. Over time, it has become clear that earlier administration of such agents is not associated with an increased rate of new or worsening intracranial hemorrhage. A commonly cited time point is 72 hours after injury or after the last stable CT scan, that is, the scan that demonstrates that intracranial hemorrhage has not progressed. Although 72 hours seems to be the interval at which many neurosurgeons now feel comfortable with pharmacologic deep venous thrombosis prophylaxis, it should be remembered that newer data indicate that this intervention can be initiated within 24 hours or even sooner. Ongoing education and discussion will progressively shorten the time at which most practitioners are comfortable with pharmacologic deep venous thrombosis prophylaxis.

It is harder to generalize about resumption of long-term anticoagulation for atrial fibrillation or other indications. In general, a waiting period of several weeks may be reasonable. Individualization of such decisions may take into account the specific anticoagulant drug, the severity of the intracranial pathology, and the nature and severity of the underlying condition that required anticoagulation in the first place.

Paroxysmal sympathetic hyperactivity (PSH), also commonly known as dysautonomia or storming, can be a difficult problem to treat in TBI and other neurocritical care patients.[37] It is characterized by episodic bursts of apparently sympathetic-mediated activity, causing such signs as tachycardia, hypertension, tachypnea, diaphoresis, increased muscle tone, fever, mydriasis, and other symptoms. Such episodes may seem to occur spontaneously, whereas others may be caused by stimulation induced by standard nursing care of critically ill patients, such as turning, bathing, or endotracheal suctioning. PSH is most commonly associated with TBI, but it can also occur after cerebral hypoxic injury or other types of cerebral insult. Acutely, as many as a third of TBI patients admitted to an ICU may exhibit this condition, an incidence that seems to decrease to roughly 10% or less at later postinjury time periods. Reported pharmacologic interventions vary so widely as to preclude solid recommendations, forcing practitioners to try specific medications on an empiric basis. Commonly used agents include opioids, benzodiazepines, baclofen, centrally acting alpha agonists, beta antagonists, bromocriptine, and others. Although the prognosis for long-term outcome is generally not good in patients with PSH, occasional good outcomes have been reported, and the authors have treated PSH patients who went on to do well.

EVALUATION OF OUTCOME

It has been stated that the outcome from severe TBI has been progressively improving in recent years. Although mortality rates often exceeded 50% in past decades, some current series report mortality rates as low as 20%. Such series, however, reflect outcomes from only selected patients. Because those studies were often designed to evaluate potential new therapies, they frequently excluded patients who demonstrated the poorest prognostic factors, such as dilated and nonreactive pupils, advanced age, extremely poor neurologic status, significant comorbidities, or prolonged time between injury and intervention.

A reasonable expectation of outcome after severe TBI was provided by the Traumatic Coma Data Bank, and it remains useful to this day.[38] Outcome was classified by the Glasgow Outcome Scale (**Table 6**).[39] Mortality can be expected in roughly one-third of patients. Only a few percent will remain indefinitely in a persistent vegetative state. Roughly 15% to 20% will have a severe disability, and a similar proportion will have a moderate disability. Approximately 25% will achieve a good outcome.

In contrast with the 5-point Glasgow Outcome Scale, an 8-point Extended Glasgow Outcome Scale has been developed to provide more detailed categorization of functional outcomes.[40]

The improvement in outcomes from decades ago to the present can be attributed to improved organization and delivery of prehospital care and to advances in delivery of hospital-based critical care services. Many clinical trials have been conducted to test the effects of medications or other potential treatments for TBI. However, no brain-specific medication or other magic bullet has been developed to improve recovery of the injured brain directly.[41] Many reasons have been put forth to explain the failure of so many clinical trials, including the heterogeneity of TBI, the difficulties of initiating treatment early enough for it to be effective, the inability of preclinical models to reproduce the full pathophysiologic spectrum of human TBI, and flawed design of clinical trials.

The recent trend in the increasing incidence of TBI among the elderly, who tend to fare worse after TBI than younger patients, will likely have a negative effect on outcome of the overall TBI population, with an increased proportion of deaths and poor outcomes. The worse overall health and decreased physiologic reserve of

Table 6 Glasgow Outcome Scale	
Score	Description
5	Good recovery
4	Moderate disability
3	Severe disability
2	Persistent vegetative state
1	Death

Severe disability: Needs assistance with activities of daily living.
Moderate disability: Some disability, but independent in activities of daily living.

most elderly patients contributes to these poorer outcomes. Another increasingly common complication results from the growing use of newer anticoagulant or anti-platelet agents in this population. Falls and other types of head impacts in these patients may precipitate significant intracranial bleeding, while at the same time the presence of these medications may contraindicate immediate surgery.

SUMMARY AND DISCUSSION

Despite tremendous effort expended in numerous clinical trials over the past several decades, moderate and severe TBI remain stubbornly resistant to treatment. Lessons learned from those trials have suggested different ways not just to conduct future studies, but also to conceptualize both the varying types of pathologies caused by TBI and the body's different responses to various types of injury.

In the meantime, the cornerstone of care remains the prevention of secondary injury by careful attention to the ABCs. Prophylactic interventions to stimulate neural recovery or to prevent secondary insults have so far been unsuccessful or even harmful. Ongoing and future work on specific types of TBI, on optimized application of imaging, and on the roles of molecular biomarkers will allow us to make the advances that have so far been elusive.

REFERENCES

1. Faul M, Xu L, Wald M, et al. Traumatic brain injury in the United States emergency department visits, hospitalizations, and deaths 2002-2006. Atlanta (GA): Centers for Disease Control and Prevention; National Center for Injury Prevention and Control; 2010.
2. Centers for Disease Control and Prevention (CDC). Report to congress on traumatic brain injury in the United States: epidemiology and rehabilitation. Atlanta (GA): National Center for Injury Prevention and Control; Division of Unintentional Injury Prevention; 2015.
3. Teasdale G, Jennett B. Assessment of coma and impaired consciousness. A practical scale. Lancet 1974;2(7872):81–4.
4. Rimel RW, Giordani B, Barth JT, et al. Moderate head injury: completing the clinical spectrum of brain trauma. Neurosurgery 1982;11:344–51.
5. Becker DP, Miller JD, Ward JD, et al. The outcome from severe head injury with early diagnosis and intensive management. J Neurosurg 1977;47:491–502.
6. Jenkins L, Moszynski K, Lyeth B, et al. Increased vulnerability of the mildly traumatized rat brain to cerebral ischemia: the use of controlled secondary ischemia as a research tool to identify common or different mechanisms contributing to mechanical and ischemic brain injury. Brain Res 1989;477:211–24.
7. Chesnut RM, Marshall LF, Klauber MR, et al. The role of secondary brain injury in determining outcome from severe head injury. J Trauma 1993;34:216–22.
8. Muizelaar JP, Marmarou A, Ward JD, et al. Adverse effects of prolonged hyperventilation in patients with severe head injury: a randomized clinical trial. J Neurosurg 1991;75:731–9.
9. Robertson CS, Valadka AB, Hannay HJ, et al. Prevention of secondary ischemic insults after severe head injury. Crit Care Med 1999;27:2086–95.
10. Brain Trauma Foundation. Guidelines for the management of severe traumatic brain injury, 3rd edition. J Neurotrauma 2007;24(Suppl 1):S1–106.
11. Shafi S, Diaz-Arrastia R, Madden C, et al. Intracranial pressure monitoring in brain-injured patients is associated with worsening of survival. J Trauma 2008; 64:335–40.

12. Chesnut RM, Temkin N, Carney N, et al. A trial of intracranial-pressure monitoring in traumatic brain injury. N Engl J Med 2012;367:2471–81.

13. Neurocritical Care Society. BOOST 2 trial study results. In: Neurocritical Care Society 2014 Annual Meeting Highlights. Available at: http://beta.neurocriticalcare.org/news/2014-annual-meeting-highlights. Accessed June 20, 2016.

14. Marshall LF, Marshall SB, Klauber MR, et al. A new classification of head injury based on computerized tomography. J Neurosurg Spec Suppl 1991;75(1S): S14–20.

15. Maas AIR, Hukkelhoven CWPM, Marshall LF, et al. Prediction of outcome in traumatic brain injury with computed tomographic characteristics: a comparison between the computed tomographic classification and combinations of computed tomographic predictors. Neurosurgery 2005;57:1173–82.

16. Lesko MM, Woodford M, White L, et al. Using abbreviated injury scale (AIS) codes to classify computed tomography (CT) features in the Marshall System. BMC Med Res Methodol 2010;10:72–81.

17. Brown CVR, Zada G, Salim A, et al. Indications for routine repeat head computed tomography (CT) stratified by severity of traumatic brain injury. J Trauma 2007;62: 1339–45.

18. Papa L, Brophy GM, Welch RD, et al. Time course and diagnostic accuracy of glial and neuronal blood biomarkers GFAP and UCH-L1 in a large cohort of trauma patients with and without mild traumatic brain injury. JAMA Neurol 2016;73:551–60.

19. Muizelaar JP, Wei EP, Kontos HA, et al. Mannitol causes compensatory cerebral vasoconstriction and vasodilation in response to blood viscosity changes. J Neurosurg 1983;59:822–8.

20. Diringer MN. New trends in hyperosmolar therapy? Curr Opin Crit Care 2013;19: 77–82.

21. Hsiang J, Chesnut RM, Crisp C, et al. Early, routine paralysis for intracranial pressure control in severe head injury: is it necessary? Crit Care Med 1994;22:1471–6.

22. Temkin NR, Dikmen S, Wilensky A, et al. A randomized, double-blind study of phenytoin for the prevention of post-traumatic seizures. N Engl J Med 1990; 323:497–502.

23. Temkin NR, Dikmen SS, Anderson GD, et al. Valproate therapy for prevention of posttraumatic seizures: a randomized trial. J Neurosurg 1999;91:593–600.

24. Edwards P, Arango M, Balica L, et al. Final results of MRC CRASH, a randomised placebo-controlled trial of intravenous corticosteroid in adults with head injury—outcomes at 6 months. Lancet 2005;365(9475):1957–9.

25. American College of Surgeons Trauma Quality Improvement Program. ACS TQIP Best Practices in the Management of Traumatic Brain Injury. Available at: https://www.facs.org/~/media/files/quality%20programs/trauma/tqip/traumatic%20brain%20injury%20guidelines.ashx. Accessed June 20, 2016.

26. Schwartz ML, Tator CH, Rowed DW, et al. The University of Toronto head injury treatment study: a prospective, randomized comparison of pentobarbital and mannitol. Can J Neurol Sci 1984;11:434–40.

27. Eisenberg HM, Frankowski RF, Contant CF, et al. High-dose barbiturate control of elevated intracranial pressure in patients with severe head injury. J Neurosurg 1988;69:15–23.

28. Ward JD, Becker DP, Miller JD, et al. Failure of prophylactic barbiturate coma in the treatment of severe head injury. J Neurosurg 1985;62:383–8.

29. Clifton GL, Miller ER, Choi SC, et al. Lack of effect of induction of hypothermia after acute brain injury. N Engl J Med 2001;344:556–63.

30. Clifton GL, Valadka A, Zygun D, et al. Very early hypothermia induction in patients with severe brain injury (the National Acute Brain Injury Study: Hypothermia II): a randomised trial. Lancet Neurol 2011;10:131–9.

31. Clifton GL, Coffey CS, Fourwinds S, et al. Early induction of hypothermia for evacuated intracranial hematomas: a post hoc analysis of two clinical trials. J Neurosurg 2012;117:714–20.

32. Andrews PJD, Sinclair HL, Rodriguez A, et al. Hypothermia for intracranial hypertension after traumatic brain injury. N Engl J Med 2015;373:2403–12.

33. Hutchinson PJ, Corteen E, Czosnyka M, et al. Decompressive craniectomy in traumatic brain injury: the randomized multicenter RESCUEicp study (www.RESCUEicp.com). Acta Neurochir Suppl 2006;96:17–20.

34. Szczygielski J, Mautes AE, Müller A, et al. Decompressive craniectomy increases brain lesion volume and exacerbates functional impairment in closed head injury in mice. J Neurotrauma 2016;33:122–31.

35. Stiver SI. Complications of decompressive craniectomy for traumatic brain injury. Neurosurg Focus 2009;26(6):E7.

36. Cooper DJ, Rosenfeld JV, Murray L, et al. Decompressive craniectomy in diffuse traumatic brain injury. N Engl J Med 2011;364:1493–502.

37. Perkes I, Baguley IJ, Nott MT, et al. A review of paroxysmal sympathetic hyperactivity after acquired brain injury. Ann Neurol 2010;68:126–35.

38. Marshall LF, Gautille T, Klauber MR, et al. The outcome of severe closed head injury. J Neurosurg Spec Suppl 1991;75(Suppl 1):S28–36.

39. Jennett B, Bond M. Assessment of outcome after severe brain damage. Lancet 1975;1(7905):480–4.

40. Jennett B, Snoek J, Bond M, et al. Disability after severe head injury: observations on the use of the Glasgow Outcome Scale. J Neurol Neurosurg Psychiatry 1981; 44:285–93.

41. Maas AI, Roozenbeek B, Manley GT. Clinical trials in traumatic brain injury: past experience and current developments. Neurotherapeutics 2010;7:115–26.

Disorders of Consciousness

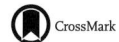

Blessen C. Eapen, MD[a],*, Jason Georgekutty, DO[b],
Bruno Subbarao, DO[a], Sheital Bavishi, DO[c], David X. Cifu, MD[d]

KEYWORDS

- Disorder of consciousness • Rehabilitation • Coma • Vegetative state
- Minimally conscious state • Traumatic brain injury

KEY POINTS

- Disorders of consciousness (DOC) are altered states of pathologic consciousness, which can be subdivided into coma, vegetative state, and minimally conscious state (MCS) based on neurobehavioral function.
- The Coma Recovery Scale-Revised assessment scale is recommended in DOC for clinical practice and research.
- Emergence from MCS is defined as reliable and consistent functional object use and functional communication.
- In a randomized, double-blinded, placebo controlled study, Amantadine improved functional recovery in patients with DOC.

INTRODUCTION

Annually, approximately 2.5 million people sustain a traumatic brain injury (TBI) in the United States, and more than 5.3 million people live with a TBI-related disability. TBI not only impacts the life of an individual and their family but also has a large societal and economic toll. The estimated economic cost of TBI in 2010, including direct and indirect medical costs, was approximately $76.5 billion. In addition, the cost of fatal TBIs and TBIs requiring hospitalization accounts for approximately 90% of the total TBI medical costs.[1] Approximately 0.3% severe TBIs can result in Disorders of Consciousness (DOC).[2] DOC is a state of prolonged altered consciousness, which can be

Disclosure Statement: The views, opinions, and/or findings expressed herein are those of the authors and do not necessarily reflect the views or the official policy of the Department of Veterans Affairs or US Government.
[a] Polytrauma Rehabilitation Center, South Texas Veterans Healthcare System, 7400 Merton Minter, San Antonio, TX 78229, USA; [b] Kessler Institute for Rehabilitation, 201 Pleasant Hill Road, Chester, NJ 07830, USA; [c] Traumatic Brain Injury Rehabilitation Program, Department of Physical Medicine and Rehabilitation, Ohio State University Wexner Medical Center, 480 Medical Center Drive, Columbus, OH 43210, USA; [d] Department of PM&R, Virginia Commonwealth University, US Department of Veterans Affairs, VA/DoD Chronic Effects of NeuroTrauma Consortium, 1223 E. Marshall Street, P.O. Box 980677, Richmond, Virginia 23284-0667, USA
* Corresponding author.
E-mail address: blessen.eapen2@va.gov

categorized into coma, vegetative state (VS), and minimally conscious state (MCS). DOC can prove difficult to diagnose and treat and can result in increased burden of care for families and facilities. In this article, the authors review the definition, diagnosis, imaging, and treatment interventions for this difficult patient population.

CONSCIOUSNESS

Historically, the concept of human consciousness has been difficult to describe on both a philosophic and a scientific level. Previous models often describe this phenomenon as a subjective experience, which consequently poses a diagnostic challenge in patients with a DOC. However, recent advances in modern medicine have allowed for improved survivability of acute brain injury and have secondarily imparted insight into the neural correlates of consciousness. Clinically, the 2 components that separate consciousness from unconsciousness are arousal and awareness.[3] Wakefulness is a state of arousal, which can be assessed by the presence of eye-opening and brainstem responses. The depth of wakefulness can be evaluated objectively using measures such as the Glasgow Coma Scale.[4] On a neuroanatomic level, arousal is mediated by the ascending reticular activating system of the upper brainstem. Activation of the cerebral cortex occurs with passage of sensory information from the upper brainstem via reticulothalamocortical and extrathalamic pathways. From a neurobiologic perspective, the conscious awake state is associated with a high energy demand and electrical activity within the corticothalamic system. This is further supported by electroencephalogram recordings (EEG), which show that increasing levels of arousal are associated with increased frequency of electrical activity in the cerebral cortex.[4] Conversely, a decline in arousal is associated with reduction in excitatory neuromodulatory influences. The global deafferentation and disruption of the corticothalamic networks could explain the dysfunction in arousal seen in severe brain injuries.[5] Awareness refers to the ability of an individual to respond to both external and internal stimuli in an integrated manner. It is inferred by command following and neurobehavioral assessment.[6] On a neuroanatomic level, the connectivity of frontoparietal regions and the thalamus appears to play a role in the maintenance of consciousness.[7] This is supported by functional MRI (fMRI) studies, which suggest dysfunctional cerebral connectivity in widespread areas of the frontoparietal networks in patients with DOC.[8] In a healthy individual, an increase in arousal is associated with an increase in awareness in a linear fashion along the continuum of conscious states.[9] A dissociation of these 2 components of consciousness is seen in pathologic states, such as in the VS and MCS.

CLINICAL ENTITIES
Brain Death

In 1995, the American Academy of Neurology (AAN) provided practice guidelines for the determination of brain death. They emphasized 3 clinical findings that indicate cessation of brain function: (1) coma (of known cause), (2) absence of brainstem reflexes, and (3) apnea. Before this determination, other causes for brainstem dysfunction should be excluded, including shock/hypotension, hypothermia, central nervous system depressants, spinal cord injury, and electrolyte and/or endocrine abnormalities. There is no consensus regarding the timing of follow-up testing, but clinicians must use judgment and perform serial evaluations to exclude the possibility for recovery. A diagnosis of brain death is ominous, and there have been no reports of neurologic recovery once determined by the 1995 AAN practice parameters.[10,11]

Coma

A coma is a state of unconsciousness characterized by a lack of arousal and awareness. The defining clinical feature is the complete loss of spontaneous or stimulus-induced arousal.[5] There is no eye opening, and EEG testing reveals the absence of sleep-wake cycles. Structural lesions usually involve diffuse cortical or white matter damage, or a brainstem lesion.[6] Those who survive this stage will begin to awaken and transition to a VS/unresponsive wakefulness state (UWS) or MCS within 2 to 4 weeks.[5,12]

Vegetative State/Unresponsive Wakefulness State

The VS is thought of as an unconscious, dissociative state of wakefulness without awareness. The patient's eyes open spontaneously, and EEG testing reveals the presence of sleep-wake cycles. Patients may arouse by provocation or external stimuli, but they show no signs of conscious perception or deliberate action.[4] Interestingly, these patients may perform stereotyped gestural movements such as yawning, chewing, crying, smiling, or moaning, but these are unrelated to context.[6] The presence of wakefulness suggests preserved brainstem functioning, but the lack of awareness suggests an underlying cortical dysfunction. Likewise, functional neuroimaging has shown sensory stimuli will activate primary cortical areas, but not the higher order cortical areas thought necessary for awareness.[4] With proper medical care, a patient in a VS can survive for many years.

Minimally Conscious State

The MCS is characterized by a severe impairment of consciousness, with evidence of wakefulness and partial preservation of awareness. Unlike the VS, there are discernible, purposeful behaviors that can be differentiated from reflexive behavior. Originally, these patients were categorized as VS, but there was evidence that they comparatively had meaningful improvement in outcomes. Therefore, in 2002 the Aspen Neurobehavioral Conference Workgroup established guidelines for MCS. The hallmark of MCS is inconsistent but reproducible, command following. The preservation of corticothalamic connections might explain why patients in MCS retain the capacity for cognitive processing. The patient may exhibit visual pursuit, emotional responses, and gestures to appropriate environmental stimuli, but are unable to functionally communicate their thoughts or feelings. Recently, a further subcategorization of the MCS was proposed by Bruno and colleagues,[13] based on the complexity of observed behavioral responses, to minimally conscious plus (MCS+) and minimally conscious minus (MCS−).

Acute Confusional State

Once emerged from the MCS, patients continue to experience a transient period of disorientation and agitation. The full array of symptoms associated with the acute confusional state can also include irritability, distractibility, anterograde amnesia, restlessness, emotional lability, impaired perception, attentional abnormalities, and a disrupted sleep-wake cycle.[14] A key pattern to this state is the day-to-day fluctuation of behavioral responses. The return of behavioral consistency despite situational stresses may indicate a resolution of this period.

Locked in Syndrome

Locked in syndrome is a rare condition characterized by intact consciousness and cognition, but with anarthria and quadriplegia.[15] It is likely caused by damage to the ventral pons and the corticospinal/corticobulbar pathways, which communicate with the brainstem.[5] Patients have intact sensation, and eye movements are spared, allowing for gaze-based communication. Over time, some patients may recover some control of the fingers, toes, or head. This atypical presentation, with lost speech and motor control, places these patients at risk for misdiagnosis as a DOC.

CLINICAL EXAMINATION AND QUANTITATIVE ASSESSMENT

A focused clinical examination is essential in distinguishing between DOC. Specifically, 7 domains should be tested and include sleep-wake cycles, awareness, motor skills, auditory function, visual function, communication, and emotional integrity (**Table 1**).[16] Sleep-wake cycles alone, detected through observation of intermittent eye-opening, will help differentiate someone in a VS from someone in a coma. The presence of awareness will further distinguish someone in a MCS from those in a vegetative one.

When testing the remainder of the domains, it is worth noting that certain caveats exist. First, yes/no responses can be given through direct verbal communication or through gestures such as a thumbs-up. These responses can be incorrect in regards to the questions asked, but they must be reproducible. Second, behavioral responses should demonstrate a definite relationship with their stimuli, such that reflexive activity cannot explain the response. For example, visual tracking of objects or persons, appropriate emotional responses to nonneutral content, and reaching for or grasping and manipulating objects. It is important to test a wide array of behavioral responses within the abilities of the patient and perform serial examinations to ensure accuracy. Last, it is imperative that a complete physical examination be done to provide insight for any findings that may obscure appropriate diagnosis, including but not limited to effects of sedative medications, aphasia, apraxia, motor impairments, or sensory deficits.[16]

As the patient continues along the spectrum of recovery, emergence from an MCS would be evidenced by 2 distinct behaviors. The first is functional interactive communication, which would have to be demonstrated through means of correct yes/no responses to 6 situational questions on 2 consecutive examinations. Examples of such questions could include, "Are you lying in bed right now?" or "Am I holding a pen in my hand?" Again, responses can be gestural, written, or verbal. The second behavior is the functional use of 2 different objects that can be validated. Examples include the patient bringing a toothbrush to their mouth or pointing a remote to a television.[16]

BEHAVIORAL ASSESSMENT SCALES

Diagnosis of DOC is based on clinical observations and standardized neurobehavioral assessments. Neurobehavioral assessment scales require standardized scoring and ability to detect subtle signs of consciousness.[5] Several scales have been developed to assess DOC patients. In 2010, a special task force, with the American Congress of Rehabilitation Medicine Special Interest Group in Disorders of Consciousness, reviewed 13 scales, of which 6 proved to be sensitive for detecting conscious awareness.[17] Of those 6 scales, the Coma Recovery Scale-Revised (CRS-R) had the strongest content validity based on the Aspen criteria.[5]

Coma Recovery Scale-Revised

The Coma Recovery Scale (CRS) was first described in 1991 and revised in 2004 (CRS-R).[18] It has had multiple studies that have proved its sensitivity and reliability in diagnosis and monitoring progress in DOC patients. The CRS-R is a 23-item scale

Table 1
Comparing features of coma, vegetative state, and minimally conscious state

	Sleep-Wake Cycles	Awareness	Motor	Auditory	Visual	Communication	Emotional
Coma	Absent	Absent	Reflexive	None	None	None	None
VS	Present	Absent	Purposeless/postures/withdraws to noxious stimuli	Startle	Startle	None	Reflexive
MCS	Present	Partial	Purposeful/localizes noxious stimuli	Localizes sound	Sustained fixation or pursuit	Intelligible verbal or gestural	Contingent responses

Adapted from Giacino JT, Ashwal S, Childs N, et al. The minimally conscious state: definition and diagnostic criteria. Neurology 2002;58(3):349–53.

comprising 6 subscales, whose items are arranged hierarchically from reflexive to cognitively mediated processes. Subscales address visual, auditory, motor, oromotor, communication, and arousal categories. Emergence criteria are assessed by the communication (yes/no accuracy) and motor subscales (functional object use).[18,19] Currently, this is the recommended scale because of its sensitivity and validity. Practitioner experience increases the interrater reliability and test-retest reliability. Training can be done by establishing interdisciplinary and particularly trained teams, using instructional videos, multicenter residency agreements, workshops, and video conferences.[20]

Sensory Modality and Rehabilitation Techniques

Sensory modality and rehabilitation techniques or SMART was developed by Occupational Therapists at the Royal Hospital for Neuro-disability in London, United Kingdom as both an assessment and a treatment tool for patients in VS or MCS.[21] SMART comprises 2 components. The formal component, conducted by the SMART assessors, includes the SMART Sensory Assessment and the SMART Behavioral Observation Assessment. The informal component consists of information from family and caregivers regarding observed behaviors and premorbid interests, likes, and dislikes.[21] The SMART requires a 5-day training course to become an assessor and prior submission of a portfolio to gain access to the assessment tool.

Western Neurosensory Stimulation Profile

Western neurosensory stimulation profile (WNSSP) consists of 32 items, which assess patients' arousal/attention, expressive communication, and response to auditory, visual, tactile, and olfactory stimulation. The WNSSP takes 20 to 40 minutes to administer and has shown internal consistency and standardized scoring and administration. It does rely on visual comprehension and tracking.[22]

Wessex Head Injury Matrix

Wessex Head Injury Matrix (WHIM) is a 62-item scale, ordered in hierarchy, that assesses communication ability, cognitive skills, and social interaction. Assessment is by observation and testing tasks used in everyday life. The WHIM was created to follow a patient from emergence from coma to emergence from posttraumatic amnesia. It could take anywhere from 30 to 120 minutes to administer. To obtain the rating scale and training manual, there is a fee and training is required because it has been noted that interrater reliability and test-retest reliability relies on experience.[23]

Sensory Stimulation Assessment Measure

Sensory stimulation assessment measure consists of presentation of standardized stimuli, including visual, auditory, tactile, olfactory, and gustatory. It is based on Glasgow Coma Scale responses of eye opening, motor, and vocalization. It is meant to follow a DOC patient long term and to be used with physical and neurological examinations. It takes 40 to 50 minutes to administer. It is useful in guiding treatment because the rater can evaluate what stimuli gives the most responses.[24]

Coma Near Coma Scale

Coma Near Coma Scale consists of an 11-item test with specific and structured sensory stimulation for auditory, visual, olfactory, and tactile modalities. Vocalization and command response are also tested. It takes 15 minutes to administer and has good interrater reliability with self-training by reviewing instructions on the back of the form. It is good for evaluation but not guiding treatment.[22,25]

Disorders of Consciousness Scale

Disorders of Consciousness Scale (DOCS) consists of 23 items with 8 subscales: auditory, visual, tactile, olfactory, proprioceptive/vestibular, taste/swallowing. It takes about 45 minutes to administer and has standardized administration. It is a free test and requires training with a 2-hour DVD and observation by a trained practitioner. It covers testing of only 3 of the 4 MCS diagnostic criteria.[17] The DOCS measure is not used by practicing clinicians.

IMAGING AND COMPLEMENTARY STUDIES

Misdiagnosis in DOC is as high as 40%, which creates an obvious need for objective measures through neuroimaging.[26] Although debate persists as to the utility of structural neuroimaging by means of computed tomography and MRI apart from initial evaluation or in the event of an acute neurologic deterioration, serial neuroimaging may be helpful in monitoring the evolution of cerebral hematomas or monitoring for brain atrophy.[27] Advanced neuroimaging, on the other hand, has shown promise through several studies that elucidated differences in comparing patients in a VS to those in a MCS.

PET Scan

Laureys and colleagues[12] demonstrated that an auditory stimulus activated secondary brain regions thought to be associated with awareness in minimally conscious patients, but which remained inactive in patients considered to be in a VS using PET scans. Similarly, in 2008, Boly and colleagues[28] used PET scanning to observe activation of the pain centers in the cortex and thalamus in minimally conscious, VS, and control groups. The study concluded that levels of neuronal activity were significantly lower in the VS group as compared with the MCS and control groups, which were essentially equivalent. Still, in 2010, Fisher and Appelbaum[29] argued that brain activity without visible corresponding behavior cannot be assumed to mean that a specific cognitive task is indeed being, or attempting to be, performed.

Functional MRI

fMRI is another modality that can play a complementary diagnostic role for patients with DOC that do not have metallic implants. This modality has the additional benefit of not exposing patients to radiation. In 2010, Monti and colleagues[26] used fMRI to study the volitional ability to create mental imagery in patients with DOC. Of 23 patients diagnosed to be in a VS, 4 were able to perform volitional imagery tasks, putting their clinical diagnoses into question. Other similar studies using fMRI with differing paradigms for testing demonstrated promising results, although most contained a small research subject pool. More research into this area is certainly warranted for diagnostic and, perhaps, communicative purposes.

Electroencephalograms

EEGs are a cheaper alternative to the fMRI, and they still retain diagnostic utility.[30] One proposed mechanism to identify changes in consciousness may be through recognition of normal sleep-wake cycles. A 2011 study by Landsness and colleagues[31] demonstrated the presence of sleep-wake cycles similar to a healthy population in MCS patients. This was in contrast to patients in a VS, that, although had observable behavioral periods of eye-opening and eye-closing, their EEGs failed to show any resemblance to normal sleep patterns.

Event-Related Potentials

Event-related potentials (ERP) can help to understand subtle responses linked to consciousness. As the name suggests, these potentials are specifically related to a stimulus, whether it be motor, sensory, or cognitive. An EEG, once averaged, will cancel out whole brain waveforms, revealing only the ERPs. ERPs can be subdivided into short-latency, where the potentials are occurring before 100 ms, and long-latency cognitive ERPs, which occur after 100 ms. In this way, one can understand where the potentials are being derived from, because potentials occurring before 100 ms most likely are from the ascending pathways and primary cortex, and those occurring after from the cortical and subcortical structures. Thus, cognitive ERPs are considered more directly related to cognitive processing, arousal, and awareness. They have been found to be useful in eliciting remaining cognitive functions, especially when using emotionally linked stimuli. Short-latency ERPs, on the other hand, show promise as a predictor of negative outcomes in patients with DOC and tout a low false-negative rate.[32]

Bispectral Index/Power Spectral Analysis

Two EEG derivatives known as bispectral index (BIS) and power spectral analysis have also been researched for utility as diagnostic tools. BIS was developed for anesthesiologists to measure the depth of sedation of their patients. In 2008, Schnakers and colleagues[33] proposed BIS as a way to distinguish the MCS from the VS by observing in their study that (1) BIS levels were demonstrably lower in VS than in MCS and (2) a strong correlation exists between BIS levels and CRS-R, especially compared with other EEG parameters. In a similar manner, power spectral analysis, a method used when there is a significant delay in the neural response after a stimulus, was studied in this same patient population. Goldfine and colleagues[34] observed 2 patients in an MCS and recorded any EEG evidence of awareness by means of asking the patients to imagine different scenarios. Although this study was small, they posit power spectral analysis as a potential for diagnostic and communicative purposes for patients with DOC.

TREATMENT INTERVENTIONS

The primary goal of DOC rehabilitation programs is to promote arousal while preventing secondary medical complications. Although there are no consensus treatment guidelines for DOC patients, there are several pharmacologic and nonpharmacologic treatments available.

Pharmacologic Treatment

Amantadine

Dopamine agonist and N-methyl-D-aspartate antagonist have been used in DOC for hypoarousal. In a large, multicenter, double-blind, placebo-controlled trial, the ability of Amantadine versus placebo to accelerate functional recovery among patients with nonpenetrating TBI in a vegetative or MCS was studied. A total of 184 patients were treated for 1 month, in the period between 4 and 16 weeks after severe TBI while they also received inpatient rehabilitation (IPR). The rate of functional recovery was measured by the Disability Rating Score (DRS), and there was a statistically significant rate of weekly improvement of 0.24 ($P = .007$) compared with the placebo group.

Patients started with Amantadine 100 mg twice daily and underwent serial escalations in daily dosage up to 400 mg depending on evidence of a positive response on DRS score. Interestingly, regardless of the interval since injury, the benefit of Amantadine appeared consistent.[35] Furthermore, although the rate of recovery diminished after a washout period, gains were sustained after cessation of the drug.

Bromocriptine
Direct agonist at the D2 receptor has limited information regarding its use in patients with DOC. A 5-patient case review series involving patients in a VS who were administered Bromocriptine 1 month after TBI exhibited encouraging results. When compared with a literature-based control group at 3, 6, and 12 months, there was an improvement in the DRS and CRS scores.[36] Unfortunately, this study had a low sample size and a lack of experimental control, which limited the significance of the findings.

Modafinil
The exact mechanism of action of Modafinil is unknown, but it is thought to stimulate adrenergic, histaminergic, glutaminergic activity and cause decreased gamma amino-buytric acid (GABA) activity in the brain. In a single-center, double-blind, placebo-controlled trial by Jha and colleagues[37] to evaluate Modafinil in the treatment of excessive daytime sleepiness in patients with chronic TBI, there was no clear evidence between treatment with Modafinil versus placebo. No clear evidence for its use in DOC currently exists, and more research is warranted.

Methylphenidate
Methylphenidate is a neurostimulant that acts synaptically by blocking the reuptake of Dopamine and Norepinephrine. In a retrospective cohort study, 8 patients who were in a post–cardiac arrest comatose state and received Methylphenidate exhibited an improvement in following commands and a higher survival rate to hospital discharge (62.5% vs 27.7%; $P = .005$) than those who did not.[38] The findings from a recent PET study suggest that Methylphenidate may help to normalize cerebral glucose metabolism and neural circuits after brain injury.[39]

Zolpidem
Zolpidem is a sedative-hypnotic and a GABA agonist. There have been several case studies in the literature describing a transient, paradoxic, awakening effect after administration of zolpidem.[40] A large, prospective, placebo-controlled, double-blind, single-dose, crossover study was designed to study the effects of Zolpidem on recovery of consciousness in vegetative and minimally conscious patients. Of the 84 total participants, only 4 definite "responders" (5% of total) were identified, which had no demographic or clinic predictors of response. Further studies are warranted to identify why and how Zolpidem is active in such a selective manner.[41]

Levodopa
Levodopa is a precursor of the neurotransmitters dopamine, norepinephrine, and adrenaline. An 8-patient, prospective study of patients in a VS, who were administered Levodopa approximately 104 days after their TBI, was performed. All of the patients made improvement in their consciousness, and 7 of 8 patients had full recovery of consciousness. Interestingly, gradual increases of Levodopa doses were associated with increasing complexity of motor responses.[42] In a study by Matsuda and colleagues,[43] patients in a VS or MCS, with symptoms of Parkinsonism and neuroradiologic evidence of damaged dopaminergic pathways, were responsive to Levodopa. Although promising, both studies are limited by their small sample size.

Nonpharmacologic Treatments

Nonpharmacologic treatments for DOC can vary from rehabilitation with specially trained therapists to noninvasive and invasive brain stimulation. More data are emerging on the benefit of early rehabilitation and interventions for this group of patients. Specialized neurorehabilitation programs in an IPR facility setting have shown improved emergence to consciousness. Noninvasive brain stimulation and neurorehabilitation when used in conjunction are synergistic and can enhance neuroplasticity more than either alone.[44,45]

Neurorehabilitation

Specialized rehabilitation protocols for DOC population are essential for improving recovery and long-term care. In 2013, National Institute on Disability and Rehabilitation Research and Traumatic Brain Injury Model Systems evaluated the functional outcomes at 5 years from patients admitted to IPR and unable to follow commands. Their study showed substantial proportions of the patients not following commands on admission to IPR recovered independent functioning over 5 years (56%–85% of patients in the early recovery group and 19%–36% of patients in the late recovery group), particularly if they followed commands before discharge (early recovery group).[46] Specialized multidisciplinary rehabilitation with acute medical management and 90 minutes or more of therapy are likely to show improved consciousness and body function. Medical management can focus on prevention and/or treatment of medical complications of TBI, including paroxysmal sympathetic hyperactivity, spasticity, respiratory insufficiency, prevention and treatment of infections, deep venous thrombosis, and wounds (pressure ulcers). Neurorehabilitation should use standardized assessments for measurement of DOC level performed by trained clinicians and the interdisciplinary team to focus on recovery of consciousness, functional communication, and positioning and mobility.[47,48] The team consists of physicians, rehabilitation nursing, physical therapy, occupational therapy, speech language pathology, rehabilitation psychology, neuropsychology, case management, and social work. It has been seen that with specialized early treatment, including acute medical care and rehabilitation, that patients may be able to transition to mainstream rehabilitation and emerge to consciousness.[47] Each member of the team is essential in the success of a DOC rehabilitation program. Families who receive comprehensive education and hands-on training with ongoing follow-up and support may be able to take care of patients with DOC at home versus facility placement.[47]

Transcranial direct current stimulation

Transcranial direct current stimulation (TDCS) is a form of neurostimulation that delivers a low constant current to an area of the brain using scalp electrodes. Anodal TDCS elicits prolonged increases in cortical excitability and facilitates underlying regional activity. Cathodal TDCS has the opposite effect.[49] Emerging data exist on the use of TDCS for transient improvement in consciousness in patients in MCS but not UWS.[50,51] TDCS when used in conjunction with rehabilitation may enhance cortical plasticity and recovery in patients with DOC. Therefore, the ease of use, minimal risk of harm, and portability may provide an additional intervention for this population.[49]

Transcranial magnetic stimulation

Transcranial magnetic stimulation (TMS) provides neuromodulation with the application of rapidly changing magnetic fields to the scalp via a copper wire coil connected to a magnetic stimulator. Repetitive trains of TMS can suppress or facilitate cortical processes depending on stimulation parameters. Effect of TMS has been seen to have modulatory effects longer than the duration of the stimulation, thereby modulating neural plasticity. Case reports have been published that improved neural conduction mediates neurobehavioral gains in coma recovery.[52]

Deep brain stimulation

Deep brain stimulation is an invasive brain stimulation that requires surgical implantation of a deep brain stimulator. Thalamic and brainstem control of forebrain arousal is not a novel concept. This neurophysiologic concept has led to the consideration of thalamic electrical stimulation to promote consciousness in DOC patients.[53]

SUMMARY

DOC presents both a scientific and a clinical challenge for clinicians caring for individuals with DOC. Currently, behavioral assessment remains the gold standard for diagnosis of these individuals, but advanced neuroimaging and electrophysiological techniques present possibilities for improvement of the current diagnostic classification systems. Future studies need to focus on diagnostic as well as therapeutic interventions to aid in the recovery from DOC.

REFERENCES

1. Severe TBI. Concussion Traumatic Brain Injury CDC Injury Center. Available at: http://www.cdc.gov/traumaticbraininjury/severe.html. Accessed August 16, 2016.
2. Gray M, Lai S, Wells R, et al. A systematic review of an emerging consciousness population: focus on program evolution. J Trauma 2011;71(5):1465–74.
3. Plum F, Posner JB. The diagnosis of stupor and coma. Philadelphia: FA Davis; 1966. p. 5–6.
4. Cavanna AE, Shah S, Eddy CM, et al. Consciousness: a neurological perspective. Behav Neurol 2011;24(1):107–16.
5. Giacino JT, Fins JJ, Laureys S, et al. Disorders of consciousness after acquired brain injury: the state of the science. Nat Rev Neurol 2014;10(2):99–114.
6. Zasler ND, Katz DI, Zafonte RD, editors. Brain injury medicine: principles and practice. 2nd edition. New York: Demos Medical Pub; 2013.
7. Laureys S. The neural correlate of (un)awareness: lessons from the vegetative state. Trends Cogn Sci 2005;9(12):556–9.
8. Crone JS, Soddu A, Höller Y, et al. Altered network properties of the fronto-parietal network and the thalamus in impaired consciousness. Neuroimage Clin 2014;4:240–8.
9. Cavanna AE, Ali F. Epilepsy: the quintessential pathology of consciousness. Behav Neurol 2011;24(1):3–10.
10. Practice parameters for determining brain death in adults (summary statement). The Quality Standards Subcommittee of the American Academy of Neurology. Neurology 1995;45(5):1012–4.
11. Wijdicks EFM, Varelas PN, Gronseth GS, et al, American Academy of Neurology. Evidence-based guideline update: determining brain death in adults: report of the Quality Standards Subcommittee of the American Academy of Neurology. Neurology 2010;74(23):1911–8.
12. Laureys S, Owen AM, Schiff ND. Brain function in coma, vegetative state, and related disorders. Lancet Neurol 2004;3(9):537–46.

13. Bruno M-A, Vanhaudenhuyse A, Thibaut A, et al. From unresponsive wakefulness to minimally conscious PLUS and functional locked-in syndromes: recent advances in our understanding of disorders of consciousness. J Neurol 2011; 258(7):1373–84.

14. Sherer M, Nakase-Thompson R, Yablon SA, et al. Multidimensional assessment of acute confusion after traumatic brain injury. Arch Phys Med Rehabil 2005;86(5): 896–904.

15. Bauer G, Gerstenbrand F, Rumpl E. Varieties of the locked-in syndrome. J Neurol 1979;221(2):77–91.

16. Giacino JT, Ashwal S, Childs N, et al. The minimally conscious state: definition and diagnostic criteria. Neurology 2002;58(3):349–53.

17. American Congress of Rehabilitation Medicine, Brain Injury-Interdisciplinary Special Interest Group, Disorders of Consciousness Task Force, Seel RT, Sherer M, et al. Assessment scales for disorders of consciousness: evidence-based recommendations for clinical practice and research. Arch Phys Med Rehabil 2010; 91(12):1795–813.

18. Kalmar K, Giacino JT. The JFK coma recovery scale–revised. Neuropsychol Rehabil 2005;15(3–4):454–60.

19. Giacino JT, Kalmar K, Whyte J. The JFK coma recovery scale-revised: measurement characteristics and diagnostic utility. Arch Phys Med Rehabil 2004;85(12): 2020–9.

20. Løvstad M, Frøslie KF, Giacino JT, et al. Reliability and diagnostic characteristics of the JFK coma recovery scale-revised: exploring the influence of rater's level of experience. J Head Trauma Rehabil 2010;25(5):349–56.

21. Gill-Thwaites H, Munday R. The Sensory Modality Assessment and Rehabilitation Technique (SMART): a valid and reliable assessment for vegetative state and minimally conscious state patients. Brain Inj 2004;18(12):1255–69.

22. O'Dell MW, Jasin P, Lyons N, et al. Standardized assessment instruments for minimally-responsive, brain-injured patients. NeuroRehabilitation 1996;6(1): 45–55.

23. Shiel A, Horn SA, Wilson BA, et al. The Wessex Head Injury Matrix (WHIM) main scale: a preliminary report on a scale to assess and monitor patient recovery after severe head injury. Clin Rehabil 2000;14(4):408–16.

24. Rader MA, Ellis DW. The Sensory Stimulation Assessment Measure (SSAM): a tool for early evaluation of severely brain-injured patients. Brain Inj 1994;8(4): 309–21.

25. Rappaport M. The disability rating and coma/near-coma scales in evaluating severe head injury. Neuropsychol Rehabil 2005;15(3–4):442–53.

26. Monti MM, Vanhaudenhuyse A, Coleman MR, et al. Willful modulation of brain activity in disorders of consciousness. N Engl J Med 2010;362(7):579–89.

27. Bernat JL. Chronic consciousness disorders. Annu Rev Med 2009;60:381–92.

28. Boly M, Faymonville M-E, Schnakers C, et al. Perception of pain in the minimally conscious state with PET activation: an observational study. Lancet Neurol 2008; 7(11):1013–20.

29. Fisher CE, Appelbaum PS. Diagnosing consciousness: neuroimaging, law, and the vegetative state. J Law Med Ethics 2010;38(2):374–85.

30. Rosenbaum AM, Giacino JT. Clinical management of the minimally conscious state. Handb Clin Neurol 2015;127:395–410.

31. Landsness E, Bruno M-A, Noirhomme Q, et al. Electrophysiological correlates of behavioural changes in vigilance in vegetative state and minimally conscious state. Brain 2011;134(Pt 8):2222–32.

32. Vanhaudenhuyse A, Schnakers C, Boly M, et al. Behavioural assessment and functional neuro-imaging in vegetative state patients. Rev Med Liège 2007; 62(Spec No):15–20 [in French].
33. Schnakers C, Ledoux D, Majerus S, et al. Diagnostic and prognostic use of bispectral index in coma, vegetative state and related disorders. Brain Inj 2008; 22(12):926–31.
34. Goldfine AM, Victor JD, Conte MM, et al. Determination of awareness in patients with severe brain injury using EEG power spectral analysis. Clin Neurophysiol 2011;122(11):2157–68.
35. Giacino JT, Whyte J, Bagiella E, et al. Placebo-controlled trial of amantadine for severe traumatic brain injury. N Engl J Med 2012;366(9):819–26.
36. Passler MA, Riggs RV. Positive outcomes in traumatic brain injury-vegetative state: patients treated with bromocriptine. Arch Phys Med Rehabil 2001;82(3): 311–5.
37. Jha A, Weintraub A, Allshouse A, et al. A randomized trial of modafinil for the treatment of fatigue and excessive daytime sleepiness in individuals with chronic traumatic brain injury. J Head Trauma Rehabil 2008;23(1):52–63.
38. Reynolds JC, Rittenberger JC, Callaway CW. Methylphenidate and amantadine to stimulate reawakening in comatose patients resuscitated from cardiac arrest. Resuscitation 2013;84(6):818–24.
39. Kim YW, Shin J-C, An Y. Effects of methylphenidate on cerebral glucose metabolism in patients with impaired consciousness after acquired brain injury. Clin Neuropharmacol 2009;32(6):335–9.
40. Tucker C, Sandhu K. The effectiveness of zolpidem for the treatment of disorders of consciousness. Neurocrit Care 2016;24(3):488–93.
41. Whyte J, Rajan R, Rosenbaum A, et al. Zolpidem and restoration of consciousness. Am J Phys Med Rehabil 2014;93(2):101–13.
42. Krimchansky B-Z, Keren O, Sazbon L, et al. Differential time and related appearance of signs, indicating improvement in the state of consciousness in vegetative state traumatic brain injury (VS-TBI) patients after initiation of dopamine treatment. Brain Inj 2004;18(11):1099–105.
43. Matsuda W, Komatsu Y, Yanaka K, et al. Levodopa treatment for patients in persistent vegetative or minimally conscious states. Neuropsychol Rehabil 2005;15(3–4):414–27.
44. Page SJ, Cunningham DA, Plow E, et al. It takes two: noninvasive brain stimulation combined with neurorehabilitation. Arch Phys Med Rehabil 2015;96(4 Suppl): S89–93.
45. Eapen BC, Murphy DP, Cifu DX. Neuroprosthetics in amputee and brain injury rehabilitation. Exp Neurol 2017;287(Pt 4):479–85.
46. Whyte J, Nakase-Richardson R, Hammond FM, et al. Functional outcomes in traumatic disorders of consciousness: 5-year outcomes from the National Institute on Disability and Rehabilitation Research Traumatic Brain Injury Model Systems. Arch Phys Med Rehabil 2013;94(10):1855–60.
47. Seel RT, Douglas J, Dennison AC, et al. Specialized early treatment for persons with disorders of consciousness: program components and outcomes. Arch Phys Med Rehabil 2013;94(10):1908–23.
48. Eapen BC, Allred DB, O'Rourke J, et al. Rehabilitation of moderate-to-severe traumatic brain injury. Semin Neurol 2015;35(1):e1–3.
49. Demirtas-Tatlidede A, Vahabzadeh-Hagh AM, Bernabeu M, et al. Noninvasive brain stimulation in traumatic brain injury. J Head Trauma Rehabil 2012;27(4): 274–92.

50. Thibaut A, Bruno M-A, Ledoux D, et al. tDCS in patients with disorders of consciousness: sham-controlled randomized double-blind study. Neurology 2014; 82(13):1112–8.
51. Angelakis E, Liouta E, Andreadis N, et al. Transcranial direct current stimulation effects in disorders of consciousness. Arch Phys Med Rehabil 2014;95(2):283–9.
52. Louise-Bender Pape T, Rosenow J, Lewis G, et al. Repetitive transcranial magnetic stimulation-associated neurobehavioral gains during coma recovery. Brain Stimul 2009;2(1):22–35.
53. Giacino J, Fins JJ, Machado A, et al. Central thalamic deep brain stimulation to promote recovery from chronic posttraumatic minimally conscious state: challenges and opportunities. Neuromodulation 2012;15(4):339–49.

Management of Medical Complications During the Rehabilitation of Moderate-Severe Traumatic Brain Injury

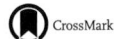

Billie A. Schultz, MD*, Erica Bellamkonda, MD

KEYWORDS

- Traumatic brain injury • Rehabilitation • Complications • Agitation • Neuroendocrine
- Spasticity • Post-traumatic hydrocephalus • Paroxysmal sympathetic hyperreflexia

KEY POINTS

- Medical complications after moderate-severe traumatic brain injury (TBI) are common and should be considered by the brain injury specialist in all patients.
- Many similar signs and symptoms exist for medical complications after TBI, making an understanding of differential diagnosis essential in ensuring appropriate treatment.
- Medical complications after moderate-severe TBI include posttraumatic seizures, paroxysmal sympathetic hyperactivity, spasticity, hydrocephalus, agitation, neuroendocrine dysfunction, heterotopic ossification, venous thromboembolism, and cranial nerve (CN) dysfunction.
- Caregiver support and education is essential during the acute and subacute period of time after a moderate-severe TBI.

Traumatic brain injury (TBI) in the United States is well publicized for the potential long-term effects. With incidence of TBI as defined by emergency department visits, hospitalization, and deaths rising ongoing attention from public and private organizations continues. These data show increasing rates of brain injury driven by emergency department visits gaining 56% from 2007 to 2010.[1] The rates of TBI-related hospitalization have been relatively stable over that period of time and associated deaths have decreased. It is postulated that deaths have decreased owing to a focus on primary prevention and improving acute management.

The management of moderate-severe TBI in the acute care setting is shared by critical care physicians, neurosurgeons, trauma surgeons, neurologists, and physiatrists.

Disclosure Statement: The authors have nothing to disclose.
Department of Physical Medicine and Rehabilitation, Mayo Clinic, 200 1st Street Southwest, Rochester, MN 55905, USA
* Corresponding author.
E-mail address: schultz.billie@mayo.edu

Phys Med Rehabil Clin N Am 28 (2017) 259–270
http://dx.doi.org/10.1016/j.pmr.2016.12.004   pmr.theclinics.com

The initial goals of acute care management are prevention of the secondary injury by surgical management, management of intracranial pressures, respiratory support, and management of concurrent injuries. The other providers typically manage these conditions while the brain injury rehabilitation specialist assists in management of many other brain injury–specific complications in the acute and subacute periods. Various domains including physical, cognitive, behavioral, and somatic can be involved.

Once the patient is stabilized medically after the brain injury, transitions to the next level of care are planned. Despite decreasing numbers of patients post-TBI transferring to acute rehabilitation in the postprospective payment system,[2] acute inpatient rehabilitation is a consideration for all patients after moderate-severe TBI. Management of medical complications after TBI continues in this setting as well. This process can include the management of posttraumatic seizures, paroxysmal sympathetic hyperactivity, spasticity, hydrocephalus, agitation, neuroendocrine dysfunction, heterotopic ossification, venous thromboembolism, and CN dysfunction.

POSTTRAUMATIC SEIZURES

Posttraumatic seizures and posttraumatic epilepsy can develop after TBI with an incidence described between 4% and 53%.[3] Risk factors for seizure development include hydrocephalus, intracranial hemorrhage, depressed skull fracture, surgical hematoma evacuations, lower Glasgow Coma Scale levels, dural penetration, parietal lesions, and focal neurologic deficits.[4–6] Additionally, late seizures—those that develop after day 7 post injury—are also associated with prolonged duration of posttraumatic amnesia and a lower Glasgow Coma score. Late seizures are defined as those seizures arising after day 7. Immediate and early seizures are described as in the first 24 hours and between 24 hours through 7 days, respectively. Classic research showed that seizure prophylaxis beyond the first 7 days does not add any additional benefit in the prevention of late posttraumatic seizures. Traditionally, phenytoin was used based on the classic studies[7]; however, recently other medications were shown to have equal/better seizure control.[8–11] Late development of seizures after TBI continues at a higher rate than the general population. Based on the veterans of the Vietnam era, this increased incidence continues decades later.[12] The treatment of seizures is recommended with the development of early and late seizures. First-line treatment is antiepileptic medication; however, for medication-refractory seizures, surgical resection of the seizure focus and vagal nerve stimulators have also been described. There is lack of consensus of timing of medication discontinuation. Withdrawal of antiepileptics after seizure development is typically delayed 1 to 2 years after the last seizure. Electroencephalography can provide more information and it is reasonable to include neurologists in this decision.

PAROXYSMAL SYMPATHETIC HYPERACTIVITY

Paroxysmal sympathetic hyperactivity is thought to result from uninhibited sympathetic outflow after a central nervous symptom insult.[13] It has been described after stroke, anoxic brain injury, and encephalitis, in addition to TBI. First described in 1954 as an "autonomic seizure,"[14] more than 30 terms for this condition have been found in review of the literature, including sympathetic storming and dysautonomia.[15] Not surprisingly, definitions and diagnostic criteria also vary and recommendations have been made to more clearly define this syndrome.[16] In general, it is agreed that the diagnosis is based on paroxysmal cycling of agitation/dystonia in association with autonomic symptoms including tachycardia, tachypnea, elevation in systolic blood pressure, hyperthermia, and diaphoresis occurring for at least 3 consecutive days, 2 weeks or greater after injury. This is a diagnosis of exclusion with a differential diagnosis including infection, agitation, and seizure, among others. The pathophysiology is still being explained with more recent literature suggesting an excitatory:inhibitory ratio where spinal cord circuits are left unopposed by the damage to the inhibitory centers in the brainstem. This allows amplification of previously nonnoxious or mildly noxious stimuli, causing the paroxysmal sympathetic hyperactivity.[17] Other theories suggest some form of disconnection through alternative pathways.[18] Incidence reported varies owing to the lack of consensus diagnostic criteria with 8% to 32% described.[19,20]

Treatment algorithms first suggest monitoring and ruling out other causes.[21] Afterward, treatment is based on inhibiting the uninhibited sympathetic outflow and blocking the end-organ responses to the uninhibited outflow. Gabapentin, baclofen, clonidine, propranolol, morphine, and bromocriptine have been described.[22–26] For prolonged symptoms of paroxysmal sympathetic hyperactivity unresponsive to noninvasive measures, intrathecal baclofen use has also been described.[27]

SPASTICITY

Muscle overactivity is one "positive" sign after TBI in contrast with weakness or loss of muscle control, which is considered a "negative" sign. Spasticity is one of those positive signs. Defined as a velocity-dependent increase in muscle tone, spasticity must be monitored closely to ensure that no complications develop secondary to spasticity, including skin alterations, muscle contractures, or pain. It is postulated that enhanced excitability of monosynaptic pathways is involved in cortically mediated spasticity. Spasticity is often measured using the modified Ashworth scale.[28] Other measurement tools include the Tardieu and Penn spasm frequency scale.[29]

The decision to treat spasticity is not always an easy one because there are some potential benefits as well as negative to spasticity. Positive effects can include assistance with ambulation/transfers, muscle bulk maintenance, deep vein thrombosis (DVT) prevention, and osteoporosis prevention. Negative effects can include pain, poor cosmesis, seating issues, skin disruption, and impaired function. Therefore, clearly identifying the goals of the patient and caregiver is vital. It is proposed that the provider assess the following concerns: is treatment needed, what are the aims of treatment, is the time needed for treatment available, and will treatment disrupt the lives of the patient and caregiver.[30] The goals should be communicated clearly to the patient and their family members.

Treatment approaches vary but include different levels of invasiveness and reversibility. They can be described as treatment for more systemic manifestations of spasticity or more generalized.[31,32] Requisite nonpharmacologic treatment includes stretching and use of orthoses. Medication management with baclofen, dantrolene, diazepam, and tizanidine has been described. Focal treatment with chemical neurolysis and denervation are also used commonly. Intrathecal baclofen has been used for the severe cases or those with significant lower extremity involvement. Legalization of medical cannabis is changing the landscape of neurologic spasticity treatment, with some states specifically defining an indication for neurologic spasticity.[33]

POSTTRAUMATIC HYDROCEPHALUS

Posttraumatic hydrocephalus (PTH) can develop after TBI at a rate of 0.7% to 51.4%.[34–38] Part of this variation results from underdiagnosis and atypical presentation. Additionally, different sets of clinical criteria are used to diagnoses PTH, depending on the study contributing to the variation in incidence. It is especially associated with the presence of subarachnoid hemorrhage. Other risk factors for development of PTH include advanced age, the timing of cranioplasty, higher score on the Fisher grading system, a low postresuscitation Glasgow Coma Scale score, cerebrospinal fluid (CSF) infection, and decompressive craniectomy.[34] Pathophysiology is related to excessive CSF accumulation through either overproduction of CSF, the blockage of normal CSF flow, or insufficient CSF absorption.[39] If the patient has a decline or plateau in function, hydrocephalus should be considered. This is in contrast with the patient without a brain injury, such as those with normal pressure hydrocephalus, where the classic triad of bladder incontinence, cognitive deficits, and gait impairment is noted. Although the symptoms of normal pressure hydrocephalus may be present in the brain injured patient, it is often impossible to disentangle the symptoms from the underlying injury. In PTH, physical examination findings can include papilledema from increased intracranial pressure, changes in level of consciousness, memory deficits, headache, or focal neurologic deficits in addition to the previous stated symptoms. When hydrocephalus is suspected, imaging should be obtained and treatment includes resolution of the underlying increase in intracranial pressure with surgical management with extraventricular drain and/or shunting.

AGITATION

Agitation has various definitions. Initially described as "combativeness, arm thrashing, truncal rocking, screaming and signs of sympathetic activation."[40] Agitation has also been defined as "subjective evidence of one or more of the following behaviors: restlessness, derogatory or threatening demands, verbal abusiveness, sexual inappropriate comments or actions or threats or attempts at physical violence of sufficient severity to disrupt nursing care or therapy,"[41] "post-traumatic amnesia plus an excess of behavior such as aggression, disinhibition and/or emotional lability,"[42] and "a subtype of delirium unique to survivors of TBI in which the survivor is in the state of posttraumatic amnesia and there are excesses of behavior that include some combination of aggression, akathisia, disinhibition and/or emotional lability."[43] Thought to be an essential part of recovery after brain injury it is also defined as Rancho Los Amigos IV- confused and agitated. A variety of definitions make research in this area very challenging.

The incidence is difficulty to define owing to the inconsistent definitions used. One study indicates an 11% incidence[44] and another describes a 41% incidence of persons hospitalized with TBI had 1 agitated behavior with 9% have significant agitation.[45] Yet another describes a 70% incidence.[46] Assuming agitation is part of the brain recovery process as suggested by the Rancho Los Amigos Scale, then 100% of patients with moderate-severe TBI should experience agitation, which should resolved concurrently with the resolution of the posttraumatic amnesia. Understandably, the wide range of incidence reported is likely owing to the lack of a definitive diagnosis.

The underlying etiology of agitation is postulated to be various causes. Structurally, frontal and temporal involvement seems to be of most interest, although also described is involvement of the interconnections between the frontal cortex and subcortical nuclei in the striatum, globus pallidus, substantia nigra and thalamus, hippocampal mesocortex and temporal neocortex, and frontal limbic cortex.[47,48] The dopaminergic, noradrenergic, cholinergic, and serotonergic systems have been implicated as playing a role in agitation after brain injury.[49–51] Multiple other factors can contribute to worsening in agitation including infection, seizures, electrolytes imbalances, drug/nicotine/alcohol withdrawal, and pain, and should be identified and addressed accordingly.

Monitoring of agitation can include the agitated behavior scale and the overt aggression scale. Unfortunately, most practitioners do not use a consistent method to monitor agitation,[52] despite its importance to follow-up treatment effects and determining if further changes need to be made for management.

When treating a patient with agitation, contributing causes of agitation should be investigated first. Investigation may include a complete blood count, electrolytes, urinalysis, and imaging including chest radiographs and computed tomography scans of the head. Other investigations should be based on likelihood within the differential.

Once investigated completely and any complicating factors treated, management should include nonpharmacologic and pharmacologic options. Nonpharmacologic treatment includes environmental modification with minimization of stimuli,[53] consistency of caregivers, and gentle reorientation.

Multiple studies suggest that agitation is time limited[44,54]; thus, one could consider watchful monitoring before considering pharmacologic intervention. However, if the patient is at risk for harming themselves or others, pharmacologic management can be considered.[55] Many medications and algorithms have been[56] suggested. Beta-blockers,[57,58] antidepressants including tricyclic antidepressants,[41] selective serotonin reuptake inhibitors,[59] valproic acid,[60] and antipsychotic agents have been used and reported in the literature for the management of agitation.

NEUROENDOCRINE DYSFUNCTION

Recognition of neuroendocrine dysfunction after TBI is becoming more common in both the acute and chronic periods. The hypothalamus and pituitary gland are both implicated in this dysfunction. The suggested pathophysiology is thought to be 3-fold. First, the pituitary gland and hypothalamus are anatomically vulnerable due to their location, structure, and blood supply. Second, the "stress response" related to the stress of injury and hospitalization may contribute. Last, in the acute period many medications used can also contribute. Despite this, screening in the postacute period remains somewhat controversial despite published guidelines.[61]

The posterior pituitary lobe releases antidiuretic hormone. Implicated in regulation of sodium and fluid status after brain injury, many people are aware of the potential for dysregulation and actively monitor for it. Acutely, seen most commonly are problems with sodium regulations—both hyponatremia and hypernatremia. Included are diabetes insipidus from posterior pituitary lobe dysfunction with 21.6% of person with moderate-severe TBI diagnosed acutely.[62] Diabetes insipidus is characterized by excessive urination and thirst. If the patient is able to drink to thirst, sodium remains within normal limits; however, if they are unable to drink or if the thirst mechanism is impaired, hypernatremia and dehydration can result. Treatment consists of trying to match input and output with the addition of desmopressin as needed. In the same study, 12.7% of patients were noted to develop the syndrome of inappropriate antidiuretic hormone, caused by the uncontrolled release of antidiuretic hormone. This release causes hyponatremia in the setting of euvolemia and is first treated with fluid restriction. Completing the discussion about sodium regulation, cerebral salt wasting is also seen. Leading to hypovolemic hyponatremia, its pathophysiology remains uncertain.[63] Cerebral salt wasting is hyponatremia as a result of inappropriate loss of sodium in the urine. Mechanisms postulated are disrupted sympathetic neural input to the kidney and increased secretion of brain natriuretic peptide, causing decreased renal sodium resorption and impaired renin–aldosterone release with subsequent volume depletion. Some authors suggest that cerebral salt wasting may not exist, whereas others consider it a distinct disease. Because cerebral salt wasting as an entity is in dispute, its incidence is unclear. Treatment includes hydration and sodium replacement. Treatment for any sodium abnormality (hyponatremia or hypernatremia) depends on the cause; therefore, identification of the etiology is essential.

Anterior pituitary lobe dysfunction is also seen after TBI, as well as gonadotrophic and somatotrophic axis disorders. Forty percent of persons had gonadotrophin deficiency acutely; however, this improved to 7.7% at 1 year.[64] Consensus guidelines for replacement in the acute period exist.[61] The most commonly deficient hormone, however, is growth hormone.[65,66] Thyroid-stimulating hormone and cortisol levels can also be abnormal after brain injury.

Screening consensus statements exist and agree that physicians should monitor for symptoms and test for a select group of abnormalities at 0, 3, and 12 months.[61] Outcomes after brain injury have been shown to be affected negatively by neuroendocrine disorders.[67] Therefore, care should be taken to evaluate for and properly manage any deficiencies.[68]

HETEROTOPIC OSSIFICATION

Heterotopic ossification (HO) is development of an inflammatory reaction in the periarticular tissues with subsequent bone matrix formation and calcification. Multiple risk factors for HO exist, including, TBI where the incidence is reported between 8% and 73%.[69,70] TBI with the addition of bone fracture can further increase the incidence of HO.[69] Other risk factors for the development of HO in persons with TBI include surgery, prolonged coma, and spasticity. Hip is most commonly involved joint. Pathophysiology remains unclear; however, 3 components are needed—an inciting event, undifferentiated precursor cells, and an environment conducive to osteogenesis. The patient may present with pain, swelling, and/or limitation in joint range of motion. A triple phase bone scan is the gold standard for diagnosis. Treatment depends on whether it is clinically significant, because a large percentage of cases are found incidentally. Gentle passive range of motion is recommended for physical therapies with nonsteroidal antiinflammatories to treat the inflammation stage. Bisphosphonates, specifically etidronate, is approved by the Food and Drug Administration for the treatment of HO. Surgical excision is reserved for those with function limitations, severe pain, or wound/hygiene issues secondary to the HO formation. There is no evidence to support early versus late excision, although a general rule of thumb is to wait, allowing bone maturation. Current recommendations are to delay excision for 1.5 years after TBI.[71]

VENOUS THROMBOEMBOLISM

Venous thromboembolism, both pulmonary embolism and DVT are seen commonly in the acute, postacute, and chronic periods for all rehabilitation patients. After TBI, the incidence varies depending on screening[72–74]; however, TBI has been described as an independent risk factor for DVT.[75] Complicating both prophylaxis and treatment is the underlying TBI and associated injuries, as well as the subsequent risk for bleeding. Most recent guidelines by the American College of Chest Physicians suggest prophylactic options, including the use of unfractionated heparin, low-molecular-weight heparin, and/or mechanical prophylaxis in persons after major trauma, including TBI. Practically, however, the risk of bleeding may be concerning to the point that pharmacologic prophylaxis is not recommended, such as in the case of craniotomy. Even in that case, guidelines advise against surveillance studies. They also note that inferior vena cava filters should not be used as the sole form of DVT prophylaxis.[76] Owing to the high risk and sometimes less than ideal prophylaxis, providers should be vigilant to the possibility of venous thromboembolism and monitor for the signs and symptoms. DVT can cause leg pain, edema, and/or erythema. Pulmonary embolism can result in chest pain, tachypnea, tachycardia, and a decrease in oxygen saturations. With a large thrombotic burden, a patient can become hemodynamically unstable, requiring intensive care. Once diagnosed, careful balance of risk and benefits of treatment should be considered and all venous thromboembolism treated accordingly.

CRANIAL NERVE DYSFUNCTION

CN dysfunction is common after TBI. Traumatic CN injuries can occur from skull fractures (particularly those that traverse over bony prominences and through bony canals), acceleration–deceleration forces, shearing, intracranial hemorrhage, uncal herniation, ischemia/infarction, or edema. The olfactory nerve (CN I) is reportedly most often injured. This is followed by the facial (CN VII) and vestibulocochlear (CN VIII) nerves. Less commonly injured nerves are the optic (CN II) and oculomotor (CN III) nerves. Rarely are the trigeminal (CN V) and lower CNs (CN IX, X, XI, XII) injured.[77] The true incidence is hard to obtain because of difficult or incomplete examinations in patients with altered sensorium that often accompanies moderate-severe TBI. CN injury identification may also be delayed owing to other life-threatening injuries. They can result in motor or sensory impairments, contributing to morbidity and impacting quality of life. Diagnosis is often based on a careful and complete clinical examination. For certain CNs, electromyography and nerve conduction studies are an extension of the physical examination and can help to localize the lesion, determine its severity, and prognosticate. Electrodiagnostic study can also help to identify those patients who would benefit from surgical intervention. Computed tomography scanning best visualizes the integrity of the skull base and bony canals/foramina that may can lead to a CN injury. Standard MRIs can readily visualize large CN, such as the ophthalmic, optic, trigeminal, oculomotor, facial, and vestibulocochlear nerves, on 4-mm T2-weighted/susceptibility sequence imaging. For smaller CN, thin section images and an intimate knowledge of the courses of the nerves are required to obtain specific MRI sequences for optimal visualization.[78] Treatment depends on the specific CN injured; sometimes surgical intervention is necessary and can improve outcomes.[79]

FAMILY AND CAREGIVER SUPPORT

Supporting family members is equally important during this time. Frank discussions about goals of care should be discussed and palliative care services and ethics services can be helpful in this. Families are usually looking for something that they can do to help their loved one. Sites such as Caring Bridge provide a platform for sharing information about the hospitalization. Child life services can be helpful for younger family members in understanding the hospitalization and injury. Multiple pieces of family education published can be helpful. Last, the Brain Injury Associations/Alliances in each state can provide more information. Social work should be consulted early. A survey of family members published in 2016 showed that more than one-half of those surveyed indicated the education was not adequate. Key themes identified were prognostic information and adequacy of discharge planning and resources.[80]

SUMMARY

Brain injury specialists are experienced providers able to identify and treat the unique medical complications after moderate-severe TBI. These complications can include

posttraumatic seizures, paroxysmal sympathetic hyperactivity, spasticity, hydrocephalus, and agitation. Owing to the potential negative impact on outcome if left un-
treated, identification and appropriate treatment of these complications is essential.
An additional role of the brain injury specialist is to education family about the potential
medical complications and the anticipated outcomes after brain injury. The provider,
patient, and family work as a team to identify and treat any potential sequelae of the
moderate-severe brain injury. Therefore, it is of utmost importance that the brain injury
medicine specialist be aware of the potential complications, impact on rehabilitation,
and treatment options.

REFERENCES

1. Centers for Disease Control and Prevention (CDC). Report to congress on traumatic brain injury in the United States: epidemiology and rehabilitation. Atlanta
(GA): National Center for Injury Prevention and Control Division of Unintentional
Injury Prevention; 2015.
2. Hoffman JM, Donoso Brown E, Chan L, et al. Change in inpatient rehabilitation
admissions for individuals with traumatic brain injury after implementation of
the Medicare inpatient rehabilitation facility prospective payment system. Arch
Phys Med Rehabil 2012;93(8):1305–12.
3. Frey LC. Epidemiology of posttraumatic epilepsy: a critical review. Epilepsia
2003;44(Suppl 10):11–7.
4. Hasan D, Schonck RS, Avezaat CJ, et al. Epileptic seizures after subarachnoid
hemorrhage. Ann Neurol 1993;33(3):286–91.
5. Jamjoom AB, Kane N, Sandeman D, et al. Epilepsy related to traumatic extradural
haematomas. BMJ 1991;302(6774):448.
6. Mazzini L, Cossa FM, Angelino E, et al. Posttraumatic epilepsy: neuroradiologic
and neuropsychological assessment of long-term outcome. Epilepsia 2003;
44(4):569–74.
7. Temkin NR, Dikmen SS, Wilensky AJ, et al. A randomized, double-blind study of
phenytoin for the prevention of post-traumatic seizures. N Engl J Med 1990;
323(8):497–502.
8. Inaba K, Menaker J, Branco BC, et al. A prospective multicenter comparison of
levetiracetam versus phenytoin for early posttraumatic seizure prophylaxis.
J Trauma Acute Care Surg 2013;74(3):766–71 [discussion: 771–3].
9. Jones KE, Puccio AM, Harshman KJ, et al. Levetiracetam versus phenytoin for
seizure prophylaxis in severe traumatic brain injury. Neurosurg Focus 2008;
25(4):E3.
10. Zafar SN, Khan AA, Ghauri AA, et al. Phenytoin versus Leviteracetam for seizure
prophylaxis after brain injury - a meta analysis. BMC Neurol 2012;12:30.
11. Thompson K, Pohlmann-Eden B, Campbell LA, et al. Pharmacological treatments
for preventing epilepsy following traumatic head injury. Cochrane Database Syst
Rev 2015;(8):CD009900.
12. Raymont V, Salazar AM, Lipsky R, et al. Correlates of posttraumatic epilepsy 35
years following combat brain injury. Neurology 2010;75(3):224–9.
13. Lemke DM. Sympathetic storming after severe traumatic brain injury. Crit Care
Nurse 2007;27(1):30–7 [quiz: 38].
14. Penfield W, Jasper H. Autonomic seizures. In: Penfield W, Jasper H, editors.
Epilepsy and the functional anatomy of the human brain. London: J & A Churchill
Ltd; 1954. p. 412–37.

15. Perkes I, Baguley IJ, Nott MT, et al. A review of paroxysmal sympathetic hyperactivity after acquired brain injury. Ann Neurol 2010;68(2):126–35.

16. Baguley IJ, Perkes IE, Fernandez-Ortega JF, et al. Paroxysmal sympathetic hyperactivity after acquired brain injury: consensus on conceptual definition, nomenclature, and diagnostic criteria. J Neurotrauma 2014;31(17):1515–20.

17. Baguley IJ. The excitatory:inhibitory ratio model (EIR model): an integrative explanation of acute autonomic overactivity syndromes. Med Hypotheses 2008;70(1): 26–35.

18. Baguley IJ, Heriseanu RE, Cameron ID, et al. A critical review of the pathophysiology of dysautonomia following traumatic brain injury. Neurocrit Care 2008;8(2): 293–300.

19. Dolce G, Quintieri M, Leto E, et al. Dysautonomia and Clinical Outcome in Vegetative State. J Neurotrauma 2008;25:1079–82.

20. Baguley IJ, Slewa-Younan S, Heriseanu RE, et al. The incidence of dysautonomia and its relationship with autonomic arousal following traumatic brain injury. Brain Inj 2007;21(11):1175–81.

21. Lump D, Moyer M. Paroxysmal sympathetic hyperactivity after severe brain injury. Curr Neurol Neurosci Rep 2014;14(11):494.

22. Patel MB, McKenna JW, Alvarez JM, et al. Decreasing adrenergic or sympathetic hyperactivity after severe traumatic brain injury using propranolol and clonidine (DASH After TBI Study): study protocol for a randomized controlled trial. Trials 2012;13:177.

23. Bullard DE. Diencephalic seizures: responsiveness to bromocriptine and morphine. Ann Neurol 1987;21(6):609–11.

24. Baguley IJ, Cameron ID, Green AM, et al. Pharmacological management of Dysautonomia following traumatic brain injury. Brain Inj 2004;18(5):409–17.

25. Baguley IJ, Heriseanu RE, Gurka JA, et al. Gabapentin in the management of dysautonomia following severe traumatic brain injury: a case series. J Neurol Neurosurg Psychiatry 2007;78(5):539–41.

26. Blackman JA, Patrick PD, Buck ML, et al. Paroxysmal autonomic instability with dystonia after brain injury. Arch Neurol 2004;61(3):321–8.

27. Hoarau X, Richer E, Dehail P, et al. 10-year follow-up study of patients with severe traumatic brain injury and dysautonomia treated with intrathecal baclofen therapy. Brain Inj 2012;26(7–8):927–40.

28. Pandyan AD, Johnson GR, Price CI, et al. A review of the properties and limitations of the Ashworth and modified Ashworth Scales as measures of spasticity. Clin Rehabil 1999;13(5):373–83.

29. Marciniak C. Poststroke hypertonicity: upper limb assessment and treatment. Top Stroke Rehabil 2011;18(3):179–94.

30. Tizard J. Cerebral palsies: treatment and prevention. The Croonian lecture 1978. J R Coll Physicians Lond 1980;14:72–80.

31. Merritt JL. Management of spasticity in spinal cord injury. Mayo Clin Proc 1981; 56(10):614–22.

32. Graham HK, Aoki KR, Autti-Ramo I, et al. Recommendations for the use of botulinum toxin type A in the management of cerebral palsy. Gait Posture 2000;11(1): 67–79.

33. A review of medical cannabis studies relating to chemical compositions and dosages for qualifying medical conditions. St Paul (MN): Minnesota Department of Health Office of Medical Cannabis; 2016.

34. De Bonis P, Pompucci A, Mangiola A, et al. Post-traumatic hydrocephalus after decompressive craniectomy: an underestimated risk factor. J Neurotrauma 2010;27(11):1965–70.
35. Groswasser Z, Cohen M, Reider-Groswasser I, et al. Incidence, CT findings and rehabilitation outcome of patients with communicative hydrocephalus following severe head injury. Brain Inj 1988;2(4):267–72.
36. Guyot LL, Michael DB. Post-traumatic hydrocephalus. Neurol Res 2000;22(1): 25–8.
37. Mazzini L, Campini R, Angelino E, et al. Posttraumatic hydrocephalus: a clinical, neuroradiologic, and neuropsychologic assessment of long-term outcome. Arch Phys Med Rehabil 2003;84(11):1637–41.
38. Mori K, Shimada J, Kurisaka M, et al. Classification of hydrocephalus and outcome of treatment. Brain Dev 1995;17(5):338–48.
39. Katz RT, Brander V, Sahgal V. Updates on the diagnosis and management of posttraumatic hydrocephalus. Am J Phys Med Rehabil 1989;68(2):91–6.
40. Levin HS, Grossman RG. Behavioral sequelae of closed head injury. A quantitative study. Arch Neurol 1978;35(11):720–7.
41. Mysiw WJ, Jackson RD, Corrigan JD. Amitriptyline for post-traumatic agitation. Am J Phys Med Rehabil 1988;67(1):29–33.
42. Fugate LP, Spacek LA, Kresty LA, et al. Definition of agitation following traumatic brain injury: I. A survey of the Brain Injury Special Interest Group of the American Academy of Physical Medicine and Rehabilitation. Arch Phys Med Rehabil 1997; 78(9):917–23.
43. Sandel ME, Mysiw WJ. The agitated brain injured patient. Part 1: definitions, differential diagnosis, and assessment. Arch Phys Med Rehabil 1996;77(6):617–23.
44. Brooke MM, Questad KA, Patterson DR, et al. Agitation and restlessness after closed head injury: a prospective study of 100 consecutive admissions. Arch Phys Med Rehabil 1992;73(4):320–3.
45. McNett M, Sarver W, Wilczewski P. The prevalence, treatment and outcomes of agitation among patients with brain injury admitted to acute care units. Brain Inj 2012;26(9):1155–62.
46. Nott MT, Chapparo C, Baguley IJ. Agitation following traumatic brain injury: an Australian sample. Brain Inj 2006;20(11):1175–82.
47. Ommaya AK, Gennarelli TA. Cerebral concussion and traumatic unconsciousness. Correlation of experimental and clinical observations of blunt head injuries. Brain 1974;97(4):633–54.
48. Derryberry D, Tucker DM. Neural mechanisms of emotion. J Consult Clin Psychol 1992;60(3):329–38.
49. McIntosh TK. Neurochemical sequelae of traumatic brain injury: therapeutic implications. Cerebrovasc Brain Metab Rev 1994;6(2):109–62.
50. Hamill RW, Woolf PD, McDonald JV, et al. Catecholamines predict outcome in traumatic brain injury. Ann Neurol 1987;21(5):438–43.
51. Mysiw WJ, Sandel ME. The agitated brain injured patient. Part 2: pathophysiology and treatment. Arch Phys Med Rehabil 1997;78(2):213–20.
52. Fugate LP, Spacek LA, Kresty LA, et al. Measurement and treatment of agitation following traumatic brain injury: II. A survey of the Brain Injury Special Interest Group of the American Academy of Physical Medicine and Rehabilitation. Arch Phys Med Rehabil 1997;78(9):924–8.
53. Donchin Y, Seagull FJ. The hostile environment of the intensive care unit. Curr Opin Crit Care 2002;8(4):316–20.

54. Kadyan V, Mysiw WJ, Bogner JA, et al. Gender differences in agitation after traumatic brain injury. Am J Phys Med Rehabil 2004;83(10):747–52.
55. Rosati DL. Early polyneuropharmacologic intervention in brain injury agitation. Am J Phys Med Rehabil 2002;81(2):90–3.
56. Lombard LA, Zafonte RD. Agitation after traumatic brain injury: considerations and treatment options. Am J Phys Med Rehabil 2005;84(10):797–812.
57. Fleminger S, Greenwood RJ, Oliver DL. Pharmacological management for agitation and aggression in people with acquired brain injury. Cochrane Database Syst Rev 2006;(4):CD003299.
58. Brooke MM, Patterson DR, Questad KA, et al. The treatment of agitation during initial hospitalization after traumatic brain injury. Arch Phys Med Rehabil 1992; 73(10):917–21.
59. Kant R, Smith-Seemiller L, Zeiler D. Treatment of aggression and irritability after head injury. Brain Inj 1998;12(8):661–6.
60. Chatham Showalter PE, Kimmel DN. Agitated symptom response to divalproex following acute brain injury. J Neuropsychiatry Clin Neurosci 2000;12(3):395–7.
61. Ghigo E, Masel B, Aimaretti G, et al. Consensus guidelines on screening for hypopituitarism following traumatic brain injury. Brain Inj 2005;19(9):711–24.
62. Agha A, Thornton E, O'Kelly P, et al. Posterior pituitary dysfunction after traumatic brain injury. J Clin Endocrinol Metab 2004;89(12):5987–92.
63. Sterns RH. Disorders of plasma sodium–causes, consequences, and correction. N Engl J Med 2015;372(1):55–65.
64. Tanriverdi F, Senyurek H, Unluhizarci K, et al. High risk of hypopituitarism after traumatic brain injury: a prospective investigation of anterior pituitary function in the acute phase and 12 months after trauma. J Clin Endocrinol Metab 2006; 91(6):2105–11.
65. Popovic V. GH deficiency as the most common pituitary defect after TBI: clinical implications. Pituitary 2005;8(3–4):239–43.
66. Lieberman SA, Oberoi AL, Gilkison CR, et al. Prevalence of neuroendocrine dysfunction in patients recovering from traumatic brain injury. J Clin Endocrinol Metab 2001;86(6):2752–6.
67. Bondanelli M, Ambrosio MR, Cavazzini L, et al. Anterior pituitary function may predict functional and cognitive outcome in patients with traumatic brain injury undergoing rehabilitation. J Neurotrauma 2007;24(11):1687–97.
68. Ripley D, Wierman M, Gerber D, et al. Testosterone replacement in hypogonadal men following traumatic brain injury: results from a double-blind, placebo controlled pilot study. PM&R 2015;7(9):S86–7.
69. Sullivan MP, Torres SJ, Mehta S, et al. Heterotopic ossification after central nervous system trauma: a current review. Bone Joint Res 2013;2(3):51–7.
70. Simonsen LL, Sonne-Holm S, Krasheninnikoff M, et al. Symptomatic heterotopic ossification after very severe traumatic brain injury in 114 patients: incidence and risk factors. Injury 2007;38(10):1146–50.
71. Chalidis B, Stengel D, Giannoudis PV. Early excision and late excision of heterotopic ossification after traumatic brain injury are equivalent: a systematic review of the literature. J Neurotrauma 2007;24(11):1675–86.
72. Cifu DX, Kaelin DL, Wall BE. Deep venous thrombosis: incidence on admission to a brain injury rehabilitation program. Arch Phys Med Rehabil 1996;77(11): 1182–5.
73. Lai JM, Yablon SA, Ivanhoe CB. Incidence and sequelae of symptomatic venous thromboembolic disease among patients with traumatic brain injury. Brain Inj 1997;11(5):331–4.

74. Meythaler JM, DeVivo MJ, Hayne JB. Cost-effectiveness of routine screening for proximal deep venous thrombosis in acquired brain injury patients admitted to rehabilitation. Arch Phys Med Rehabil 1996;77(1):1–5.

75. Reiff DA, Haricharan RN, Bullington NM, et al. Traumatic brain injury is associated with the development of deep vein thrombosis independent of pharmacological prophylaxis. J Trauma 2009;66(5):1436–40.

76. Guyatt GH, Akl EA, Crowther M, et al. Executive summary: antithrombotic therapy and prevention of thrombosis, 9th ed: American College of Chest Physicians Evidence-Based Clinical Practice Guidelines. Chest 2012;141(Suppl 2):7s–47s.

77. Hammond F, Msael T. Cranial nerve disorders. In: Zasler N, editor. Brain injury medicine principles and practice. 2nd edition. New York: Demos Medical; 2013. p. 680–92.

78. Tomandi B, Sommer N, Egan P, et al. Imaging of disease of the cranial nerves: tips and tricks. Available at: http://clinical-mri.com/wp-content/uploads/new_technologies/Flash_51_Cranial_Nerves_Tomandl_final.pdf. Accessed July 23, 2016.

79. Roofe S, Kolb C, Seibert J. Cranial nerve injuries. In: Banks D, editor. Otolaryngology/head and neck combat casualty care in Operation Iraqi Freedom and Operation Enduring Freedom. Falls Church (VA): Office of the Surgeon General, United States Army; 2015. p. 213–25.

80. Biester RC, Krych D, Schmidt MJ, et al. Individuals with traumatic brain injury and their significant others' perceptions of information given about the nature and possible consequences of brain injury: analysis of a national survey. Prof Case Manag 2016;21(1):22–33 [quiz: E23–4].

Diagnosis and Management of Acute Concussion

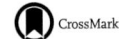
CrossMark

Michael A. McCrea, PhD[a],*, Lindsay D. Nelson, PhD[a],
Kevin Guskiewicz, PhD[b]

KEYWORDS

- Concussion • Mild traumatic brain injury • Acquired brain injury • Sports injuries

KEY POINTS

- An estimated 80% to 90% of all traumatic brain injuries are classified as mild traumatic brain injury, or concussion.
- Recent reports suggest that a high percentage of concussions go undiagnosed and unidentified in the acute care setting (eg, hospital emergency department, sports).
- Over the past 20 years, there has been great progress toward standardized definition, diagnosis, assessment, and management of acute concussion.
- Consensus guidelines now provide guidance regarding injury management and approaches to ensure safe return to activity after acute concussion.

INTRODUCTION

Mild traumatic brain injury (mTBI), or concussion, is now recognized as a major public health problem in the United States and around the world. Each year in the United States, there are approximately 2.5 million visits to hospital emergency departments (EDs) for traumatic brain injury (TBI), with an estimated 80% to 90% classified as mild based on traditional case definitions and acute injury characteristics.[1–3] The World Health Organization Collaborating Centre Task Force on Mild Traumatic Brain Injury cited the incidence of hospital-treated mTBI to be 100 to 300 per 100,000.[4] These figures likely significantly underestimate the true incidence of mTBI, because most patients with concussion do not receive hospital treatment and many do not seek any form of medical attention after their injury.

[a] Department of Neurosurgery, Medical College of Wisconsin, 8701 Watertown Plank Road, Milwaukee, WI 53226, USA; [b] Department of Exercise and Sport Science, College of Arts & Sciences, University of North Carolina – Chapel Hill, 2207 Stallings, Chapil Hill, NC 27599, USA
* Corresponding author. Department of Neurosurgery, Medical College of Wisconsin, 8701 Watertown Plank Road, Milwaukee, WI 53226.
E-mail address: mmccrea@mcw.edu

Phys Med Rehabil Clin N Am 28 (2017) 271–286
http://dx.doi.org/10.1016/j.pmr.2016.12.005
1047-9651/17/© 2017 Elsevier Inc. All rights reserved.
pmr.theclinics.com

For many reasons, identification and diagnosis of mTBI in the ED and other acute trauma settings has proved challenging. First, there has been great variability in operational definitions and criteria for diagnosis of mTBI. Second, there have been no systematic, standardized processes for assessing patients with probable or suspected mTBI. Third, other more severe or life-threatening injuries understandably take priority during triage, and the effects of mTBI are often uncovered later. In addition, several comorbidities that either mask or mimic the effects of concussion often complicate the routine examination of patients with mTBI.[5] The collective result is that a high percentage (50%–90%) of patients with mTBI often go unidentified and undiagnosed in the hospital ED.[6,7]

Over the past 2 decades, there has been considerable progress toward advancing the basic and clinical science of concussion in all populations at risk, including civilians, athletes, and military service members. As a result, there is now a new understanding of the defining characteristics of concussion, on which current definitions of injury and diagnostic criteria are based.[8] These research advances have directly affected the development of evidence-based, best-practice guidelines for the diagnosis, assessment, and management of concussion, including protocols that drive the decision-making process regarding an individual's fitness to return to activity (eg, work, play, duty) after concussion. This article provides a brief, high-level overview of evidence-based approaches to best practice in diagnosis, assessment, and management of acute concussion.

DEFINITION AND DIAGNOSIS OF ACUTE CONCUSSION

There has been a large amount of variability in concussion definitions developed over the past 30 years, but more recent progress toward greater consensus based on the latest evidence. Central to all concussion definitions is the rapid onset of impairment of neurologic function, which most often and typically resolves spontaneously over a short time frame.

Historically, the definition of mTBI developed by the Mild Traumatic Brain Injury Committee of the Head Injury Interdisciplinary Special Interest Group of the American Congress of Rehabilitation Medicine (ACRM)[9] was commonly used in both research and clinical settings. The ACRM definition required a single criterion of unconsciousness, amnesia, or alteration in mental status for the diagnosis of mTBI. More recently, the US Centers for Disease Control and Prevention (CDC), US Department of Defense (DoD), and the World Health Organization (WHO) have developed operational definitions of mTBI, which place varied emphasis on acute injury characteristics and other signs and symptoms to establish a diagnosis. **Box 1** shows the clinical definition of mTBI developed by the CDC mTBI Working Group.[10]

Published definitions specific to sport-related concussion have also gained consensus. The 4th International Consensus Conference on Concussion in Sport (Zurich 2012) consensus statement defines concussion as a brain injury characterized by a complex pathophysiologic process affecting the brain, induced by biomechanical forces.[11] Similarly, the American Medical Society for Sports Medicine (AMSSM) defines concussion as a traumatically induced transient disturbance of brain function involving a complex pathophysiologic process.[12]

Ultimately, concussion is a clinical diagnosis based on the combination of injury mechanism and acute symptoms and signs.[8,11,12] The mechanism of injury is an important consideration showing a causal link between injury and clinical signs and symptoms, as well as ruling out other causes of more nonspecific signs or symptoms. Once the mechanism is better delineated, the signs and symptoms essentially represent the clinical criteria used to diagnose concussion.

Box 1
Centers for Disease Control and Prevention conceptual definition of mild traumatic brain injury

Experts from the CDC's mTBI Working Group define mTBI as the occurrence of injury to the head arising from blunt trauma or acceleration or deceleration forces with 1 or more of the following conditions attributable to the head injury:

Any period of observed or self-reported:
- Transient confusion, disorientation, or impaired consciousness
- Dysfunction of memory around the time of injury
- Loss of consciousness lasting less than 30 minutes

Observed signs of other neurologic or neuropsychological dysfunction, such as:
- Seizures acutely following injury to the head
- Irritability, lethargy, or vomiting following head injury, especially among infants and very young children
- Headache, dizziness, irritability, fatigue, or poor concentration, especially among older children and adults

From National Center for Injury Prevention and Control. Report to congress on mild traumatic brain injury in the United States. Atlanta (GA): Centers for Disease Control and Prevention; 2003.

Evident from research over the past 2 decades is the finding that concussion often occurs in the absence of unconsciousness or measurable posttraumatic amnesia, once considered defining characteristics of acquired brain injury.[13] Rather, concussion is characterized by a common set of physical, cognitive, behavioral, and other symptoms. **Table 1** provides a listing of common signs and symptoms observed in the setting of acute concussion.[14]

It should be noted that several symptoms of concussion are considered nonspecific, meaning that they commonly occur in the context of health conditions other than concussion that are commonly encountered by patients. Symptoms of concussion may also be common in other comorbid conditions, such as mood disorders,

Table 1
Common signs and symptoms of concussion

Physical	Cognitive	Emotional	Sleep
• Headache • Nausea • Vomiting • Balance problems • Dizziness • Visual problems • Fatigue • Sensitivity to light • Sensitivity to noise • Numbness/tingling • Dazed • Stunned	• Feeling mentally foggy • Feeling slowed down • Difficulty concentrating • Difficulty remembering • Forgetful of recent information and conversations • Confused about recent events • Answers questions slowly • Repeats questions	• Irritable • Sadness • More emotional • Nervousness	• Drowsiness • Sleep more than usual • Sleep less than usual • Difficulty falling asleep

Adapted from Harmon KG, Drezner JA, Gammons M, et al. American Medical Society for Sports Medicine position statement: concussion in sport. Br J Sports Med 2013;47(1):15–26.

learning disabilities, or other developmental cognitive disorders other than concussion. Therefore, it is essential for clinicians to link the onset of suspected concussion signs and symptoms with an apparent mechanism of injury in order to more precisely isolate concussion as the probable cause of those signs and symptoms. Infrequently, there is a delayed onset of symptoms after concussion, but most often these abnormalities manifest immediately or very soon after the injury event.

ACUTE CONCUSSION ASSESSMENT AND MANAGEMENT

For patients who present to a hospital after injury, the ED is typically the first and only point of medical contact, because an estimated 90% of patients are treated and released without hospital admission.[3] A vast number of individuals with mTBI are treated in urgent care, primary care, or other specialty outpatient settings, without hospital evaluation or admission.

Regardless of setting, during the acute injury phase, the first priority in the acute setting is to rule out the occurrence of more severe injury (eg, cervical spine injury, severe brain injury, airway obstruction) that may represent a medical emergency.[15] Ideally, the diagnosis is formulated by a health care provider with expertise and knowledge in the recognition and evaluation of concussion. Although the odds may seem low, this rule also applies in nonemergency settings (eg, urgent care, clinic).

In a sports setting, both consensus guidelines and legislation in most states indicate that any athlete suspected of having a concussion should be immediately removed from play and assessed by a qualified health care provider, and any athlete with suspected concussion is prohibited from returning to competition or participation on the day of the injury.[11]

Most individuals with concussion do not require or undergo neuroimaging studies. When indicated, CT is the preferred technology to rule out structural or more severe underlying brain injury that may represent or escalate to a neurosurgical emergency (eg, skull fracture, intracranial bleed, contusion, cerebral swelling, brain stem herniation). In the subacute setting, brain MRI may be helpful in identifying any underlying structural abnormalities that correlate with persistent symptoms, prolonged recovery, or poor outcome. Newer, innovative neuroimaging technologies show promise in identifying changes in brain structure and function associated with concussion, but require further study before being considered a central component of clinical practice.

MULTIDIMENSIONAL ASSESSMENT OF ACUTE CONCUSSION

Once other or more severe injuries have been ruled out and all first aid issues have been addressed, then a formal concussion assessment should be initiated. Individuals, to varying degrees, experience a complex combination of symptoms and show deficits across multiple domains of functioning after concussion. Therefore, the acute evaluation should include a survey of common concussion signs, assessment of symptoms, and multidimensional testing of functions known to be affected by concussion (eg, cognition, balance).[14] Reliance on a single test or multiple measures in a single assessment domain are likely to be less accurate than a multimodal assessment.

Over the past 10 years or more, several standardized tests have been developed to aid in acute concussion assessment.[14] Concussion symptom checklists can provide clinicians with a systematic way to document the presence and severity of concussion symptoms, as well as a method for tracking changes in symptom levels on serial assessment over the course of the patient's postinjury recovery.[14] Several of these tools are available for clinical use in a variety of settings (eg, hospital ED, outpatient clinic, sports medicine).

In addition, several functional tests have been validated for use in the assessment of acute concussion.[14] These measures may form a more accurate and reliable assessment than simply relying on patients' self-reporting of symptoms. Standardized tools are intended to provide a more objective, performance-based method of detecting the acute effects of injury, measuring postinjury recovery and determining a patient's fitness to return to activity. These tests provide important data on symptoms and functional impairments that clinicians can incorporate into their diagnostic formulation, but should not solely be used to diagnose concussion or drive clinical decision making. The specific tests selected to form the multidimensional assessment approach not only need to be reliable and valid but also may vary depending on the situational constraints of the clinical environment, population, and the experience of the assessor.

Various multidimensional assessment tools have been developed and validated for clinical use. The CDC has developed the Acute Concussion Evaluation (ACE), including multiple versions adopted for various clinical environments (eg, outpatient clinic, ED).[16] The tool integrates a survey of information on the injury event and acute injury characteristics with assessment of physical, cognitive, emotional, and sleep symptoms (**Fig. 1**). Risk factors and red flags to warrant emergent intervention are also documented. The ACE derives a clinical diagnosis and action plan for diagnostic testing, referral, or other follow-up based on the presenting signs and symptoms. This tool is versatile for use across a variety of settings and patient populations.

In the setting of sport-related concussion, the Sport Concussion Assessment Tool, Third Edition (SCAT3), from the 4th Consensus Statement on Concussion in Sport[11] provides a multimodal assessment model that integrates several assessments recommended by the American Academy of Neurology (AAN) into a singular assessment package (**Fig. 2**).[8,11] The SCAT3 has a graded symptom checklist, the Standardized Assessment of Concussion (SAC), and the Balance Error Scoring System (BESS) all embedded in a unified, multidimensional assessment tool appropriate for use in a competitive sporting environment. The individual components of the SCAT3 (symptom checklist, SAC, BESS) have all been well validated in the acute assessment of athletes affected by sports concussion, but further research is required to determine the overall utility of the integrated SCAT3.[14] Tools such as the SCAT3 can easily be adapted for use in clinical environments outside of sports.

FOLLOW-UP EVALUATION AND MANAGEMENT OF ACUTE CONCUSSION

Research over the last decade has shown that most individuals achieve a complete recovery in symptoms, cognitive functioning, postural stability, and other functional impairments over a period of 1 to 3 weeks following concussion.[17–21] The rate of recovery varies across individuals and may be influenced by several modifiers, including severity of injury, patient age and gender, prior concussion and health history, and presence of comorbidities or vulnerabilities.

Ideally, patients with concussion should have medical follow-up with a qualified health care professional knowledgeable in the evaluation and management of acute

ACUTE CONCUSSION EVALUATION (ACE)
Emergency Department (ED) Version v1.4
Gerard Gioia, PhD[1] & Micky Collins, PhD[2]
[1]Children's National Medical Center
[2]University of Pittsburgh Medical Center

Patient Name_____
DOB: _____ Age:_____
Date:_____ ID/MR#_____

A. Injury Characteristics   Date/Time of Injury_____   Reporter: __Patient __Parent __Spouse __Other_____

1. Injury Description _____

1a. Is there evidence of a forcible blow to the head (direct or indirect)?   __Yes __No __Unknown
1b. Is there evidence of intracranial injury or skull fracture?   __Yes __No __Unknown
1c. Location of Impact: __Frontal __Lft Temporal __Rt Temporal __Lft Parietal __Rt Parietal __Occipital __Neck __Indirect Force
2. **Cause:** __MVC __Pedestrian-MVC __Fall __Assault __Sports (specify)_____ Other_____
3. **Amnesia Before (Retrograde)** Are there any events just BEFORE the injury that you/ person has no memory of (even brief)? __ Yes __No Duration_____
4. **Amnesia After (Anterograde)** Are there any events just AFTER the injury that you/ person has no memory of (even brief)? __ Yes __No Duration_____
5. **Loss of Consciousness:** Did you/ person lose consciousness?   __ Yes __No Duration_____
6. EARLY SIGNS: __Appears dazed or stunned __Is confused about events __Answers questions slowly __Repeats Questions __Forgetful (recent info)
7. **Seizures:** Were seizures observed? No__ Yes__ Detail_____

B. Symptom Check List* Since the injury, has the person experienced any of these symptoms any more than usual today or in the past day?
Indicate presence of each symptom (0=No, 1=Yes).   *Lovell & Collins, 1998 JHTR

PHYSICAL (10)			COGNITIVE (4)			SLEEP (4)			Other Observations
Headache	0	1	Feeling mentally foggy	0	1	Drowsiness	0	1	
Nausea	0	1	Feeling slowed down	0	1	Sleeping less than usual	0 1 N/A		_____
Vomiting	0	1	Difficulty concentrating	0	1	Sleeping more than usual	0 1 N/A		_____
Balance problems	0	1	Difficulty remembering	0	1	Trouble falling asleep	0 1 N/A		_____
Dizziness	0	1	COGNITIVE Total (0-4)			SLEEP Total (0-4) ____			_____
Visual problems	0	1	EMOTIONAL (4)						_____
Fatigue	0	1	Irritability	0	1				_____
Sensitivity to light	0	1	Sadness	0	1				_____
Sensitivity to noise	0	1	More emotional	0	1				_____
Numbness/Tingling	0	1	Nervousness	0	1				_____
PHYSICAL Total (0-10) ____			EMOTIONAL Total (0-4) ____						_____
(Add Physical, Cognitive, Emotion, Sleep totals) Total Symptom Score (0-22) ____									

Patient Participation: Full__ Partial __ None __
Reason for Partial/None: Young Age__ Confused__ Inattentive__ Low arousal__ Emotional Upset__ In Pain__ Other_____

C. Concussion History: *Previous#* 0 1 2 3 4 5 Date(s)_____
Headache History: Prior treatment for headache N___ Y___ Details_____

D. Diagnosis (ICD): __Concussion w/o LOC 850.0 __Concussion w/ LOC 850.1 __Concussion (Unspecified) 850.9 __Other (854)_____
__No diagnosis

E. Follow-Up Action Plan _√_ Referral to PCP for Office Monitoring   MD Name_____
___ Neuropsychological Testing (recommended for Return to Sport decisions and academic/ behavioral management)
___ Physician: Neurosurgery____ Neurology____ Sports Medicine____ Physiatry____ Psychiatry____
___ Other_____

ACE-ED Completed by: _____MD RN NP DO

Fig. 1. CDC ACE. (*From* McCrory P, Meeuwisse WH, Aubry M, et al. Consensus statement on concussion in sport: the 4th International Conference on Concussion in Sport held in Zurich, 2012. Br J Sports Med 2013;47(5):250–8.)

concussion. Follow-up should include serial monitoring of postconcussive symptoms, in addition to performance-based measures of recovery at the appropriate point in the patient's recovery. Ideally, a standardized symptom checklist should be used to quantify the presence and severity of common postconcussive symptoms, which also allows the clinician to then quantitatively track the patient's level of symptom recovery over time. Although a rare occurrence, any indication of rapidly worsening symptoms or deterioration in the patient's neurologic status should prompt emergent medical evaluation and work-up.

A concussion is an injury to the brain as a result of a force or jolt applied directly or indirectly to the head, which produces a range of possible symptoms, and may or may not involve a loss of consciousness. It is a complex pathophysiologic process affecting the brain, induced by traumatic biomechanical forces secondary to direct or indirect forces to the head. Disturbance of brain function is related to neurometabolic dysfunction, rather than structural injury, and is typically associated with normal structural neuroimaging findings (i.e., CT scan, MRI). Concussion may or may not involve a loss of consciousness (LOC). Concussion results in a constellation of cognitive, somatic, emotional and sleep-related symptoms. Duration of symptoms are variable and may last for as short as several minutes and last as long as several days, weeks, months or even longer in some cases.

ACE ED Instructions

A. Injury Characteristics

1. **Injury Description:** Ask for **description of events** resulting in the injury; how the injury occurred, type of force, location on head.
2. **Cause:** Indicate the cause of injury or write in Other cause.
3/4. **Amnesia:** Determine whether child was not registering memories (amnesia) – before (retrograde) and after (anterograde) injury. Estimate length of time for each (Retrograde amnesia "What is the last thing you remember before your injury?" Anterograde amnesia "What is the first thing you remember after your injury?")
5. **Loss of consciousness (LOC)** - If occurs, determine length of LOC.
6. **Early signs observed by others.** Ask the individuals who know the patient (parent, spouse, friend, etc.) about signs of the concussion/ mTBI that they may have observed. Signs are typically observed early after the injury.
7. **Seizures:** Inquire whether seizures were observed or not.

B. Symptom Check List:

- Ask patient (and/ or parent, if child) to report presence of the 4 categories of symptoms since injury. It is important to assess all listed symptoms as different parts of the brain control different functions. One or all symptoms may be present depending upon mechanisms of injury. If the symptom is not present, circle "0" on the scale. Circle "1" if present.
- Note: Most sleep symptoms are only applicable after a night has passed since the injury. If not applicable, circle N/A. Drowsiness may be present on the day of injury.
- Since symptoms can be present premorbidly/ at baseline (e.g., inattention, headaches, sleep, sadness), it is important to assess change from its typical presentation. For any symptom - if Patient/ Parent indicates "I/ He usually has that problem/symptom" – Ask "Are you/ they experiencing this symptom more than usual or in a different manner than usual?" If "Yes" circle "1".

Scoring: Sum total number of symptoms present per area, and sum all 4 areas into Total Symptom Score. (Note: Most sleep symptoms are only applicable after a night has passed since the injury. Drowsiness may be present on the day of injury.) If symptoms are new and present, there is no lower limit symptom score. Any score > 0 indicates positive symptom history.

- **General Impression:** Ask how different the person is acting than usual. Circle 0 (No difference) to 6 (Major) to rate degree.
- **Patient Participation:** Indicate the extent to which the patient is able to participate in the evaluation and, if less than fully, give reason for Partial or No participation.

C. Concussion history:
Assess the number and date(s) of prior concussions.[4-8] History of prior concussions, especially recent (within past several weeks or months) would suggest the need for more conservative decision-making regarding Return to Play, and general post-injury management.

Headache history: Assess personal history of diagnosis/treatment for headaches. Recent research indicates headache (migraine in particular) can result in protracted recovery from concussion.[8-11]

D. Diagnosis:
Assign the most appropriate diagnosis given the following:

850.0 (Concussion, with no loss of consciousness) – Positive Injury Description (A1), i.e., forcible direct/ indirect blow to the head; plus evidence of active symptoms (B) of any type and number related to the trauma; no evidence of LOC (A5), skull fracture, or other intracranial injury.

850.1 (Concussion, with brief loss of consciousness < 1 hour) - Positive Injury Description (A1), i.e., forcible direct/ indirect blow to the head; plus evidence of active symptoms (B) of any type and number related to the trauma; positive evidence of LOC (A5); no skull fracture, or other intracranial injury.

850.9 (Concussion, unspecified) - Positive Injury Description (A1), i.e., forcible direct/ indirect blow to the head; plus evidence of active symptoms (B) of any type and number related to the trauma; unclear/unknown injury details; unclear evidence of LOC (A5), no skull fracture, or other intracranial injury.

NOTE: If there is evidence of skull fracture of structural intracranial injury to the brain, consider 854 (Intracranial injury of other and unspecified nature; 854.0 Without mention of open intracranial wound, 854.1 With open intracranial wound). Avoid using nonspecific Head injury NOS (959.01) whenever possible.

E. Follow-Up Action:
Determine a plan of action for follow-up of symptomatic patients. Serial evaluation of the concussion is critical as symptoms may resolve, worsen, or ebb and flow depending upon a variety of factors (e.g., cognitive/ physical exertion, comorbidities). Referral to a specialist can be particularly valuable to help manage certain aspects of the patient's condition.

(a) Patient monitoring in the primary care physician office.

(b) Referral to a specialist: particularly valuable to help manage certain aspects of the patient's condition.

- Neuropsychological Testing is particularly relevant for cognitive and/or behavioral dysfunction affecting school, home or work activities, for purpose of treatment planning. Testing is also recommended when a patient may be returning to sports or other at-risk activities.
- Physician Evaluation is particularly relevant for medical evaluation and management of concussion. Also, critical for evaluation and management of focal neurologic, sensory, vestibular, and motor concerns. May be useful for medication management (e.g., headaches, sleep disturbance, depression) if post-concussive problems persist.

Fig. 1. (continued).

Brief repeatable assessments can be used to monitor symptoms, cognitive status, and other impairment associated with mTBI. In collaboration with medical and rehabilitation staff, the goal of a brief evaluation is to track physical and cognitive recovery, educate patients and families about the normal course of recovery after TBI, and generate referrals as needed to services such as cognitive/speech therapy, physical/ vestibular therapy, and psychology/psychiatry. Feedback at this time is often a useful intervention, designed to reassure individuals that they are still recovering and have not yet reached their healing plateau, as well as to facilitate treatment of secondary issues that may impede recovery (eg, sleep disturbance, emotional distress, and pain).

Further out from injury, more comprehensive outpatient neuropsychological testing is more appropriate to address a diverse range of issues related to specific

SCAT3™

FIFA° ❋ ⊕⊕⊕ ⊕ ℱℰℐ

Sport Concussion Assessment Tool – 3rd Edition

For use by medical professionals only

Name   Date/Time of Injury: Examiner:
                              Date of Assessment:

What is the SCAT3?[1]

The SCAT3 is a standardized tool for evaluating injured athletes for concussion and can be used in athletes aged from 13 years and older. It supersedes the original SCAT and the SCAT2 published in 2005 and 2009, respectively[2]. For younger persons, ages 12 and under, please use the Child SCAT3. The SCAT3 is designed for use by medical professionals. If you are not qualified, please use the Sport Concussion Recognition Tool[1]. Preseason baseline testing with the SCAT3 can be helpful for interpreting post-injury test scores.

Specific instructions for use of the SCAT3 are provided on page 3. If you are not familiar with the SCAT3, please read through these instructions carefully. This tool may be freely copied in its current form for distribution to individuals, teams, groups and organizations. Any revision or any reproduction in a digital form requires approval by the Concussion in Sport Group.
NOTE: The diagnosis of a concussion is a clinical judgment, ideally made by a medical professional. The SCAT3 should not be used solely to make, or exclude, the diagnosis of concussion in the absence of clinical judgement. An athlete may have a concussion even if their SCAT3 is "normal".

What is a concussion?

A concussion is a disturbance in brain function caused by a direct or indirect force to the head. It results in a variety of non-specific signs and/or symptoms (some examples listed below) and most often does not involve loss of consciousness. Concussion should be suspected in the presence of **any one or more** of the following:

- Symptoms (e.g., headache), or
- Physical signs (e.g., unsteadiness), or
- Impaired brain function (e.g. confusion) or
- Abnormal behaviour (e.g., change in personality).

SIDELINE ASSESSMENT

Indications for Emergency Management

NOTE: A hit to the head can sometimes be associated with a more serious brain injury. Any of the following warrants consideration of activating emergency procedures and urgent transportation to the nearest hospital:

- Glasgow Coma score less than 15
- Deteriorating mental status
- Potential spinal injury
- Progressive, worsening symptoms or new neurologic signs

Potential signs of concussion?

If any of the following signs are observed after a direct or indirect blow to the head, the athlete should stop participation, be evaluated by a medical professional and **should not be permitted to return to sport the same day** if a concussion is suspected.

Any loss of consciousness?	Y	N
"If so, how long?"		
Balance or motor incoordination (stumbles, slow/laboured movements, etc.)?	Y	N
Disorientation or confusion (inability to respond appropriately to questions)?	Y	N
Loss of memory:	Y	N
"If so, how long?"		
"Before or after the injury?"		
Blank or vacant look:	Y	N
Visible facial injury in combination with any of the above:	Y	N

1 Glasgow coma scale (GCS)

Best eye response (E)	
No eye opening	1
Eye opening in response to pain	2
Eye opening to speech	3
Eyes opening spontaneously	4

Best verbal response (V)	
No verbal response	1
Incomprehensible sounds	2
Inappropriate words	3
Confused	4
Oriented	5

Best motor response (M)	
No motor response	1
Extension to pain	2
Abnormal flexion to pain	3
Flexion/Withdrawal to pain	4
Localizes to pain	5
Obeys commands	6

Glasgow Coma score (E + V + M)	of 15

GCS should be recorded for all athletes in case of subsequent deterioration.

2 Maddocks Score[3]

"I am going to ask you a few questions, please listen carefully and give your best effort."

Modified Maddocks questions (1 point for each correct answer)

What venue are we at today?	0	1
Which half is it now?	0	1
Who scored last in this match?	0	1
What team did you play last week/game?	0	1
Did your team win the last game?	0	1
Maddocks score		of 5

Maddocks score is validated for sideline diagnosis of concussion only and is not used for serial testing.

Notes: Mechanism of Injury ("tell me what happened"?):

Any athlete with a suspected concussion should be REMOVED FROM PLAY, medically assessed, monitored for deterioration (i.e., should not be left alone) and should not drive a motor vehicle until cleared to do so by a medical professional. No athlete diagnosed with concussion should be returned to sports participation on the day of Injury.

Fig. 2. SCAT3. (*From* McCrory P, Meeuwisse WH, Aubry M, et al. Consensus statement on concussion in sport: the 4th International Conference on Concussion in Sport held in Zurich, 2012. Br J Sports Med 2013;47(5):250–8.)

accommodations for return to work or school, recommendations for vocational rehabilitation, and determination of neurocognitive residuals for disability application or personal injury litigation. In this setting, test batteries can be tailored to more completely assess the cognitive residuals of mTBI, as well as the contribution of emotional symptoms or personality characteristics.

BACKGROUND

Name: _____ Date: _____
Examiner: _____
Sport/team/school: _____ Date/time of injury: _____
Age: _____ Gender: ☐ M ☐ F
Years of education completed: _____
Dominant hand: ☐ right ☐ left ☐ neither
How many concussions do you think you have had in the past? _____
When was the most recent concussion? _____
How long was your recovery from the most recent concussion? _____
Have you ever been hospitalized or had medical imaging done for a head injury? ☐ Y ☐ N
Have you ever been diagnosed with headaches or migraines? ☐ Y ☐ N
Do you have a learning disability, dyslexia, ADD/ADHD? ☐ Y ☐ N
Have you ever been diagnosed with depression, anxiety or other psychiatric disorder? ☐ Y ☐ N
Has anyone in your family ever been diagnosed with any of these problems? ☐ Y ☐ N
Are you on any medications? If yes, please list: ☐ Y ☐ N

SCAT3 to be done in resting state. Best done 10 or more minutes post excercise.

SYMPTOM EVALUATION

3

How do you feel?

"You should score yourself on the following symptoms, based on how you feel now".

	none		mild		moderate		severe
Headache	0	1	2	3	4	5	6
"Pressure in head"	0	1	2	3	4	5	6
Neck Pain	0	1	2	3	4	5	6
Nausea or vomiting	0	1	2	3	4	5	6
Dizziness	0	1	2	3	4	5	6
Blurred vision	0	1	2	3	4	5	6
Balance problems	0	1	2	3	4	5	6
Sensitivity to light	0	1	2	3	4	5	6
Sensitivity to noise	0	1	2	3	4	5	6
Feeling slowed down	0	1	2	3	4	5	6
Feeling like "in a fog"	0	1	2	3	4	5	6
"Don't feel right"	0	1	2	3	4	5	6
Difficulty concentrating	0	1	2	3	4	5	6
Difficulty remembering	0	1	2	3	4	5	6
Fatigue or low energy	0	1	2	3	4	5	6
Confusion	0	1	2	3	4	5	6
Drowsiness	0	1	2	3	4	5	6
Trouble falling asleep	0	1	2	3	4	5	6
More emotional	0	1	2	3	4	5	6
Irritability	0	1	2	3	4	5	6
Sadness	0	1	2	3	4	5	6
Nervous or Anxious	0	1	2	3	4	5	6

Total number of symptoms (Maximum possible 22)
Symptom severity score (Maximum possible 132)

Do the symptoms get worse with physical activity? ☐ Y ☐ N
Do the symptoms get worse with mental activity? ☐ Y ☐ N

☐ self rated   ☐ self rated and clinician monitored
☐ clinician interview   ☐ self rated with parent input

Overall rating: If you know the athlete well prior to the injury, how different is the athlete acting compared to his/her usual self?
Please circle one response:

no different	very different	unsure	N/A

Scoring on the SCAT3 should not be used as a stand-alone method to diagnose concussion, measure recovery or make decisions about an athlete's readiness to return to competition after concussion. Since signs and symptoms may evolve over time, it is important to consider repeat evaluation in the acute assessment of concussion.

COGNITIVE & PHYSICAL EVALUATION

4

Cognitive assessment
Standardized Assessment of Concussion (SAC) [4]

Orientation (1 point for each correct answer)

What month is it?	0	1
What is the date today?	0	1
What is the day of the week?	0	1
What year is it?	0	1
What time is it right now? (within 1 hour)	0	1
Orientation score		of 5

Immediate memory

List	Trial 1	Trial 2	Trial 3	Alternative word list		
elbow	0 1	0 1	0 1	candle	baby	finger
apple	0 1	0 1	0 1	paper	monkey	penny
carpet	0 1	0 1	0 1	sugar	perfume	blanket
saddle	0 1	0 1	0 1	sandwich	sunset	lemon
bubble	0 1	0 1	0 1	wagon	iron	insect
Total						

Immediate memory score total   of 15

Concentration: Digits Backward

List	Trial 1	Alternative digit list		
4-9-3	0 1	6-2-9	5-2-6	4-1-5
3-8-1-4	0 1	3-2-7-9	1-7-9-5	4-9-6-8
6-2-9-7-1	0 1	1-5-2-8-6	3-8-5-2-7	6-1-8-4-3
7-1-8-4-6-2	0 1	5-3-9-1-4-8	8-3-1-9-6-4	7-2-4-8-5-6
Total of 4				

Concentration: Month in Reverse Order (1 pt. for entire sequence correct)

Dec-Nov-Oct-Sept-Aug-Jul-Jun-May-Apr-Mar-Feb-Jan	0	1
Concentration score		of 5

5

Neck Examination:
Range of motion   Tenderness   Upper and lower limb sensation & strength
Findings: _____

6

Balance examination
Do one or both of the following tests.
Footwear (shoes, barefoot, braces, tape, etc.) _____

Modified Balance Error Scoring System (BESS) testing [5]
Which foot was tested (i.e. which is the **non-dominant** foot) ☐ Left ☐ Right
Testing surface (hard floor, field, etc.) _____
Condition

Double leg stance:	Errors
Single leg stance (non-dominant foot):	Errors
Tandem stance (non-dominant foot at back):	Errors

And/Or

Tandem gait [6,7]
Time (best of 4 trials): _____ seconds

7

Coordination examination
Upper limb coordination
Which arm was tested: ☐ Left ☐ Right
Coordination score   of 1

8

SAC Delayed Recall [4]
Delayed recall score   of 5

SCAT3 SPORT CONCUSSION ASSESMENT TOOL 3 | **PAGE 2**   © 2013 Concussion in Sport Group

Fig. 2. (*continued*).

INSTRUCTIONS

Words in *Italics* throughout the SCAT3 are the instructions given to the athlete by the tester.

Symptom Scale

"You should score yourself on the following symptoms, based on how you feel now".

To be completed by the athlete. In situations where the symptom scale is being completed after exercise, it should still be done in a resting state, at least 10 minutes post exercise.
For total number of symptoms, maximum possible is 22.
For Symptom severity score, add all scores in table, maximum possible is 22 x 6 = 132.

SAC [4]

Immediate Memory

"I am going to test your memory. I will read you a list of words and when I am done, repeat back as many words as you can remember, in any order."

Trials 2 & 3:

"I am going to repeat the same list again. Repeat back as many words as you can remember in any order, even if you said the word before."

Complete all 3 trials regardless of score on trial 1 & 2. Read the words at a rate of one per second. **Score 1 pt. for each correct response.** Total score equals sum across all 3 trials. Do not inform the athlete that delayed recall will be tested.

Concentration
Digits backward

"I am going to read you a string of numbers and when I am done, you repeat them back to me backwards, in reverse order of how I read them to you. For example, if I say 7-1-9, you would say 9-1-7."

If correct, go to next string length. If incorrect, read trial 2. **One point possible for each string length.** Stop after incorrect on both trials. The digits should be read at the rate of one per second.

Months in reverse order

"Now tell me the months of the year in reverse order. Start with the last month and go backward. So you'll say December, November ... Go ahead"

1 pt. for entire sequence correct

Delayed Recall

The delayed recall should be performed after completion of the Balance and Coordination Examination.

"Do you remember that list of words I read a few times earlier? Tell me as many words from the list as you can remember in any order."

Score 1 pt. for each correct response

Balance Examination

Modified Balance Error Scoring System (BESS) testing [5]

This balance testing is based on a modified version of the Balance Error Scoring System (BESS)[5]. A stopwatch or watch with a second hand is required for this testing.

"I am now going to test your balance. Please take your shoes off, roll up your pant legs above ankle (if applicable), and remove any ankle taping (if applicable). This test will consist of three twenty second tests with different stances."

(a) Double leg stance:

"The first stance is standing with your feet together with your hands on your hips and with your eyes closed. You should try to maintain stability in that position for 20 seconds. I will be counting the number of times you move out of this position. I will start timing when you are set and have closed your eyes."

(b) Single leg stance:

"If you were to kick a ball, which foot would you use? [This will be the dominant foot] Now stand on your non-dominant foot. The dominant leg should be held in approximately 30 degrees of hip flexion and 45 degrees of knee flexion. Again, you should try to maintain stability for 20 seconds with your hands on your hips and your eyes closed. I will be counting the number of times you move out of this position. If you stumble out of this position, open your eyes and return to the start position and continue balancing. I will start timing when you are set and have closed your eyes."

(c) Tandem stance:

"Now stand heel-to-toe with your non-dominant foot in back. Your weight should be evenly distributed across both feet. Again, you should try to maintain stability for 20 seconds with your hands on your hips and your eyes closed. I will be counting the number of times you move out of this position. If you stumble out of this position, open your eyes and return to the start position and continue balancing. I will start timing when you are set and have closed your eyes."

Balance testing – types of errors

1. Hands lifted off iliac crest
2. Opening eyes
3. Step, stumble, or fall
4. Moving hip into > 30 degrees abduction
5. Lifting forefoot or heel
6. Remaining out of test position > 5 sec

Each of the 20-second trials is scored by counting the errors, or deviations from the proper stance, accumulated by the athlete. The examiner will begin counting errors only after the individual has assumed the proper start position. **The modified BESS is calculated by adding one error point for each error during the three 20-second tests. The maximum total number of errors for any single condition is 10.** If a athlete commits multiple errors simultaneously, only one error is recorded but the athlete should quickly return to the testing position, and counting should resume once subject is set. Subjects that are unable to maintain the testing procedure for a minimum of **five seconds** at the start are assigned the highest possible score, ten, for that testing condition.

OPTION: For further assessment, the same 3 stances can be performed on a surface of medium density foam (e.g., approximately 50 cm x 40 cm x 6 cm).

Tandem Gait [6,7]

Participants are instructed to stand with their feet together behind a starting line (the test is best done with footwear removed). Then, they walk in a forward direction as quickly and as accurately as possible along a 38mm wide (sports tape), 3 meter line with an alternate foot heel-to-toe gait ensuring that they approximate their heel and toe on each step. Once they cross the end of the 3m line, they turn 180 degrees and return to the starting point using the same gait. A total of 4 trials are done and the best time is retained. Athletes should complete the test in 14 seconds. Athletes fail the test if they step off the line, have a separation between their heel and toe, or if they touch or grab the examiner or an object. In this case, the time is not recorded and the trial repeated, if appropriate.

Coordination Examination

Upper limb coordination
Finger-to-nose (FTN) task:

"I am going to test your coordination now. Please sit comfortably on the chair with your eyes open and your arm (either right or left) outstretched (shoulder flexed to 90 degrees and elbow and fingers extended), pointing in front of you. When I give a start signal, I would like you to perform five successive finger to nose repetitions using your index finger to touch the tip of the nose, and then return to the starting position, as quickly and as accurately as possible."

Scoring: 5 correct repetitions in < 4 seconds = 1
Note for testers: Athletes fail the test if they do not touch their nose, do not fully extend their elbow or do not perform five repetitions. **Failure should be scored as 0.**

References & Footnotes

1. This tool has been developed by a group of international experts at the 4th International Consensus meeting on Concussion in Sport held in Zurich, Switzerland in November 2012. The full details of the conference outcomes and the authors of the tool are published in The BJSM Injury Prevention and Health Protection, 2013, Volume 47, Issue 5. The outcome paper will also be simultaneously co-published in other leading biomedical journals with the copyright held by the Concussion in Sport Group, to allow unrestricted distribution, providing no alterations are made.

2. McCrory P et al., Consensus Statement on Concussion in Sport – the 3rd International Conference on Concussion in Sport held in Zurich, November 2008. British Journal of Sports Medicine 2009; 43: i76-89.

3. Maddocks, DL; Dicker, GD; Saling, MM. The assessment of orientation following concussion in athletes. Clinical Journal of Sport Medicine. 1995; 5(1): 32 – 3.

4. McCrea M. Standardized mental status testing of acute concussion. Clinical Journal of Sport Medicine. 2001; 11: 176 – 181.

5. Guskiewicz KM. Assessment of postural stability following sport-related concussion. Current Sports Medicine Reports. 2003; 2: 24 – 30.

6. Schneiders, A.G., Sullivan, S.J., Gray, A., Hammond-Tooke, G. & McCrory, P. Normative values for 16-37 year old subjects for three clinical measures of motor performance used in the assessment of sports concussions. Journal of Science and Medicine in Sport. 2010; 13(2): 196 – 201.

7. Schneiders, A.G., Sullivan, S.J., Kvarnstrom. J.K., Olsson, M., Yden. T. & Marshall, S.W. The effect of footwear and sports-surface on dynamic neurological screening in sport-related concussion. Journal of Science and Medicine in Sport. 2010; 13(4): 382 – 386

Fig. 2. *(continued).*

ATHLETE INFORMATION

Any athlete suspected of having a concussion should be removed from play, and then seek medical evaluation.

Signs to watch for

Problems could arise over the first 24–48 hours. The athlete should not be left alone and must go to a hospital at once if they:

- Have a headache that gets worse
- Are very drowsy or can't be awakened
- Can't recognize people or places
- Have repeated vomiting
- Behave unusually or seem confused; are very irritable
- Have seizures (arms and legs jerk uncontrollably)
- Have weak or numb arms or legs
- Are unsteady on their feet; have slurred speech

Remember, it is better to be safe.
Consult your doctor after a suspected concussion.

Return to play

Athletes should not be returned to play the same day of injury.
When returning athletes to play, they should be **medically cleared and then follow a stepwise supervised program**, with stages of progression.

For example:

Rehabilitation stage	Functional exercise at each stage of rehabilitation	Objective of each stage
No activity	Physical and cognitive rest	Recovery
Light aerobic exercise	Walking, swimming or stationary cycling keeping intensity, 70 % maximum predicted heart rate. No resistance training	Increase heart rate
Sport-specific exercise	Skating drills in ice hockey, running drills in soccer. No head impact activities	Add movement
Non-contact training drills	Progression to more complex training drills, eg passing drills in football and ice hockey. May start progressive resistance training	Exercise, coordination, and cognitive load
Full contact practice	Following medical clearance participate in normal training activities	Restore confidence and assess functional skills by coaching staff
Return to play	Normal game play	

There should be at least 24 hours (or longer) for each stage and if symptoms recur the athlete should rest until they resolve once again and then resume the program at the previous asymptomatic stage. Resistance training should only be added in the later stages.

If the athlete is symptomatic for more than 10 days, then consultation by a medical practitioner who is expert in the management of concussion, is recommended.

Medical clearance should be given before return to play.

CONCUSSION INJURY ADVICE

(To be given to the **person monitoring** the concussed athlete)

This patient has received an injury to the head. A careful medical examination has been carried out and no sign of any serious complications has been found. Recovery time is variable across individuals and the patient will need monitoring for a further period by a responsible adult. Your treating physician will provide guidance as to this timeframe.

If you notice any change in behaviour, vomiting, dizziness, worsening headache, double vision or excessive drowsiness, please contact your doctor or the nearest hospital emergency department immediately.

Other important points:

- Rest (physically and mentally), including training or playing sports until symptoms resolve and you are medically cleared
- No alcohol
- No prescription or non-prescription drugs without medical supervision. Specifically:
   · No sleeping tablets
   · Do not use aspirin, anti-inflammatory medication or sedating pain killers
- Do not drive until medically cleared
- Do not train or play sport until medically cleared

Clinic phone number

Scoring Summary:

Test Domain	Score		
	Date:	Date:	Date:
Number of Symptoms of 22			
Symptom Severity Score of 132			
Orientation of 5			
Immediate Memory of 15			
Concentration of 5			
Delayed Recall of 5			
SAC Total			
BESS (total errors)			
Tandem Gait (seconds)			
Coordination of 1			

Notes:

Patient's name

Date/time of injury

Date/time of medical review

Treating physician

Contact details or stamp

Fig. 2. (*continued*).

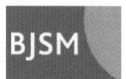

SCAT3

Br J Sports Med 2013 47: 259

Updated information and services can be found at:
http://bjsm.bmj.com/content/47/5/259.citation

These include:

Email alerting service	Receive free email alerts when new articles cite this article. Sign up in the box at the top right corner of the online article.

Notes

Fig. 2. (*continued*).

INJURY MANAGEMENT AND RETURN TO ACTIVITY AFTER CONCUSSION

Consensus guidelines call for a brief initial period of physical and cognitive rest as a cornerstone of acute concussion management. Although there is a dearth of empirical research in this area, it is thought that an initial period of rest in the order of 24 to 48 hours may be of benefit to the patient.[22,23] At the same time, lengthy or indefinite periods of complete rest are not supported by the literature and are thought by some to even be detrimental to overall recovery.

Following the initial rest period, the prevailing approach to injury management calls for a graded return to activity (eg, work, school, sports participation). The Zurich consensus statement outlines a graded exertion protocol specifically designed for athletes, which has become the standard (**Table 2**) (http://bjsm.bmj.com). Similar guidelines have been developed for return to activity after civilian or military mTBI. Although these are the accepted standards, research-based evidence supporting the timing and specifics of return to play is lacking and rehabilitation should be tailored to each individual's needs and progress.

This approach provides the combined advantages of allowing adequate time for recovery, enabling the patient to reacclimate to demanding physical and cognitive activity, and reducing the known risk of reinjury. With this stepwise progression, the patients should continue to proceed to the next level as long as they are able to remain asymptomatic during activities at the prescribed level. In most cases, each step requires a minimum of 24 hours for the patient to accommodate to the level of exertion, without any recurrent or worsening symptoms. Many patients are able to progress through all stages of the rehabilitation process in the order of approximately 5 to 10 days, beginning the process only after they have become asymptomatic. Should the patient experience any recurrent or worsening symptoms or other setbacks once the process has begun, the patient is then recommended to return to the prior rehabilitation stage for another 24-hour trial before graduating to the next stage of exertion.

Table 2
Concussion in sport group graduated return-to-activity protocol

Rehabilitation Stage	Functional Exercise at Each Stage of Rehabilitation	Objective of Each Stage
(1) No activity	Symptom limited physical and cognitive rest	Recovery
(2) Light aerobic exercise	Walking, swimming, or stationary cycling keeping intensity <70% of maximum permitted heart rate. No resistance training	Increase heart rate
(3) Sport-specific exercise	Skating drills in ice hockey, running drills in soccer. No head impact activities	Add movement
(4) Noncontact training drills	Progression to more complex training drills; for example, passing drills in football and ice hockey. May start progressive resistance training	Exercise, coordination, and cognitive load
(5) Full-contact practice	Following medical clearance, participate in normal training activities	Restore confidence and assess functional skills by coaching staff
(6) Return to play	Normal game play	—

From McCrory P, Meeuwisse WH, Aubry M, et al. Consensus statement on concussion in sport: the 4th International Conference on Concussion in Sport held in Zurich, 2012. Br J Sports Med 2013;47(5):250–8.

Table 3
Modified return-to-activity protocol for individuals with prolonged or atypical recovery

Rehabilitation Stage	Objective	Activity Examples and Exertional Range	Activity Duration	Restrictions	Predicted Timeline[a]	Indicator to Proceed to Next Stage
Light, low-intensity aerobic exercise	Gradually increase heart rate as tolerated without symptoms	Walking, elliptical machine, or stationary bike up to 60% of MPHR	15 min maximum	No contact or head impact activities (eg, treadmill) No loud or hectic environments (eg, sporting events, dances)	3–5 d	Tolerating this level of activity without symptoms for 3 d
Moderate-intensity aerobic exercise	Gradually increase heart rate as tolerated without symptoms	Walking, elliptical machine, or stationary bike up to 70% of MPHR	30 min maximum	No contact or head impact activities No loud or hectic environments (eg, sporting events, dances)	3–5 d	Tolerating this level of activity without symptoms for 3 d
High-intensity aerobic exercise	Gradually increase heart rate as tolerated without symptoms	Jogging, elliptical machine, or stationary bike up to 80% of MPHR	30 min maximum	No head impact activities. Limited social activity, as tolerated	3–5 d	Tolerating this level of activity without symptoms for 3 d
Noncontact training drills	Progression to normal sporting activity without symptoms	Volleyball-specific drills without risk of head impact	60 min	No head impact activities	3–5 d	Tolerating this level of activity without symptoms for 3 d
Full participation	Full participation without symptoms	Normal sport-related activities	NA	None	NA	NA

Abbreviations: MPHR, maximum predicted heart rate; NA, not applicable.

[a] The predicted timeline for this graduated program is extended from a minimum of 24 hours per stage to 3 to 5 days per stage to allow adequate accommodation without symptoms at each rehabilitation stage.

Adapted from McCrory P, Meeuwisse WH, Aubry M, et al. Consensus statement on concussion in sport: the 4th International Conference on Concussion in Sport held in Zurich, 2012. Br J Sports Med 2013;47(5):250–8.

In instances of atypical or prolonged recovery, a lengthier rehabilitative process may be recommended. In these situations, an adaptation to the graded exertion protocol may be appropriate. The authors have commonly used such an approach, typically extending the trial period of each rehabilitative stage from a minimum of 24 hours to 3 to 5 days, on average. An example of this modified graded exertion protocol is contained in **Table 3**.

SUMMARY

Major advances in the basic and clinical science of concussion over the past 20 years have taken much of the guesswork out of this injury and now provide clinicians with a fairly mature evidence base to guide the diagnosis, evaluation, and management of acute concussion. Although there remains some debate about certain nuances of concussion evaluation (eg, which tests are most sensitive and specific in detecting clinically meaningful change resulting from concussion) and management (eg, how long patients should observe total rest after concussion) of injury, there is a great deal of agreement on general principles of injury management recommendations across current-day consensus guidelines that are based on the latest evidence.

Clinicians who provide care for patients with concussion should be familiar with the latest evidence-based guidelines for the evaluation and management of acute concussion. Institutions and clinicians should have a systematic protocol for acute injury evaluation and management, tracking and determining the patient's level of postinjury recovery, and criteria for clearing patients for return to activity (eg, work, school, sports). Although the specific details of a concussion management protocol vary to some degree across clinicians and institutions, the key is for all care providers to be well prepared and familiar with their respective concussion protocol. This advanced preparation improves the consistency, efficiency, and effectiveness of care delivery for patients with concussion.

Beyond the scope of conventional concussion assessment and management, current research is exploring new frontiers in treatment interventions to facilitate recovery after concussion. Although several treatment and rehabilitation modalities (eg, vestibular therapy, multimodal rehabilitation, cognitive behavior therapy, pharmacologic agents) are often used in various clinical settings, the efficacy of these methods remains unclear. Scientific advances that drive evidence-based approaches to injury assessment, diagnosis, treatment, and rehabilitation are in the best interests of improving outcome and reducing risk of long-term disability in all populations affected by concussion and mTBI.

REFERENCES

1. Cassidy JD, Carroll LJ, Peloso PM, et al. Incidence, risk factors and prevention of mild traumatic brain injury: results of the WHO Collaborating Centre Task Force on Mild Traumatic Brain Injury. J Rehabil Med 2004;(Suppl 43):28–60.

2. Bazarian JJ, McClung J, Shah MN, et al. Mild traumatic brain injury in the United States, 1998–2000. Brain Inj 2005;19(2):85–91.

3. Centers for Disease Control and Prevention. Report to congress on traumatic brain injury in the United States: epidemiology and rehabilitation. Atlanta (GA): Centers for Disease Control and Prevention; 2014.

4. Carroll LJ, Cassidy JD, Holm L, et al. Methodological issues and research recommendations for mild traumatic brain injury: the WHO Collaborating Centre Task Force on Mild Traumatic Brain Injury. J Rehabil Med 2004;(Suppl 43):113–25.

5. Furger RE, Nelson LD, Brooke Lerner E, et al. Frequency of factors that complicate the identification of mild traumatic brain injury in level I trauma center patients. Concussion 2016;1(2).

6. Powell JM, Ferraro JV, Dikmen SS, et al. Accuracy of mild traumatic brain injury diagnosis. Arch Phys Med Rehabil 2008;89(8):1550–5.

7. Delaney JS, Abuzeyad F, Correa JA, et al. Recognition and characteristics of concussions in the emergency department population. J Emerg Med 2005;29(2):189–97.

8. Giza CC, Kutcher JS, Ashwal S, et al. Summary of evidence-based guideline update: evaluation and management of concussion in sports: report of the guideline development subcommittee of the American Academy of Neurology. Neurology 2013;80(24):2250–7.

9. Kay T, Harrington DE, Adams R, et al. Definition of mild traumatic brain injury. J Head Trauma Rehabil 1993;8(3):86–7.

10. National Center for Injury Prevention and Control. Report to congress on mild traumatic brain injury in the United States. Atlanta (GA): Centers for Disease Control and Prevention; 2003.

11. McCrory P, Meeuwisse WH, Aubry M, et al. Consensus statement on concussion in sport: the 4th International Conference on Concussion in Sport held in Zurich, 2012. Br J Sports Med 2013;47(5):250–8.

12. Harmon KG, Drezner JA, Gammons M, et al. American Medical Society for Sports Medicine position statement: concussion in sport. Br J Sports Med 2013;47(1):15–26.

13. McCrea M, Guskiewicz KM, Marshall SW, et al. Acute effects and recovery time following concussion in collegiate football players: the NCAA Concussion Study. JAMA 2003;290(19):2556–63.

14. McCrea M, Iverson GL, Echemendia RJ, et al. Day of injury assessment of sport-related concussion. Br J Sports Med 2013;47(5):272–84.

15. Putukian M, Raftery M, Guskiewicz K, et al. Onfield assessment of concussion in the adult athlete. Br J Sports Med 2013;47(5):285–8.

16. Zuckerbraun NS, Atabaki S, Collins MW, et al. Use of modified acute concussion evaluation tools in the emergency department. Pediatrics 2014;133(4):635–42.

17. Belanger HG, Vanderploeg RD. The neuropsychological impact of sports-related concussion: a meta-analysis. J Int Neuropsychol Soc 2005;11(4):345–57.

18. Collins MW, Grindel SH, Lovell MR, et al. Relationship between concussion and neuropsychological performance in college football players. JAMA 1999;282(10):964–70.

19. Guskiewicz KM, McCrea M, Marshall SW, et al. Cumulative effects associated with recurrent concussion in collegiate football players: the NCAA Concussion Study. JAMA 2003;290(19):2549–55.

20. Macciocchi SN, Barth JT, Alves W, et al. Neuropsychological functioning and recovery after mild head injury in collegiate athletes. Neurosurgery 1996;39(3):510–4.

21. Broglio SP, Puetz TW. The effect of sport concussion on neurocognitive function, self-report symptoms and postural control: a meta-analysis. Sports Med 2008;38(1):53–67.

22. Schneider KJ, Iverson GL, Emery CA, et al. The effects of rest and treatment following sport-related concussion: a systematic review of the literature. Br J Sports Med 2013;47(5):304–7.

23. Silverberg ND, Iverson GL. Is rest after concussion "the best medicine?": recommendations for activity resumption following concussion in athletes, civilians, and military service members. J Head Trauma Rehabil 2013;28(4):250–9.

Rehabilitation of Persistent Symptoms After Concussion

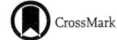

Rebecca N. Tapia, MD[a,*], Blessen C. Eapen, MD[b]

KEYWORDS

- Postconcussion syndrome • Rehabilitation • Concussion • Treatment • Chronic

KEY POINTS

- Early education about potential symptoms and expected recovery patterns is a mainstay of prevention.
- Headaches are the most common physical symptom and most common persisting symptom after mild traumatic brain injury.
- Clinical presentation is multifactorial and may be resistant to routine approaches, necessitating an individualized plan of care.
- A symptom-based approach with particular attention to sleep regulation is recommended.
- Utilize regular follow-up with realistic and measurable patient-centered goals.

INTRODUCTION

One of the more challenging aspects beyond acute concussion management occurs when symptoms do not resolve as anticipated over time, which may occur in upwards of 15% of all mild traumatic brain injury (mTBI) patients.[1] The term postconcussion syndrome generally refers to a presentation of multiple ongoing symptoms months to years from injury, typically comprised of physical, cognitive, and emotional complaints such as headaches, poor sleep, poor concentration, dizziness, and irritability.

Notably, these symptoms are common in the general healthy population and not necessarily specific to mTBI.[2,3] Although individual factors vary, the condition is often regarded as multifactorial including biological, psychological, and social factors.[4]

Disclosure Statement: The views, opinions, and/or findings expressed herein are those of the authors and do not necessarily reflect the views or the official policy of the Department of Veterans Affairs or US government.

[a] Polytrauma Service, Polytrauma Network Site, South Texas Veterans Healthcare System, 7400 Merton Minter, San Antonio, TX 78229, USA; [b] Polytrauma Service, Polytrauma Rehabilitation Center, South Texas Veterans Healthcare System, 7400 Merton Minter, San Antonio, TX 78229, USA
* Corresponding author.
E-mail address: rebecca.tapia@va.gov

Persistent issues can pose a threat to full community reintegration following concussion and reduce overall quality of life; thus early recognition and treatment are essential to optimize long term outcomes.

GENERAL APPROACH
Prevention

The mainstay of prevention of chronic symptoms following concussion is early education focused on expectations of recovery and symptom management.[5,6] Patients should be advised that most will experience a full recovery of symptoms.[7] An individualized plan for gradual return to activity with guidance about avoidance of symptom exacerbation is an effective step that can be implemented during initial concussion management.

Identification

Issues with ongoing symptoms are usually identified in a scheduled follow-up visit or through patient request for reassessment. Full history and physical examination are warranted to assess possible contributors to symptom presentation.

There are multiple tools that may be utilized to track postconcussion symptoms (**Box 1**).

Early Intervention

Education about coping strategies and expectation of recovery at time of injury has been associated with less stress and fewer symptoms at 3 months after injury.[12] This can begin at the time of initial concussion evaluation, and accomplished through conversation, handouts, or referral to online sources such as Defense and Veterans Brain Injury Center.[13]

Communication

Current verbiage regarding the event (eg, mild traumatic brain injury [mTBI], concussion, brain damage) can be confusing for both patients and providers, potentially increasing the perception that these injuries are associated with ongoing disability.[14] It is important to frame the conversation in terms of multiple contributing factors, many of which are modifiable, with positive expectations of recovery. Validating patient distress and subjective experience is important and does not have to be immediately coupled with attribution to brain dysfunction or damage. Important points include

- Consider concussion as a descriptor of the event versus mTBI[15]
- Build an early and strong alliance with patient through active listening
- Design symptom-based treatment plan focused on patient-centered priorities
- Structured follow-up with realistic and measurable goals

Box 1
Tools for assessment of postconcussion symptoms

Neurobehavioral Symptom Inventory[8]

Postconcussion Syndrome Checklist[9]

Concussion Symptom Checklist[10]

Rivermead Post Concussion Symptoms Questionnaire[11]

Conceptualizing Cocontributing Factors

It is well established that symptoms persisting after concussion are multifactorial, including factors such as genetics, personality, mental health disorders, and psychosocial stressors.[16] Premorbid history of anxiety is particularly predictive of development of postconcussive symptoms.[17] A full psycho-social assessment will help uncover conditions that may be contributing to ongoing symptoms and possibly interfering with recovery. **Fig. 1** displays a biopsychosocial conceptualization of poor outcomes after mTBI.

Caveats for Pharmacologic Treatment Options

Symptom-based interventions often include pharmacologic options. Given that persistent symptoms often occur as a group (sleep plus mood plus concentration problems), use of pharmacotherapies may quickly produce a new condition of polypharmacy; thus careful consideration of each symptom and a comprehensive approach will help dictate the medication component of any treatment plan.[18] Particular concerns include

- Be aware that many central nervous system (CNS)-acting medications have adverse effects that mimic other postconcussion symptoms (such as tricyclic antidepressants used for insomnia possibly worsening the dizziness symptom).
- Consider prioritizing the symptom that is most bothersome or most contributory to the overall presentation, such as insomnia.
- Educate the patient as to risks and benefits, including how this may impact (better or worse) other co-occurring symptoms.
- Estimate duration of pharmacotherapy and discuss with patient. Most of these medications are meant for temporary symptom reduction and not intended for life-long use.
- Ensure that the trial includes upward titration (as tolerated) to minimally effective dosing for the recommended minimum treatment duration prior to considering treatment failure. Premature assessment of any intervention as ineffective may reduce overall options in an already difficult and often refractory symptom complex.
- Track measurable and meaningful goals for each medication, weighing efficacy versus risk during the follow-up discussions. There are multiple widely available free applications for symptom tracking such as the Concussion Coach Mobile App.[19]
- Special considerations
  - Seizures: many medications will lower the seizure threshold
  - Cardiac history: some have potential for cardiac adverse effects, such as stimulants and tricyclic antidepressants (TCAs)
  - Substance abuse: general caution with the use of medication in patients with ongoing substance abuse, particularly use of alcohol, amphetamines and benzodiazapines
  - Avoid long-term use of opioid medications

Nonpharmacological Approach

Individual symptoms can be targeted with a variety of pharmacologic and nonpharmacological approaches, but it is important to understand the overarching themes of successful rehabilitation for persistent symptoms after mTBI (**Box 2**).

Rest versus return to activity

There is a fine balance between activity and rest following mTBI. Too much activity too soon or prolonged activity restriction may both have negative consequences during

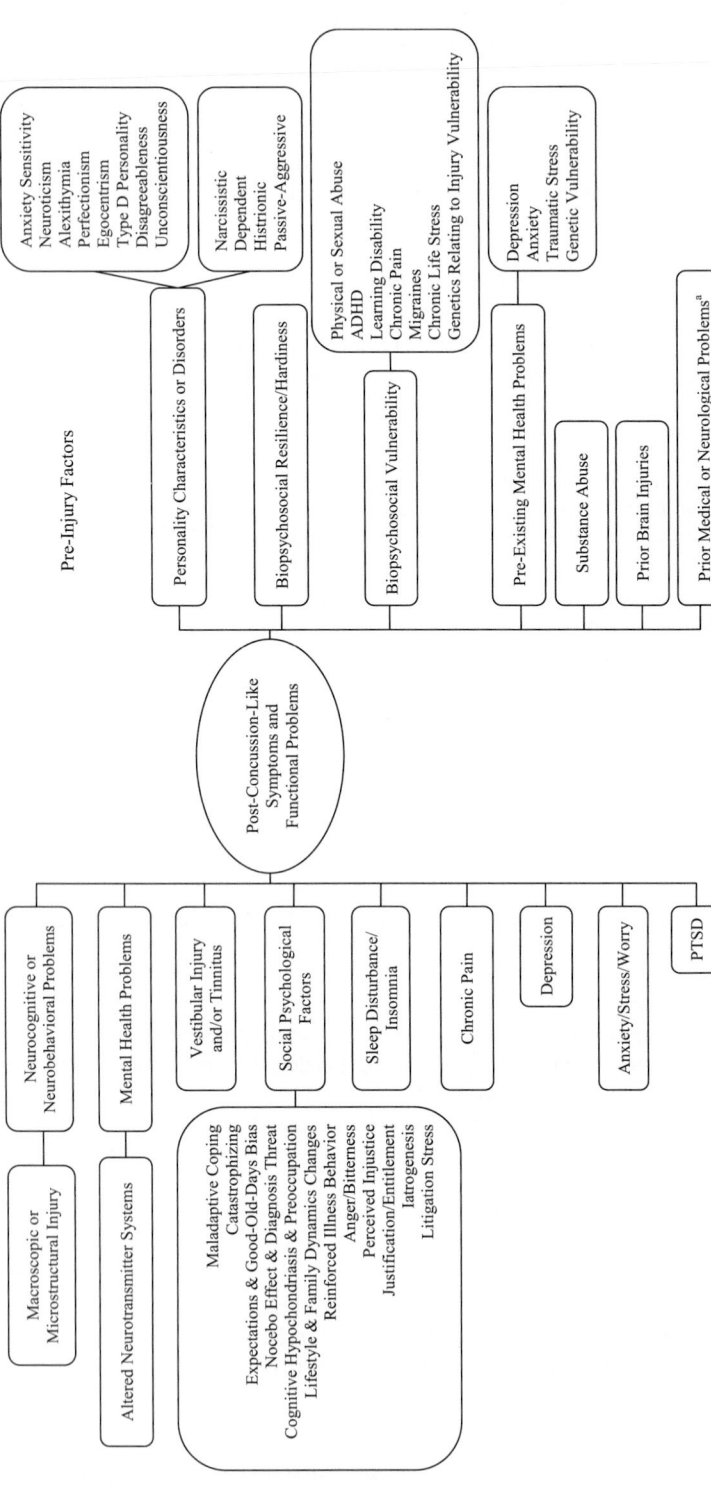

Fig. 1. A biopsychosocial conceptualization of poor outcome from mTBI. [a] For example, hypertension, heart disease, cardiac surgery, diabetes, thyroid problems, and small vessel ischemic disease. (*Courtesy of* Grant L. Iverson, PhD; with permission.)

Box 2
Treatment strategies for postconcussion syndrome

Education about mild traumatic brain injury, including natural course of recovery

Reassurance of positive outcomes

Avoidance of hazardous behaviors during acute recovery

Gradual return to activity and life roles as symptoms improve

Careful monitoring and early intervention for adverse emotional response

Symptom specific treatment

Ready access to providers during acute and subacute recovery periods

From Nelson Sheese AL, Hammeke TA. Rehabilitation from postconcussion syndrome: nonpharmacological treatment. Prog Neurol Surg 2014;28:149–60.

---

the recovery period. An individualized plan for gradual return to activity guided by symptom resolution is recommended to promote optimal function[20]:

- One to two days of rest following acute mTBI was recommended by the 2012 Zurich Consensus Statement on Concussion in Sport.[21]
- Excessive, early cognitive activity may prolong recovery from concussion.[22]
- Bedrest has not proven to be an effective strategy following mTBI.[23]

For chronic or persistent symptoms, engagement with regular aerobic exercise that does not cause symptom exacerbation is regarded as an effective method for reducing postconcussion symptoms and improving activity tolerance.[24]

SYMPTOM-SPECIFIC REHABILITATION INTERVENTIONS
Headaches

Considerations

- Headaches are the most common physical symptom reported after mTBI, and the most common persisting symptoms, with prevalence rates over 90% in concussed athletes.[25–27]
- The International Classification of Headache Disorders, third edition-beta (ICHD-III) defines post-traumatic headaches (PTH) as a secondary headache disorder attributed to head and/or neck trauma in close temporal relationship to the traumatic event (ie, within 7 days of injury to the head or within 7 days of regaining consciousness after injury or of discontinuation of any medication that could impair perception or experience of the headache).[28]
- PTH symptoms can present similarly to primary headache conditions like migraine or tension-type headache, but the onset or exacerbation of the headache symptoms must be secondary to trauma exposure.
- PTH is identified as either acute or chronic based on the duration and persistence of the post-traumatic headaches (**Table 1**).

Table 1
Acute versus chronic post-traumatic headache

Acute Post-traumatic headache	Headache resolves within 3 mo or trauma exposure was <3 mo ago
Chronic post-traumatic headache	Headache persists beyond 3 mo

- Most patients with PTH recover within 1 to 2 weeks of injury, but PTH can last for years.[29] Chronic PTH is associated with decreased quality of life, impaired activities of daily living, loss of work, and impaired societal functioning.[30]
- Begin with a focused headache history and full physical examination to identify the headache subtypes and to rule out other serious intracranial pathology, which may require emergent management.

Management

The management of PTH is empiric and is based on the primary headache phenotypes, which include migraine, tension-type, cervicogenic, neuralgic, or mixed headaches.[31] The initial management should provide education on the headache type and simple lifestyle modifications (eg, improve sleep hygiene, regular meals, improved hydration, minimizing stress, identification and avoidance of triggers, and exercise) to help mitigate reoccurrence of headaches.[32]

Nonpharmacological management of PTH may include use of

- Physical therapy
- Biofeedback
- Cognitive behavioral therapy
- Acupuncture
- Hot/cold packs
- Cranial analgesic electrotherapeutic devices
- Massage therapy
- Relaxation training

Pharmacologic management of PTH includes both medication and interventional procedures to help alleviate headaches symptoms. Clinicians should also be aware of medication overuse headaches (MOH), which may result from the use of analgesics, opioids, ergot alkaloids, and triptans, which can be used for the treatment of PTH. The treatment of MOH includes removal of the offending agents and subsequent treatment of the primary headache disorder.[33]

Pharmacologic management for PTH can be divided in abortive and prophylactic management (**Table 2**).

Table 2 Pharmacologic options for management of migraine headaches	
Abortive	**Prophylaxis**
Over the counter	AEDs (topiramate, Divlproex sodium)
Nonsteroidal anti-inflammatory drugs (NSAIDs)[a]	Beta blockers (propranolol, metoprolol)
Acetaminophen[a]	Alpha blockers (prazosin)
Aspirin[a]	TCAs (amitriptyline, nortriptyline, desipramine)
Aspirin plus caffeine plus acetaminophen[a]	Supplements (magnesium oxide, vitamin B2)
Prescription	
NSAIDs (higher dose)[a]	
Ketorolac IM	
Triptans	
Antiemetics	
Butalbital plus caffeine plus acetaminophen or aspirin	

[a] May also be considered for management of tension type headaches.

Mood

Considerations

A re-evaluation of psychiatric symptoms or comorbid psychiatric disorders is warranted for patients experiencing persistent mood symptoms following mTBI.[15] Preinjury depressed mood is a significant contributor to the severity of postinjury anxiety and postconcussion symptoms in general.[34] Depression has also been tied to poorer functional outcome following mTBI.[35]

Management

Mood symptoms should be conceptualized as part of the greater clinical presentation, in particular how mood disorders may drive or be a product of co-occurring conditions such as insomnia and pain.

Nonpharmacologic options Cognitive behavioral therapy (CBT) is the mainstay of management of persistent mood symptoms after concussion.[20] Where available, alternative medicine approaches may also be integrated into the overall treatment plan, including options such as

- Biofeedback
- Breathing techniques
- Acupuncture
- Relaxation training
- Cranioelectric stimulation
- Mindfulness

Pharmacologic options There are a host of pharmacologic options available for treatment of mood symptoms, but due to the nature of co-occurring conditions, it is highly important to individualize pharmaceutical selection to address either the primary driving issue (such as insomnia) or to address multiple issues such as pain and headaches. Options include use of selective serotonin reuptake inhibitors (SSRIs), serotonin and norepinephrine reuptake inhibitors (SNRIs), and TCAs.

Sleep

Considerations

Poor sleep is a common complaint following mTBI, occurring in 92% participants of a recent study.[36] Sleep is notoriously difficult to assess objectively even with wearable technology. Sleep impairments are an independent modifiable risk factor for ongoing neurobehavioral symptoms; therefore early recognition and intervention could improve the overall clinical outcome.[37]

Management

Nonpharmacologic options include

- Sleep hygiene education
- Environmental modifications
- Cognitive behavioral therapy

Pharmacologic options include

- Prazosin
- Antidepressants (Trazodone, TCAs, Doxepin, Mirtazapine)
- Hypnotics ("z" drugs Eszopiclone, zaleplon, zolpidem)
- Melatonin agonists (Melatonin, Ramelteon)

Over the counter antihistamine sleep aids, while effective in some patients, may exacerbate other symptoms such as dizziness or cognitive complaints.

Fatigue

Considerations

Fatigue is a common symptom following mTBI, occurring in 45% of individuals 1 year following mild-to-moderate TBI.[38] Fatigue occurs independently and at a higher rate than insomnia. Similar to insomnia, it is related to sleep disturbance, sleep hygiene, satisfaction with life, anxiety, and depression; additionally, it has a higher association with disability and sleepiness.[39]

Further characterize the fatigue (eg, physical, mental) and consider pertinent contributors such as sleep apnea or endocrine disturbances as part of the approach.

Management

Nonpharmacologic options include

- Psychoeducation, including the importance of physical activity, nutrition, and sleep hygiene
- Cognitive behavioral therapy
- Compensatory strategies
- Energy conservation
- Light therapy

Pharmacologic options include

- Modafinil
- Melatonin[40]

Stimulants in co-occurring anxiety should be used with caution, as they may worsen sleep issues.

Cognitive Dysfunction

Considerations

Cognitive impairments after mTBI can occur immediately after the initiating event and typically recover within days to months.[41,42] There is a subset of individuals who have a persistence of cognitive deficits that can last for months to years after the initial event.[43] The cognitive impairments include deficits with[44]

- Attention
- Concentration
- Processing speed
- Memory
- Executive function
- Communication
- Visuospatial

Management

Individuals who have persistence of symptoms that do not resolve and continue to affect work/school or activities of daily living should be referred for full neuropsychological evaluation to provide further insight into current deficits and help guide cognitive rehabilitation treatment programs.[45] Treatment of cognitive deficits after mTBI can be multifactorial, and individuals may benefit from an interdisciplinary team approach for evaluation and management). Initial management should include education on normal recovery trajectories after mTBI to help avoid misattribution of symptoms and to promote normalization of societal functions and to provide reassurance (**Box 3**).

There are currently limited studies that show efficacy of pharmacologic management for persistence cognitive deficits after TBI. Methylphenidate is the most studied medication and has shown modest improvement with attention and concentration.[46,47] Donepezil has showed some improvement with memory and sustained attention, but large randomized clinical trials are currently underway.

Vestibular Dysfunction

Considerations

Vestibular dysfunction following mTBI is thought to be a product of both central and peripheral dysfunction.[48]

Assessment can be challenging, as these symptoms are primarily subjective. Investigating how the patient describes the dizziness, inciting factors, and duration may help differentiate among possible causes.

Rule-out medication adverse effect (consider TCAs, antiepileptic drugs [AEDs], SSRIs, anti-cholinergics, stimulants, or benzodiazapines) and orthostasis as common factors for this symptom.

Audiological evaluation may aid in identification of etiology.

Management

Nonpharmacologic options include

Vestibular rehabilitation (or balance rehabilitation therapy) is the mainstay intervention for dizziness complaints following mTBI. A short trial may be indicated

---

Box 3
Cognitive rehabilitation strategies

Cognitive rehabilitation strategies are tailored to the individual deficits includes:

Attention/concentration
  Metacognitive strategies: focus on improved deficit awareness, self-regulation
  Self-monitoring and self-regulation
  Attention processing training

Processing speed

Memory

Compensatory strategies
  External: day calendars, notebooks, post-it notes, cellular phones, global positioning systems
  Internal: mnemonics, imagery, associations

Executive function
  Metacognitive strategies for emotion and behavior

Communication
  Social communication training

Visuospatial
  Visual scanning techniques

From Cicerone KD, Langenbahn DM, Braden C, et al. Evidence-based cognitive rehabilitation: updated review of the literature from 2003 through 2008. Arch Phys Med Rehabil 2011;92(4):519–30; and Cooper DB, Bunner AE, Kennedy JE, et al. Treatment of persistent post-concussive symptoms after mild traumatic brain injury: a systematic review of cognitive rehabilitation and behavioral health interventions in military service members and veterans. Brain Imaging Behav 2015;9(3):403–20.

as the initial intervention with close monitoring and discontinuation if no improvement.[15]

For patients who have symptoms of benign positional vertigo, consider the Dix-Hallpike maneuver for assessment, and if positive, implementation of canalith reposition therapy.

Pharmacologic options include a short trial of meclizine or other vestibular suppressants. These may be provided for symptoms that are bothersome and interfering with function; however use of this meclizine is limited by sedating adverse effects, recovery may be delayed.

Audiological Dysfunction

Considerations

Hearing loss, sensitivity to noise, and tinnitus problems are typically self-limited after mTBI. Damage to central auditory acuity is extremely rare with mTBI, with pre-injury hearing deficits begin relatively common.[15]

Management

Consider referral to an audiologist. Other options may include

- White noise generators
- Tinnitus cognitive behavioral therapy
- Reassurance
- Environmental modifications

Visual Dysfunction

Considerations

The visual consequences of mTBI are not well understood.[49] Complaints of light sensitivity, blurry vison, or eye fatigue may occur immediately following exposure to mTBI.

Management

Persistent symptoms typically require evaluation by an optometry or a vision rehabilitation specialist. A recent review article identified scanning as an effective compensatory strategy for computer visual search fields in patients with visual field deficits, but for this and various other interventions, the long-term functional improvement was not substantiated.[50]

SUMMARY

Management of patients with ongoing symptoms after mTBI can be challenging due to the multifactorial nature of the clinical presentation and the breadth of interventions typically necessary to address the issues. Focusing on modifiable risk factors such as insomnia, guiding return to activity, encouraging stress reduction, avoiding polypharmacy, and building a therapeutic alliance with the patient are solid principles for comprehensive management.

The following clinical practice guidelines are regularly updated with evidence-based recommendations and can serve as a resource for comprehensive management of persistent symptoms after concussion:

http://onf.org/documents/guidelines-for-concussion-mtbi-persistent-symptoms-second-edition

http://www.healthquality.va.gov/guidelines/Rehab/mtbi/

REFERENCES

1. Rutherford WH, Merrett JD, McDonald JR. Symptoms at one year following concussion from minor head injuries. Injury 1979;10(3):225–30.
2. Meares S, Shores EA, Taylor AJ, et al. Mild traumatic brain injury does not predict acute postconcussion syndrome. J Neurol Neurosurg Psychiatr 2008;79(3): 300–6.
3. Dean PJA, O'Neill D, Sterr A. Post-concussion syndrome: prevalence after mild traumatic brain injury in comparison with a sample without head injury. Brain Inj 2012;26(1):14–26.
4. Hou R, Moss-Morris R, Peveler R, et al. When a minor head injury results in enduring symptoms: a prospective investigation of risk factors for postconcussional syndrome after mild traumatic brain injury. J Neurol Neurosurg Psychiatr 2012;83(2):217–23.
5. Mittenberg W, Tremont G, Zielinski RE, et al. Cognitive-behavioral prevention of postconcussion syndrome. Arch Clin Neuropsychol 1996;11(2):139–45.
6. Bell KR, Hoffman JM, Temkin NR, et al. The effect of telephone counselling on reducing post-traumatic symptoms after mild traumatic brain injury: a randomised trial. J Neurol Neurosurg Psychiatr 2008;79(11):1275–81.
7. Marshall S, Bayley M, McCullagh S, et al. Updated clinical practice guidelines for concussion/mild traumatic brain injury and persistent symptoms. Brain Inj 2015; 29(6):688–700.
8. Meyers JE, English J, Miller RM, et al. Normative data for the neurobehavioral symptom inventory. Appl Neuropsychol Adult 2015;22(6):427–34.
9. Gouvier WD, Cubic B, Jones G, et al. Postconcussion symptoms and daily stress in normal and head-injured college populations. Arch Clin Neuropsychol 1992; 7(3):193–211.
10. Miller LJ, Mittenberg W. Brief cognitive behavioral interventions in mild traumatic brain injury. Appl Neuropsychol 1998;5(4):172–83.
11. King NS, Crawford S, Wenden FJ, et al. The rivermead post concussion symptoms questionnaire: a measure of symptoms commonly experienced after head injury and its reliability. J Neurol 1995;242(9):587–92.
12. Ponsford J, Willmott C, Rothwell A, et al. Impact of early intervention on outcome following mild head injury in adults. J Neurol Neurosurg Psychiatr 2002;73(3): 330–2.
13. TBI Basics | DVBIC. Available at: http://dvbic.dcoe.mil/about-traumatic-brain-injury/article/tbi-basics. Accessed June 4, 2016.
14. Wood RL. Understanding the "miserable minority": a diasthesis-stress paradigm for post-concussional syndrome. Brain Inj 2004;18(11):1135–53.
15. Management of concussion—mild traumatic brain injury (mTBI) (2016) - VA/DoD clinical practice guidelines. Available at: http://www.healthquality.va.gov/guidelines/Rehab/mtbi/. Accessed June 8, 2016.
16. Wäljas M, Iverson GL, Lange RT, et al. A prospective biopsychosocial study of the persistent post-concussion symptoms following mild traumatic brain injury. J Neurotrauma 2015;32(8):534–47.
17. Ponsford J, Cameron P, Fitzgerald M, et al. Predictors of postconcussive symptoms 3 months after mild traumatic brain injury. Neuropsychology 2012;26(3): 304–13.
18. Collett GA, Song K, Jaramillo CA, et al. Prevalence of central nervous system polypharmacy and associations with overdose and suicide-related behaviors in iraq

and afghanistan war veterans in VA care 2010-2011. Drugs Real World Outcomes 2016;3:45–52.

19. Concussion Coach Mobile App—polytrauma/TBI system of care. Available at: http://www.polytrauma.va.gov/ConcussionCoach.asp. Accessed June 10, 2016.

20. Al Sayegh A, Sandford D, Carson AJ. Psychological approaches to treatment of postconcussion syndrome: a systematic review. J Neurol Neurosurg Psychiatr 2010;81(10):1128–34.

21. McCrory P, Meeuwisse WH, Aubry M, et al. Consensus statement on concussion in sport: the 4th International Conference on Concussion in Sport held in Zurich, November 2012. Br J Sports Med 2013;47(5):250–8.

22. Brown NJ, Mannix RC, O'Brien MJ, et al. Effect of cognitive activity level on duration of post-concussion symptoms. Pediatrics 2014;133(2):e299–304.

23. de Kruijk JR, Leffers P, Meerhoff S, et al. Effectiveness of bed rest after mild traumatic brain injury: a randomised trial of no versus six days of bed rest. J Neurol Neurosurg Psychiatr 2002;73(2):167–72.

24. Leddy J, Hinds A, Sirica D, et al. The role of controlled exercise in concussion management. PM R 2016;8(Suppl 3):S91–100.

25. Lew HL, Otis JD, Tun C, et al. Prevalence of chronic pain, posttraumatic stress disorder, and persistent postconcussive symptoms in OIF/OEF veterans: polytrauma clinical triad. J Rehabil Res Dev 2009;46(6):697.

26. Nampiaparampil DE. Prevalence of chronic pain after traumatic brain injury: a systematic review. JAMA 2008;300(6):711–9.

27. Meehan WP, d'Hemecourt P, Comstock RD. High school concussions in the 2008-2009 academic year: mechanism, symptoms, and management. Am J Sports Med 2010;38(12):2405–9.

28. Headache Classification Committee of the International Headache Society (IHS). The International Classification of Headache Disorders, 3rd edition (beta version). Cephalalgia 2013;33(9):629–808.

29. Lucas S. Posttraumatic headache: clinical characterization and management. Curr Pain Headache Rep 2015;19(10):48.

30. Lipton RB, Hamelsky SW, Kolodner KB, et al. Migraine, quality of life, and depression a population-based case–control study. Neurology 2000;55(5):629–35.

31. Zasler ND. Pharmacotherapy and posttraumatic cephalalgia. J Head Trauma Rehabil 2011;26(5):397–9.

32. Obermann M, Naegel S, Bosche B, et al. An update on the management of posttraumatic headache. Ther Adv Neurol Disord 2015;8(6):311–5.

33. Diener H-C, Katsarava Z. Medication overuse headache. Curr Med Res Opin 2001;17(Suppl 1):s17–21.

34. McCauley SR, Wilde EA, Miller ER, et al. Preinjury resilience and mood as predictors of early outcome following mild traumatic brain injury. J Neurotrauma 2013; 30(8):642–52.

35. Scott KL, Strong C-AH, Gorter B, et al. Predictors of post-concussion rehabilitation outcomes at three-month follow-up. Clin Neuropsychol 2016;30(1):66–81.

36. Towns SJ, Silva MA, Belanger HG. Subjective sleep quality and postconcussion symptoms following mild traumatic brain injury. Brain Inj 2015;29(11):1337–41.

37. Sullivan KA, Berndt SL, Edmed SL, et al. Poor sleep predicts subacute postconcussion symptoms following mild traumatic brain injury. Appl Neuropsychol Adult 2016;23:1–10.

38. van der Naalt J, van Zomeren AH, Sluiter WJ, et al. One year outcome in mild to moderate head injury: the predictive value of acute injury characteristics related

to complaints and return to work. J Neurol Neurosurg Psychiatr 1999;66(2): 207–13.

39. Cantor JB, Bushnik T, Cicerone K, et al. Insomnia, fatigue, and sleepiness in the first 2 years after traumatic brain injury: an NIDRR TBI model system module study. J Head Trauma Rehabil 2012;27(6):E1–14.

40. Ponsford JL, Ziino C, Parcell DL, et al. Fatigue and sleep disturbance following traumatic brain injury–their nature, causes, and potential treatments. J Head Trauma Rehabil 2012;27(3):224–33.

41. Levin HS, Mattis S, Ruff RM, et al. Neurobehavioral outcome following minor head injury: a three-center study. J Neurosurg 1987;66(2):234–43.

42. McCrea M, Guskiewicz KM, Marshall SW, et al. Acute effects and recovery time following concussion in collegiate football players: the NCAA Concussion Study. JAMA 2003;290(19):2556–63.

43. Mittenberg W, Strauman S. Diagnosis of mild head injury and the postconcussion syndrome. J Head Trauma Rehabil 2000;15(2):783–91.

44. Barth JT, Macciocchi SN, Giordani B, et al. Neuropsychological sequelae of minor head injury. Neurosurgery 1983;13(5):529–33.

45. Cicerone KD, Langenbahn DM, Braden C, et al. Evidence-based cognitive rehabilitation: updated review of the literature from 2003 through 2008. Arch Phys Med Rehabil 2011;92(4):519–30.

46. Bhatnagar S, Iaccarino MA, Zafonte R. Pharmacotherapy in rehabilitation of post-acute traumatic brain injury. Brain Res 2016;1640(Pt A):164–79.

47. Arciniegas DB, Silver JM. Pharmacotherapy of posttraumatic cognitive impairments. Behav Neurol 2006;17(1):25–42.

48. Franke LM, Walker WC, Cifu DX, et al. Sensorintegrative dysfunction underlying vestibular disorders after traumatic brain injury: a review. J Rehabil Res Dev 2012;49(7):985–94.

49. Cockerham GC, Goodrich GL, Weichel LED, et al. Eye and visual function in traumatic brain injury. J Rehabil Res Dev 2009;46(6):811.

50. Berger S, Kaldenberg J, Selmane R, et al. Effectiveness of interventions to address visual and visual-perceptual impairments to improve occupational performance in adults with traumatic brain injury: a systematic review. Am J Occup Ther 2016;70(3). 7003180010p1–7003180010p7.

Chronic Traumatic Encephalopathy
Known Causes, Unknown Effects

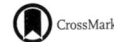

Diego Iacono, MD, PhD[a,b], Sharon B. Shively, MD, PhD[a,b,c],
Brian L. Edlow, MD[d,e], Daniel P. Perl, MD[a,c],*

KEYWORDS

- Traumatic brain injury • Chronic traumatic encephalopathy • Tau • β-Amyloid
- Diffuse axonal injury • Acute and long-term effects • Neurodegeneration
- Neuropsychiatric disorders

KEY POINTS

- Immediate and delayed neuropathologic consequences of traumatic brain injury (TBI).
- Single TBI, repetitive TBI, combat TBI, blast TBI.
- Chronic traumatic encephalopathy (CTE), tau disorder, neurodegeneration.
- CTE, aging, dementias, parkinsonisms.

INTRODUCTION

Chronic traumatic encephalopathy (CTE) is a recently defined neuropathologic entity (although, probably, a very old but unrecognized pathologic entity) that describes a constellation of brain lesions associated with a history of previous head trauma.[1] Sudden and injurious events affecting the central nervous system (CNS) are clinically termed, altogether, traumatic brain injury (TBI). TBIs are events known since human beings have been able to report accidents of the head or how people have changed

Disclosure: The opinions expressed herein are those of the authors and not necessarily representative of those of the Uniformed Services University of the Health Sciences (USUSH), the Department of Defense (DOD); or, the United States Army, Navy, or Air Force.
a Brain Tissue Repository & Neuropathology Core, Center for Neuroscience and Regenerative Medicine (CNRM), Uniformed Services University of the Health Sciences (USUHS), 4301 Jones Bridge Road, Bethesda, MD 20814, USA; b The Henry M. Jackson Foundation for the Advancement of Military Medicine (HJF), 6720A Rockledge Dr #100, Bethesda, MD 20817, USA; c Department of Pathology, F. Edward Hébert School of Medicine, Uniformed Services University of the Health Sciences (USUHS), 4301 Jones Bridge Road, Bethesda, MD 20814, USA; d Department of Neurology, Massachusetts General Hospital, 175 Cambridge Street – Suite 300, Boston, MA 02114, USA; e Athinoula A. Martinos Center for Biomedical Imaging, Massachusetts General Hospital, 149 13th Street, Charlestown, MA 02129, USA
* Corresponding author. 4301 Jones Bridge Road, Bethesda, MD 20814.
E-mail address: daniel.perl@usuhs.edu

after such traumatic events.[2–4] Although not always reported, TBIs have affected humanity because accidents to the head have been possible either as naturally occurring accidents (eg, casual cranial fractures, falls)[5] or human-created connected risks (eg, automobiles, weapons).[6] Peculiar types of TBI, especially for their association with specific neuropsychiatric consequences, are represented by traumatic brain events that cause immediate and often delayed motor, cognitive, and behavioral changes in war veterans coming back from war zones and combat operations.[7] Although an antique issue present in human society for millennia,[8] it was only during the late nineteenth century that TBIs and their medical sequelae were considered possibly linked to specific neuropathologic phenomena.[9–13] Moreover, it was not until the 1920s and 1930s that systematic attempts, although still sporadic, were made to analyze the neuropathologic effects of single TBI (sTBI) and repetitive TBI (rTBI).[14–16]

Considering the enormous long-lasting personal and socioeconomic impact of TBI for civilians and military personnel, it is surprising that, apart from those initial sporadic studies performed more than a century ago, the possible spectrum of brain disorders associated with TBI has scarcely been investigated in both civilians and military personnel until recent years. For example, the first systematic criteria to define CTE (a term initially introduced by Critchley[17] in 1957) were only published in 2016[1] based on multiple collaborative efforts of a team of investigators participating in the First National Institutes of Health Consensus Conference to Define the Neuropathological Criteria for the Diagnosis of Chronic Traumatic Encephalopathy (http://www.ninds.nih.gov/research/tbi/ReportFirstNIHConsensusConference.htm). These multi-institutional decennial efforts to develop preliminary postmortem diagnostic criteria for CTE represent an important landmark in the study of TBI neuropathology. TBI investigators began then to systematically analyze and better describe those possible neuropathologic lesions that could be exclusively, or primarily, associated with TBI. Furthermore, the long-term clinicopathologic consequences of TBI as subjacent to CTE and other possible modifying cofactors (ie, aging, genetic background, environmental risks) also started to be more carefully considered.[18–20]

The rapidly growing focus on CTE in the scientific and clinical communities as a disorder subjacent to TBI (and more specifically to mild TBI cases)[21,22] has been stimulated by 2 recent historical events:

1. The unusual presence (for age, anatomic localization, and histologic distribution) of intracellular hyperphosphorylated tau–positive lesions in an autopsy brain of a professional American football player reported by Omalu and colleagues[23] in 2005. Omalu and colleagues[23] report, and its relevant mediatic and sociopolitical impact (even to the point of stimulating the making of a movie concerning contact sports activities and related brain issues: Concussion [http://www.sonypictures.com/movies/concussion, 2016]), led other investigators to reconsider prior reports describing findings similar to the so-called punch-drunk syndrome described by Harrison S. Martland almost 90 years ago.[16] Martland[16] referred to previous studies published by Cassasa[14] in 1924 and Osnato and Giliberti[15] in 1927, which already described peculiar neuropathologic lesions in patients with concussion and hypothesized possible explanatory pathophysiologic mechanisms. Osnato and Giliberti[15] had referred to even earlier works published by Tanzi and Lugaro[24] in 1914, who began, for the first time in the published medical literature, to inquire about the possible chronic effects of concussion on the human brain. The reconsideration of the punch-drunk syndrome,[16] followed by sporadic clinical and pathologic investigations on TBI,[25–30] and of the more recent Omalu and colleagues[23] report, triggered a series of studies designed to analyze possible clinical and pathologic

consequences of various contact sports practices.[31–35] For more than half a century, the prototype of all contact sports–related neurodegenerative syndromes has been dementia pugilistica (DP), a term coined first in 1937 by JA Millspaugh,[36] a lieutenant of the Medical Corp of the US Navy. In his original manuscript, Millspaugh[36] recognized that Jokl and Guttmann[37] had already proposed a distinct form of dementia caused by pugilism. However, DP has been considered for many decades to be a unique posttraumatic brain syndrome almost, if not exclusively, confined to retired professional boxers and so reducing the chance for it to be considered and analyzed as part of a wider spectrum of possible TBI-related disorders.

2. The second relevant historical event linked to the renaissance of TBI-related neuropathologic studies has been the increased number of United States and United States allies' veterans returning home from long-lasting war operations, namely Operation Enduring Freedom (OEF), Operation Iraqi Freedom (OIF), and Operation New Dawn (OND). Some of these veterans have experienced a wide range of postwar disorders, possibly related to TBI and posttraumatic stress disorder (PTSD).[38–42] Specifically, these recent war conflicts have been characterized by the widespread use of improvised explosive devices (IEDs).[43,44] Veterans from OEF/OIF/OND, although better protected and more likely to survive TBI than soldiers in past wars, are now facing different types of long-term sequelae possibly caused by IEDs and other related blast-type explosives.[45–47] Blast TBI is considered the signature injury of current warfare, which has also been referred to as an invisible wound.[48] The original invisibility of this wound has been mainly attributable to the fact that in most of these veterans, the medical and neuropsychiatric consequences are not associated with any specific serologic, neurophysiologic, or neuroimaging biomarker. Moreover, initial neuropsychiatric signs and symptoms may not appear until soldiers exposed to IED/blasts return home.[45,49] Whether and how IEDs, and blast TBI in general, directly affect the CNS in humans is the main topic of ongoing intense clinical, neuroimaging, and neuropathologic investigations.[50–52]

The 2 events described earlier have stimulated the scientific community to increase the investigative efforts to define the neuropathologic consequences of TBI either in terms of short-term or long-term effects. The renewed and growing interest in TBI-related disorders research has also been reinforced by recent epidemiologic studies showing a significant association between a history of TBI and an increased risk of dementia,[53] parkinsonism,[54] and more general neurodegenerative disorders.[18,53]

This article summarizes the neuropathologic knowledge about CTE as acquired until June 2016.

TRAUMATIC BRAIN INJURY

Although the clinical definition of TBI has been revised and updated many times during the last 2 centuries, the most clinically useful definition considers TBI to be an acquired injury provoked by energy forces applied suddenly to the brain.[55] In its essence, TBI occurs when a transient impact or acceleration-deceleration forces (mechanical or other type) are applied to the brain causing cellular (neuronal and glial), axonal, vascular, meningeal, or lymphatic impairment that can result in a permanent damage or in a transient dysfunction (concussive episodes with loss of consciousness are not necessarily associated with a permanent damage) of the neurovascular unit.[56] Permanent damage can trigger cascades of pathologic events that produce neurohistopathologic marks that are detectable exclusively at the microscopic level. Such lesions may occur in any region of the CNS (cerebrum, cerebellum, brainstem, spinal cord, cranial nerves). However, cerebral sites of particular pathologic predilection can be recognized in relation to the stereotypical patterns of impact, especially in the case of rTBI. The stereotypical sequence of dynamic events that characterize each type of repetitive trauma (eg, professional boxing and American football) seems to allow, in most cases, the individuation of long-term specific pathologic features in terms of (1) brain lesions (eg, hyperphosphorylated tau–positive perivascular neurofibrillary tangles [tau-NFT] in professional boxers and American football players); (2) anatomic localization (eg, frontal and occipital lobes in motor vehicle accidents [MVAs]); and (3) histologic topography (eg, NFTs in the depths of cortical sulci in CTE).[57]

It is important to emphasize that the definition of acute and chronic TBI can refer either to the cause or to the temporal dimension. Although TBI can be described as single, multiple, or repetitive events for their causes, each type of event (or a combination of them) can trigger acute, subacute, and long-term persistent (chronic) effects that could respectively trigger and propagate pathologic processes in the brain. Fundamental questions about the pathogenesis and risk factors for these processes remain, because there are limited human data showing whether age, sex, genotype, environmental risks, nutrition, medications, or substance abuse (eg, alcohol consumption), and others, can negatively or positively modify acute, subacute, or long-term neuropathologic effects (and their clinical neuropsychiatric manifestations). Moreover, acute, subacute, and long-term neuropathologic lesions do not necessarily or directly correspond with acute, subacute, and long-term clinical symptoms and signs. Thus, when studying TBI and CTE, for example, it is important to consider that any type of clinicopathologic correlation needs to account for the different types of traumatic causes (eg, CTE has been mainly, if not exclusively, associated with rTBI, so far) and for specific biological, nonbiological (environmental), and timing factors. For each specific type of TBI cause and severity, the time interval between the traumatic events and formation of specific neuropathologic lesions should be better and more accurately defined. Moreover, most of the knowledge about lesion formation timing, molecular mechanisms of pathologic processes, neuroanatomical spreading (if any), genotype influences, environmental modulators, brain plasticity, and neuroglia regenerative capacities relies on experimental animal models that have mostly failed to be validated in humans. In addition, there is also the possibility that TBI cofactors, which are still unrecognized, may explain the frequently observed discrepancy between clinical symptoms and imaging analyses as well as between clinical records and pathologic findings.[58–60]

Epidemiology

In the United States 2.5 million cases of TBI are reported every year. Of these 2.5 million TBI cases, 50,000 result in death and 300,000 require hospitalization. Importantly, more than 5 million people annually live with TBI-related long-term disabilities.[61] The social and economic implications of these epidemiologic data are impressive and the annual estimated cost is approximately $60 billion in the United States alone. Nevertheless, it is not currently possible to estimate with precision the real socioeconomic burden of TBI and its consequences on the general population, because the recognition of TBI as a cause of late neurodegeneration is still in its infancy. In addition, whether these post-TBI long-term neurodegenerative effects have a potentiating or accelerating effect on other genetic and sporadic aging-related neurodegenerative diseases is mostly unknown. The absence of well-established knowledge on TBI-related long-term neurodegenerative effects is caused by the absence of large clinicopathologic postmortem correlation studies performed using unbiased general population cohorts and the lack of accurate lifetime TBI data collection. Such studies are necessary to elucidate the full spectrum of neurodegenerative consequences of TBI and to more accurately define the prevalence of CTE in civilians as well as military personnel (war veterans). However, given their autoexplanatory names (punch-drunk syndrome[16] and DP[36]) and those similar neurologic syndromes and pathologic lesions previously described,[62] they have scarcely been considered before and have been relegated to peculiar medical manifestations of specific contact sports practices,[63] thereby preventing a more general consideration (eg, of CTE and its prevalence) as a more general neuropathologic entity that can also be observed in other types of TBI.

CHRONIC TRAUMATIC ENCEPHALOPATHY

Using classic clinicopathologic methods, rTBI has been shown to be associated with neuropathologic lesions whose histopathologic characteristics and neuroanatomical distribution are distinct from those associated with other (aging-related) neurodegenerative diseases, such as Alzheimer disease (AD).[57] For this reason, the neuropathologic features associated with rTBI have been considered to be a separate neuropathologic entity termed CTE. Furthermore, studies of CTE and its potential interactions with other neurodegenerative processes also have the merit of providing intriguing new neuropathophysiologic perspectives on how the human brain reacts to different types of traumatic events; in contrast with, for example, nontraumatic disorders.[64,65]

Chronic Traumatic Encephalopathy Macroscopy

The most common observation on brains obtained from individuals with a history of rTBI (professional boxers and American football players being the most commonly analyzed) is a mild to moderate level of generalized cortical atrophy.[26,66–71] Although this atrophy may diffusely involve both cerebral hemispheres and the cerebellum, it is common to observe a more localized distribution of atrophy involving frontal > than temporal > than parietal lobes, mammillary bodies, and cerebellar tonsils. Other peculiar macroscopic autopsy findings can include mild to moderate ventricular enlargements (more frequently the third than the fourth ventricle, accounting for the patient's age), thinning of the corpus callosum, and cavum septum pellucidum, which can also be accompanied by septal fenestrations (**Fig. 1**A). Reduction of neuromelanin-containing neurons in the midbrain (commonly described as pallor of the substantia nigra and/or locus coeruleus) may also be evident. Most of these macroscopic features have been described mainly in cases of blunt-impact rTBI,

A   **B**

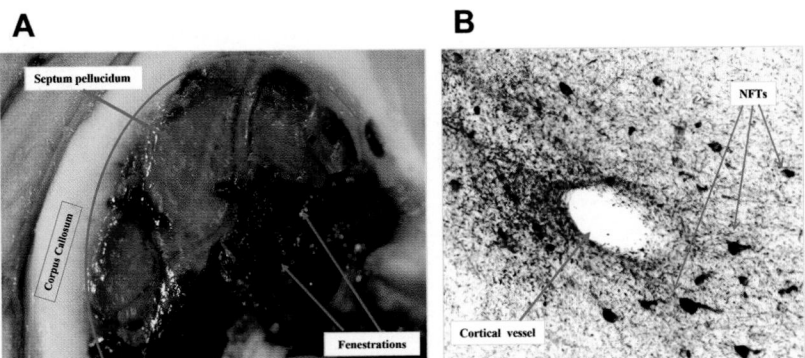

Fig. 1. Typical macroscopic and microscopic lesions observed in rTBI. (*A*) Fenestrations in the septum pellucidum of a 73-year-old patient with a history of rTBI. (*B*) Perivascular tau-NFTs in the neocortex of a 20-year-old college football player with diagnosis of CTE (modified Bielschowsky stain, original magnification ×320).

and it is not known whether they, or some of them, are also specific features of sTBI and blast-TBI cases.

Chronic Traumatic Encephalopathy Microscopy

Thus far, the only type of pathognomonic lesion established to diagnose CTE[1] is the aggregation of hyperphosphorylated tau (p-tau)–positive lesions in neuronal soma, neurites, and astrocytes (**Fig. 1**B) in the depths of cortical sulci with prevalent perivascular localization (**Fig. 2**). Other types of p-tau and non–p-tau brain lesions may be present in CTE cases, but they represent, at the moment, only supportive observations for a diagnosis of CTE. Intriguingly, p-tau lesions (similar to some of those observed in CTE cases) have been hypothesized to be associated, at least partially, with the formation of aging-related tau astrogliopathy (ARTAG).[1,72] It is not clear yet whether ARTAG is just a parallel and incidental aging-related neuropathologic phenomenon without a real pathogenetic role in neurodegeneration, or whether it is associated with pathophysiologic mechanisms related to CTE formation or progression.

Current CTE criteria are essentially based on systematic neuropathologic observations performed on the brains of people with a history of rTBI (most of which were from contact sports athletes, and, among these, most were American football players). So

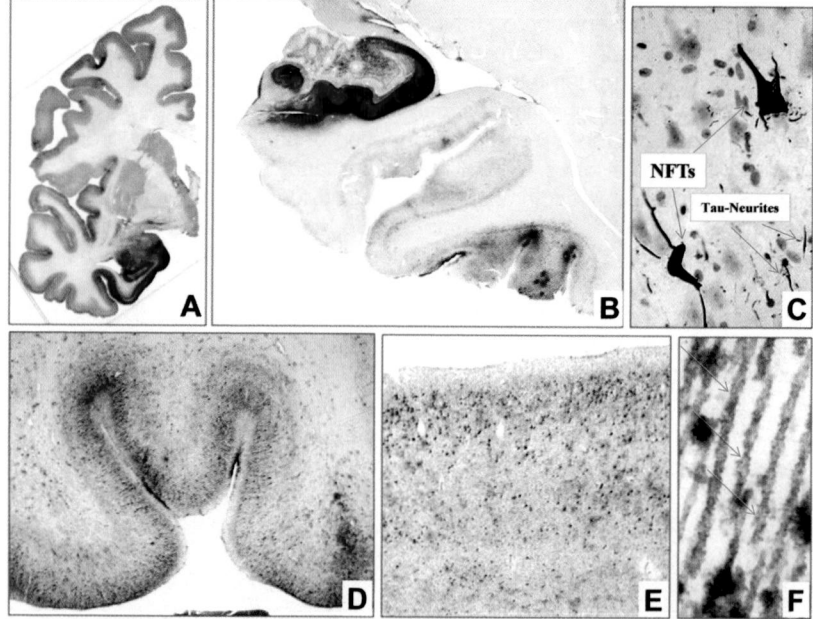

Fig. 2. Typical cerebral regions and cortical localization of tau-NFTs in rTBI. (*A*) Hemispheric section of a 46-year-old former professional American football player showing severe abnormal tau deposition (NFTs) in amygdala, parahippocampal cortex, and insular cortex (AT8/cresyl violet immunostain). (*B*) Severe hippocampal and parahippocampal abnormal tau (NFTs) accumulation (same specimen as in *A*). (*C*) High-power photomicrograph of NFTs in neocortex (AT-8 immunostain). (*D*) Insular cortex of a 48-year-old former professional football player showing severe layer II/III NFT formation (AT-8/cresyl violet immunostain). (*E*) Higher power view of *D*. (*F*) Electron microscopy details of hippocampal NFT of 46-year-old former professional football player showing (*arrows*) paired helical filaments (ultrastructural appearance of an NFT).

far, only a few CTE cases have been analyzed from military personnel (on duty or veterans) without a reported history of concomitant contact sports practices. Consequently, these epidemiologic considerations suggest that the ongoing CTE criteria may not be directly applicable to the neuropathologic assessment of brains from people with a history of sTBI or blast-TBI, or to TBI directly and exclusively related to military activities "sensu stricto", such as those present in a combat/war setting. However, the absence of specific descriptions for brain lesions exclusively, or typically, linked to sTBI or blast-TBI cases does not exclude the possible activation of neuropathologic responses triggering pathologic events resulting in the formation of CTE-like lesions, which are basically the expression of chronic pathologic phenomena.

Single Traumatic Brain Injury and Blast Traumatic Brain Injury

Little is known about the possible immediate macroscopic neuropathologic consequences associated with any type or severity of sTBI (the authors are not aware, for example, of the formation of a cavum in the septum pellucidum in sTBI or blast-TBI cases). sTBI and blast-TBI cases have rarely been assessed in detail at autopsy. At autopsy, most sTBI cases have been characterized by severe traumatic events, which caused death within a time interval usually too short to develop any evident macroscopic brain lesions. With the exception of macroscopic brain features such as cortical contusions and hemorrhagic phenomena (which may be immediately present and observable at autopsy) from coup/contracoup dynamics (mainly related to MVAs and falls),[73] no other specific macroscopic brain disorders are well established for sTBI. Detailed neuropathologic analyses focusing on the macroscopic acute effects of sTBI (of any type), and especially of mild sTBI, remain very rare.[74–79]

Chronic Traumatic Encephalopathy Prevalence

The prevalence of CTE in the general population and its potential variations with age, sex, ethnicity, and/or genotype is unknown. Thus far, only 1 study has attempted to estimate the prevalence of CTE by analyzing brains banked for neurodegenerative diseases studies.[80] Although meritorious, this study was biased by the prevalence of CTE being assessed on brains stored in a tissue repository collecting aging-related neurodegenerative diseases and without an adequate number of age-matched control brains. Moreover, this investigation was published before the current recommendations to diagnose CTE,[1] such that fewer cerebral regions were analyzed. Nonetheless, if larger unbiased autopsy studies of the general population confirm the findings from Bieniek and colleagues[80] (1.2% of collected brains were diagnosed with CTE, with 32% of CTE cases derived from people with a history of contact sports), the consequent implications in terms of medical, socioeconomic, and regulatory aspects of contact sports practicing in the adult and pediatric general population are potentially enormous. Intriguingly, there are also studies showing that CTE can be absent in some retired football players, even with the presence of multiple concussions and neurologic symptoms.[58] However, these findings, do not necessarily imply a specificity of CTE, but could reinforce the idea that CTE risk relates to the type of exposure to TBI (eg, frequency, intensity, cofactors) rather than the type of contact sport per se.

Chronic Traumatic Encephalopathy–Related Long-Term Effects

DP (the syndrome that includes acute and chronic cognitive and extrapyramidal deficits in former professional boxing players) was the focus of a series of cases analyzed by Brandenburg and Hallervorden[26] first in 1954 and then by Corsellis and Brierley[28] in 1959. Although representing an intriguing and natural model of TBI-induced chronic neurodegeneration, and probably a natural model of CTE formation and progression,

DP and related syndromes have been sporadically described[17,18,26,66,67] and never considered as the focus of longitudinal clinicopathologic investigations, thus contributing to the knowledge gap on CTE-related long-term effects. At the time of this writing, it is not definitively established whether and how CTE determines long-term neurodegenerative effects culminating in a specific form of dementia or in a typical clinical spectrum of specific cognitive and noncognitive disorders.[18,81]

CHRONIC TRAUMATIC ENCEPHALOPATHY: TAUOPATHY, OTHER PROTEINOPATHIES, AND GENETICS
Tau (Hyperphosphorylated)

CTE is currently considered a brain disorder that is mainly linked to the focal formation of hyperphosphorylated tau–positive aggregates in neurons, astrocytes, and cell processes (neurites) and having a unique perivascular and anatomic distribution. In the context of CTE, hyperphosphorylated tau–positive cells (ie, NFTs) are typically localized around the cortical vessels, in the depths of the cortical sulci, and predominantly in layers II and III of the neocortex.[52,82–84] These features are in contrast, for example, with NFTs localization in AD, which are initially localized in the deeper neocortical layers. Another topographic difference between CTE and AD is the prevalence of NFTs (and glial-tau disorder) in sector CA2 of the hippocampus and mammillary bodies in CTE compared with AD, in which they are rarely observed even in advanced cases. These and other peculiar topographic and pathologic features of tau disorder enable the conceptualization of an initial CTE staging system.[85] Furthermore, the CTE staging system represents a potential guide to study the possible progression of more subtle pathophysiologic and molecular mechanisms associated with CTE. It is also important to emphasize that the ongoing proposed CTE staging has not been validated yet in terms of clinicopathologic correlations.[86,87] As for the macroscopic descriptions of CTE, most, if not all, of what is referred to microscopic features of CTE are based on rTBI cases. There are only rare studies that describe microscopic aspects of chronic disorder after sTBI.[74,75] Because of this paucity of detailed neuropathologic studies on the chronic neuropathologic effects of sTBI, it is currently not possible to characterize similarities and differences with CTE caused by rTBI.

β-Amyloid

Biomechanical forces traumatically applied to the skull (directly or indirectly) act on intrinsic viscoelastic properties of the neural tissue, causing phenomena of axonal distortions.[43] Diffuse axonal injury (DAI) has been considered for many years[88–90] as providing postmortem evidence (now also detectable by in vivo neuroimaging techniques)[91] of brain trauma. For this reason, DAI has frequently been used in medicolegal settings.[92] However, DAI is not pathognomonic for TBI because the abuse of opiates also seems to generate similar axonal damage.[93–95] DAI, essentially, signifies abnormal, or completely interrupted, axonal transport. DAI can easily be detected by immunohistochemistry protocols using antibodies against the β-amyloid precursor protein (β-APP) **(Fig. 3)**. This protein is the precursor protein linked (in genetic and sporadic cases) to the formation of neuritic amyloid plaques in AD.[96–98] Diffuse amyloid plaques (which have been hypothesized to be the initial stage of the formation of more mature neuritic plaques in AD) have also been detected in perilesional areas of brains from some individuals with either sTBI or rTBI.[99–102] The presence of β-amyloid (βA) plaque formation, and in general of insoluble extracellular βA deposition, may represent seeds of the amyloid cascade progression that can eventually induce more generalized neurodegenerative events, which can culminate in the clinical

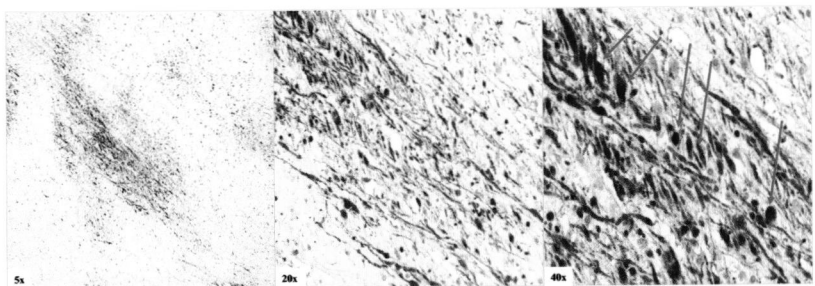

Fig. 3. An example of DAI in the white matter of a patient with a history of multiple TBI. The same DAI area has been pictured at a progressive magnification (using 5×, 20×, 40× lenses). The brain tissue section was immunostained against the β-APP, a precursor molecule that generates (by proteolysis) β-amyloid, which is one of the main molecular components of β-amyloid plaques typically associated with AD. Note the axonal swelling in the 40× image (the red arrows show just some of them).

manifestation of AD and similar neurodegenerative disorders. It is not known whether the βA-plaque formation following TBI is correlated with the age at the time of the trauma and whether other genetic and environmental factors should be also considered. Intriguingly, increased levels of various molecules (eg, βA, tau, glial fibrillary acidic protein [GFAP]) detectable in the plasma of patients with acute TBI at different time points after the trauma[103] could be signals of different, and even opposite, mechanisms of brain response (degenerative vs reparative processes), and ultimately of different prognostic clinical outcomes.

Transactive Response DNA-binding Protein

Intraneuronal lesions with immunoreactivity to transactive response DNA-binding protein (TDP43) have been reported across all stages of CTE.[104,105] TDP43-positive lesions colocalize with the tau-positive lesions in the later stages of CTE. However, to the best of our knowledge, TBI brains showing intranuclear inclusions positive to phosphorylated TDP43 (pTDP43), which is the pathologic type, have not been observed.[106] The presence of pTDP43 inclusions therefore needs to be confirmed, or excluded, by future larger clinicopathologic studies. The potential relationship between CTE and pTDP43 could acquire a special pathogenetic relevance because pTDP43 intraneuronal inclusions (lesions typically associated with specific forms of frontotemporal dementia [FTD] and FTD/amyotrophic lateral sclerosis [ALS]) might explain the increased incidence of ALS among participants of specific sports.[107]

α-Synuclein

α-Synuclein (α-syn) is the main molecular constituent of Lewy bodies (LBs) and Lewy neurites (LNs).[108] LB and LN intracellular lesions are observed in nigral and non-nigral neurons in patients with LB disease, mainly Parkinson disease (PD) and dementia with LBs. The other main pathologic feature of patients with PD, if not the major neuropathologic characteristic, is the neuronal loss of pigmented neurons in the pars compacta of the substantia nigra. Intriguingly, nigral neuronal loss in the absence of LB disorder (but often in the presence of tau-NFTs) has been observed in retired professional boxers.[109] There is ongoing debate about the possibility of a direct correlation between LB formation and neuronal loss in the substantia nigra. In the initial stages of PD, there is no correlation between the extent of LB disorder and nigral neuronal loss, which needs to reach 50% or more to cause clinical extrapyramidal manifestations.[110] To date, there are no quantitative studies analyzing possible correlations between number and type of TBI and nigral neuronal loss in sTBI or rTBI. However, animal models suggest that α-syn could also participate in pathogenetic phenomena linking TBI and PD.[111,112]

Genetics

Multiple genes have been associated with an increased risk of dementia (eg, AD) and more severe disorders (eg, βA deposition).[113] Among those, one of the most studied is the E4 allele of apolipoprotein E (APOE4).[114] Because of the presence of amyloid disorder in a subset of CTE cases, several studies have investigated the potential link between APOE4 and CTE, and more specifically APOE4 and rTBI.[115–117] No definitive conclusions can currently be made between specific genes and TBI or, more specifically, CTE. Other genes, such as neuroglobulin,[118] PPP3CC (protein phosphatase 3 catalytic subunit gamma gene),[119] COMT (catechol-O-methyltransferase gene), and ANKK1 (ankyrin repeat and kinase domain containing 1 gene),[120] glutamate transporter[121] have also been associated with modulatory effects on the clinical consequences and outcomes of TBI. However, it is not known whether these genes are directly linked to CTE pathogenesis.

CHRONIC TRAUMATIC ENCEPHALOPATHY: ASTROCYTES, MICROGLIA, BLOOD-BRAIN BARRIER, AND NEUROINFLAMMATION
Astrocytes

Astrocytes have historically been considered supporting cells for neurons.[122] However, there is now strong evidence for the essential role of astrocytes in the development and function of neurons, and it is now widely accepted that astrocytes are also involved in numerous essential physiologic functions. The neuron-astrocyte unit can therefore be considered as comprising a cellular system able to integrate various housekeeping and physiologic functions of the brain.[123] Similar to neurons, astrocytes respond to different causes and energy impacts of TBI. Among the pathophysiologic effects related to TBI, astrocytes undergo an increase in cellular volume (a signal of metabolic hyperactivation) that corresponds with increased levels of astrocyte microfilaments such as the GFAP.[124] Similar to the torsional effects of TBI on neurons, the astrocytic reaction is more pronounced in the white matter (ie, corpus callosum), which is one of the anatomic regions that, in humans, absorbs most of rotational shear-strain forces.[125]

Microglia

Microglia are immune cells in the brain that are quiescent under normal conditions.[126] Microglial cells can be activated by brain tissue changes, including episodes of TBI. Activated microglia express a series of molecules (ie, CD68 [cluster of differentiation molecule 68]), which (apart from their physiologic roles) provide excellent antigens for their identification using immunohistochemistry techniques. The chronic activation of microglia is part of the neurodegenerative processes[127,128] and has been observed to be involved in the post-TBI long-term consequences, especially related to DAI.[128]

Blood-Brain Barrier and Neuroinflammation

There is initial evidence that chronic alterations in blood-brain barrier (BBB) permeability may be caused by TBI.[129,130] BBB permeability alterations (transient or permanent) are among the fundamental components of the brain edema pathogenesis and neuroinflammatory initiatory process. Neuroinflammatory phenomena in neurodegenerative diseases such as AD and PD have long been recognized,[131] whereas much less is known in the context of CTE. Although often considered an effect of the disease, neuroinflammation events can trigger phenomena that can perpetuate the initial pathologic events, especially in rTBI.[132,133]

Chronic Traumatic Encephalopathy and Brain Polypathology

Although CTE is currently considered to be primarily a tauopathy, other proteins, such as β-amyloid, pTDP43, and α-syn, can synergistically aggregate in the form of extracellular accumulations (ie, βA plaques) or intraneuronal inclusions (ie, intracytoplasmic pTDP43 inclusions) in relation to TBI.[134–136] Each type of these brain lesions described in the context of TBI could be part of a more complex cascade of pathologic events determining acute and chronic pathologic effects on the CNS, and together could be part of more complex CTE-related phenomena that extend beyond deep sulcal and perivascular tau accumulation. Moreover, little is known about possible potentiating and modifying effects of co-occurring disorders (or brain polypathology) in the human brain.[137] Even less is known about the possible effects of brain polypathology on specific aspects of motor, cognitive, and behavioral decline or changes during aging.[138] To date, there are no published data on possible interactions among co-occurring disorders after rTBI, sTBI, or blast TBI and their contributions to CTE formation and related clinical outcomes.

COMBAT TRAUMATIC BRAIN INJURY AND BLAST TRAUMATIC BRAIN INJURY: CHRONIC TRAUMATIC ENCEPHALOPATHY?
Historical Perspective

During World War I (WWI) the use of high explosives, such as trinitrotoluene, was introduced, representing the first known widespread exposure to blast-TBI (high explosives had already been used in a limited fashion during the Russo-Japanese War in 1904). One of the initial terms used to describe the clinical consequences of closed-head blast injuries was shell shock.[12] However, the British War Office[139] (*Report of the War Office Committee of Enquiry into "Shell Shock"*) banned the use of the term because the shell shock syndrome was thought to not have a biological basis. The syndrome was considered an indecorous sign of weakness among British soldiers. Nevertheless, the British medical commission ultimately recognized some element of organicity in most of the evaluated shell shock cases because they did have some blast-related effects. The commission also recognized that there were behavioral (emotional) and mental (cognitive) alterations in these blast-injured soldiers (partially resembling what is now called PTSD [Diagnostic and Statistical Manual of Mental Disorders, Fifth Edition]).[140] However, at that time, military authorities decided to proscribe the shell shock term. This decision of the British Army "de facto" removed the opportunity to study and characterize a biological component of shell shock and shell shock–like syndromes for almost a century.

Nonetheless, after WWI a significant number of British retired soldiers were diagnosed with neurasthenia and treated for consequences of mild to moderate blast-related TBI. However, no substantial clinical or pathologic reports have been published since WWI. As a result, what has been known until very recent years about possible blast-TBI related syndromes, such as the shell shock syndrome, is largely anecdotal.[141] A few rare exceptions were the blast-TBI related reports published during WWI by Frederick W. Mott[13,142] in 1916 and 1917. These pathologic observations represent the first systematic studies on blast TBI–related consequences ever described in the English language and published in an international medical journal. A few years later, in 1942, other blast-related pathologic consequences were described by Fulton and colleagues.[42,143] These investigators described the possible effects of blast waves on animals and humans, as well as concussive and shock phenomena as mainly linked to German attacks with shelling during WWII. Curiously, in 1941, brain injuries caused by blast were described in a pheasant: probably the precursor of all blast-TBI animal models.[144] Since the 1940s, international medical literature describing possible effects of blast on the human nervous system have been extremely rare. Only in recent years, with the current conflicts in the Middle East, has there been increased attention to this matter. The increased interest has also been caused by the increasing appearance of new types of explosive devices, the IEDs, and their long-term consequences on exposed combatants.

Traumatic Brain Injury, Chronic Encephalopathy, and Posttraumatic Stress Disorder

CTE is a pathologic entity linked to rTBI-induced mechanical phenomena. However, it is not currently known whether CTE represents the pathologic substrate of blast-TBI (nonmechanical impacts) as well. A recent study[145] started to show specific types of brain lesions that could be directly linked to the consequences of blast-TBI phenomena (**Fig. 4**). This study describes previously unrecognized scarring patterns of GFAP neocortical lesions in subjects with a history of blast TBI compared with subjects with a history of nonblast TBI (ie, impact) and age-matched control subjects. These newly recognized lesions have been termed interface astroglial scarring.[145] Intriguingly, these GFAP lesions were recognized mainly in chronic cases; that is, in

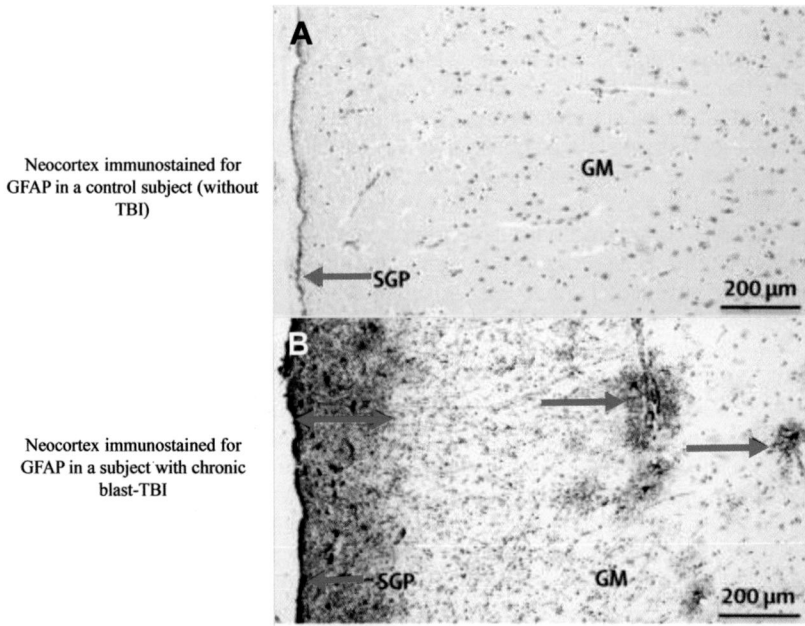

Neocortex immunostained for GFAP in a control subject (without TBI)

Neocortex immunostained for GFAP in a subject with chronic blast-TBI

Fig. 4. GFAP-positive scars in chronic blast-TBI and non-TBI control subject. (*A*) A 5-μm-thick section of neocortical brain tissue (frontal cortex) immunostained for GFAP, a marker of neuroinflammation. Control patient without a history of TBI. (*B*) A 5-μm-thick tissue section of neocortical brain tissue (frontal cortex) immunostained for GFAP. Patient with a chronic history of TBI. Single red arrows show perivascular and subpial astrogliosis; double red arrows show the thickness of the GFAP scar in a chronic blast-TBI case compared with the control (*A*). GM, gray matter; SGP, subpial glial plate.

patients who died 6 months or longer after the blast episodes. Whether there is a pathogenetic link between CTE (rTBI) and interface astroglial scarring (blast TBI) is currently not known and larger prospective autopsy studies are needed to definitively establish such a link.

In addition, whether the interface astroglial scarring without CTE could represent some of the neuropathologic substrates found in the brains of patients with a diagnosis of PTSD, or a specific subgroup of patients with PTSD (eg, rTBI and/or blast TBI), is under ongoing and intense investigation.[146,147]

FUTURE DIRECTIONS
Chronic Traumatic Encephalopathy and Clinicopathologic Studies

Postmortem evaluations from longitudinal cohort studies should be performed at a very large scale to estimate the prevalence of CTE in rTBI, sTBI, and blast/combat TBI. These prospective clinical studies should include multiple and periodic physical, neurologic, and psychiatric examinations; neuroimaging analyses; genetic and environmental assessment, followed by detailed neuropathologic evaluations of any death in the cohort. To do so, very large longitudinal studies should be prioritized and include multiple centers across different countries using identical investigative tools, harmonized assessment trainings, and well-established protocols for all personnel and investigators involved in the studies and sharing all available data across participating institutions.

Chronic Traumatic Encephalopathy and Pathology-Imaging Correlation Studies

Advanced neuroimaging techniques have significant potential to elucidate the pathophysiologic processes that link TBI to CTE and other possible posttraumatic neurodegenerative disorders.[148] These tools, which include diffusion tensor imaging,[149] resting-state functional MRI,[150] and tau-PET[151] are now being used to study in vivo biomarkers of CTE and other types of posttraumatic neurodegeneration. Similarly, structural imaging methods such as diffusion tensor imaging are being performed postmortem for correlations with histopathologic autopsy findings, and specifically for TBI investigations.[152–154] These techniques are being used to identify subtle lesions (eg, alterations in white matter connectivity),[155] as well as their differential temporal pathways and anatomic localization in relation to the type of trauma (ie, rTBI vs sTBI, or sTBI vs blast-TBI), clinical severity, and prognosis.

However, advanced imaging techniques still offer 10000-fold less spatial resolution than light microcopy, which remains by consequence an essential tool for the discovery of possible TBI-related brain lesions. Importantly, although diffusion tensor imaging[156,157] and tau-PET have shown some potential respectively for identifying blast-disorder and CTE disorder, neither blast-disorder nor CTE can currently be diagnosed by clinically available imaging techniques. Brain donations from all these longitudinally followed patients with TBI will be needed to discover and validate pathologic biomarkers that will enable the development of targeted therapies to halt or delay the progression of CTE and other CTE-related disorders.[158]

ACKNOWLEDGMENTS

We thank all families that consented for the brain donation of their family members for the better understanding of TBI and its possible treatments. We also thank Mrs. Patricia Lee and Mrs. Nichelle Gray for their technical support and Mr. Harold Anderson ("Kramer") for his writing assistance and editing skills.

REFERENCES

1. McKee AC, Cairns NJ, Dickson DW, et al. The first NINDS/NIBIB consensus meeting to define neuropathological criteria for the diagnosis of chronic traumatic encephalopathy. Acta Neuropathol 2016;131(1):75–86.
2. Panourias IG, Skiadas PK, Sakas DE, et al. Hippocrates: a pioneer in the treatment of head injuries. Neurosurgery 2005;57(1):181–9.
3. Kshettry VR, Mindea SA, Batjer HH. The management of cranial injuries in antiquity and beyond. Neurosurg Focus 2007;23(1):E8.
4. Missios S. Hippocrates, Galen, and the uses of trepanation in the ancient classical world. Neurosurg Focus 2007;23(1):E11.
5. Dart RA. The predatory implemental technique of Australopithecus. Am J Phys Anthropol 1949;7(1):1–38.
6. Gross CG. Trepanation from the Palaeolithic to the internet. In: Arnott A, Smith CUM, Finger S, editors. Trepanation: history, discovery, theory. Exton (PA): Swets & Zeitlinger; 2003. p. 307–22.
7. DePalma RG. Combat TBI: history, epidemiology, and injury modes. In: Kobeissy FH, editor. SourceBrain neurotrauma: molecular, neuropsychological, and rehabilitation aspects. Boca Raton (FL): CRC Press/Taylor & Francis; 2015. p. 5–14.
8. Rose FC. The history of head injuries: an overview. J Hist Neurosci 1997;6(2):154–80.
9. Erichsen JE. On concussion of the spine, nervous shock and other obscure injuries to the nervous system in their clinical and medico-legal aspects. London: Longmans, Green; 1875. p. 15–21.
10. Oppenheim H. Die traumatischen Neurosen. In: Nach den in der Nervenklinik der Charité in den letzten 5 Jahren gesammelten Beobachtungen. 2nd edition. Berlin (Germany): Hirschwald; 1889. 1892.
11. Forsyth D. Functional nerve disease and the shock of battle. Lancet 1915;186(4817):1399–403.
12. Myers CS. A contribution to the study of shellshock: being an account of the three cases of loss of memory, vision, smell and taste admitted to the Duchess of Westminster's War Hospital, Le Touquet. Lancet 1915;2:316–20.
13. Mott FW. The effects of high explosives upon the central nervous system. Lecture I. Lancet 1916;187(4824):331–8.
14. Cassasa CB. Multiple traumatic cerebral hemorrhages. Proc New York Pathological Soc 1924;24:101–6.
15. Osnato M, Giliberti V. Postconcussion neurosis-traumatic encephalitis – a conception of postconcussion phenomena. Arch Neurpsych 1927;6:181–214.
16. Martland H. Punch drunk. JAMA 1928;91:1103–7.
17. Critchley M. Medical aspects of boxing, particularly from a neurological standpoint. Br Med J 1957;1(5015):357–62.
18. Stern RA, Riley DO, Daneshvar DH, et al. Long-term consequences of repetitive brain trauma: chronic traumatic encephalopathy. PM R 2011;3(10 Suppl 2):S460–7.
19. Tartaglia MC, Hazrati LN, Davis KD, et al. Chronic traumatic encephalopathy and other neurodegenerative proteinopathies. Front Hum Neurosci 2014;8:30.
20. Daneshvar DH, Goldstein LE, Kiernan PT, et al. Post-traumatic neurodegeneration and chronic traumatic encephalopathy. Mol Cell Neurosci 2015;66(Pt B):81–90.

21. Carroll LJ, Cassidy JD, Holm L, et al. Methodological issues and research recommendations for mild traumatic brain injury: the WHO Collaborating Centre Task Force on Mild Traumatic Brain Injury. J Rehabil Med 2004;43(Suppl): 113–25.

22. West TA, Marion DW. Current recommendations for the diagnosis and treatment of concussion in sport: a comparison of three new guidelines. J Neurotrauma 2014;31(2):159–68.

23. Omalu BI, DeKosky ST, Minster RL, et al. Chronic traumatic encephalopathy in a National Football League player. Neurosurgery 2005;57(1):128–34 [discussion: 128–34].

24. Tanzi E, Lugaro E. Trattato delle malattie mentali 1914;2:325 [in Italian].

25. Parker HL. Traumatic encephalopathy ('punch drunk') of professional pugilists. J Neurol Psychopathol 1934;15(57):20–8.

26. Brandenburg W, Hallervorden J. Dementia pugilistica with anatomical findings. Virchows Arch 1954;325(6):680–709 [in German].

27. Grahmann H, Ule G. Diagnosis of chronic cerebral symptoms in boxers (dementia pugilistica & traumatic encephalopathy of boxers). Psychiatr Neurol (Basel) 1957;134:261–83 [in German].

28. Corsellis JA, Brierley JB. Observations on the pathology of insidious dementia following head injury. J Ment Sci 1959;105:714–20.

29. Wolowska J. Encephalopathia pugilistica (boxer's disease). Neurol Neurochir Psychiatr Pol 1960;10:787–93 [in Polish].

30. Mendez MF. The neuropsychiatric aspects of boxing. Int J Psychiatry Med 1995; 25(3):249–62.

31. Sortland O, Tysvaer AT. Brain damage in former association football players. An evaluation by cerebral computed tomography. Neuroradiology 1989;31(1):44–8.

32. Aotsuka A, Kojima S, Furumoto H, et al. Punch drunk syndrome due to repeated karate kicks and punches. Rinsho Shinkeigaku 1990;30(11):1243–6 [in Japanese].

33. Matser JT, Kessels AG, Jordan BD, et al. Chronic traumatic brain injury in professional soccer players. Neurology 1998;51(3):791–6.

34. Collins MW, Grindel SH, Lovell MR, et al. Relationship between concussion and neuropsychological performance in college football players. JAMA 1999; 282(10):964–70.

35. Erlanger DM, Kutner KC, Barth JT, et al. Neuropsychology of sports-related head injury: dementia pugilistica to post concussion syndrome. Clin Neuropsychol 1999;13(2):193–209.

36. Millspaugh JA. Dementia pugilistica. U S Navy Med Bull 1937;35:297–303.

37. Jokl E, Guttmann E. Neurologische-Psychiatrische Untersuchung On Boxern. Munch Med Woch 1933;15:560 [in German].

38. Jones E, Hodgins-Vermaas R, McCartney H, et al. Post-combat syndromes from the Boer War to the Gulf War: a cluster analysis of their nature and attribution. BMJ 2002;324(7333):321–4.

39. Cifu DX, Taylor BC, Carne WF, et al. Traumatic brain injury, posttraumatic stress disorder, and pain diagnoses in OIF/OEF/OND veterans. J Rehabil Res Dev 2013;50(9):1169–76.

40. Minshall D. Gulf War syndrome: a review of current knowledge and understanding. J R Nav Med Serv 2014;100(3):252–8.

41. Mohanty AF, Muthukutty A, Carter ME, et al. Chronic multisymptom illness among female veterans deployed to Iraq and Afghanistan. Med Care 2015; 53(4 Suppl 1):S143–8.

42. Fulton JJ, Calhoun PS, Wagner HR, et al. The prevalence of posttraumatic stress disorder in Operation Enduring Freedom/Operation Iraqi Freedom (OEF/OIF) veterans: a meta-analysis. J Anxiety Disord 2015;31:98–107.

43. Bass CR, Panzer MB, Rafaels KA, et al. Brain injuries from blast. Ann Biomed Eng 2012;40(1):185–202.

44. Singh AK, Ditkofsky NG, York JD, et al. Blast injuries: from improvised explosive device blasts to the Boston Marathon bombing. Radiographics 2016;36(1): 295–307.

45. Hoge CW, Castro CA, Messer SC, et al. Combat duty in Iraq and Afghanistan, mental health problems and barriers to care. US Army Med Dep J 2008;Jul-Sep:7–17.

46. Young L, Rule GT, Bocchieri RT, et al. When physics meets biology: low and high-velocity penetration, blunt impact, and blast injuries to the brain. Front Neurol 2015;6:89.

47. Ling G, Ecklund JM, Bandak FA. Brain injury from explosive blast: description and clinical management. Handb Clin Neurol 2015;127:173–80.

48. Vick K. Life after war. Veterans of Iraq and Afghanistan are battling lasting wounds–both visible and invisible. Time 2014;184(19):46–55.

49. Rosenfeld JV, McFarlane AC, Bragge P, et al. Blast-related traumatic brain injury. Lancet Neurol 2013;12(9):882–93.

50. Magnuson J, Leonessa F, Ling GS. Neuropathology of explosive blast traumatic brain injury. Curr Neurol Neurosci Rep 2012;12(5):570–9.

51. Bandak FA, Ling G, Bandak A, et al. Injury biomechanics, neuropathology, and simplified physics of explosive blast and impact mild traumatic brain injury. Handbook Clin Neurol 2015;127:89–104.

52. Hetherington H, Bandak A, Ling G, et al. Advances in imaging explosive blast mild traumatic brain injury. Handb Clin Neurol 2015;127:309–18.

53. Perry DC, Sturm VE, Peterson MJ, et al. Association of traumatic brain injury with subsequent neurological and psychiatric disease: a meta-analysis. J Neurosurg 2016;124(2):511–26.

54. Gardner RC, Burke JF, Nettiksimmons J, et al. Traumatic brain injury in later life increases risk for Parkinson disease. Ann Neurol 2015;77(6):987–95.

55. Available at: https://www.gpo.gov/fdsys/pkg/PLAW-104publ166/html/PLAW-104publ166.htm. Accessed July 28, 2015.

56. Del Zoppo GJ. Toward the neurovascular unit. A journey in clinical translation: 2012 Thomas Willis Lecture. Stroke 2013;44(1):263–9.

57. Hof PR, Bouras C, Buee L, et al. Differential distribution of neurofibrillary tangles in the cerebral cortex of dementia pugilistica and Alzheimer's disease cases. Acta Neuropathol 1992;85(1):23–30.

58. Hazrati LN, Tartaglia MC, Diamandis P, et al. Absence of chronic traumatic encephalopathy in retired football players with multiple concussions and neurological symptomatology. Front Hum Neurosci 2013;7:222.

59. McCrory P, Meeuwisse WH, Kutcher JS, et al. What is the evidence for chronic concussion-related changes in retired athletes: behavioural, pathological and clinical outcomes? Br J Sports Med 2013;47(5):327–30.

60. Casson IR, Viano DC, Haacke EM, et al. Is there chronic brain damage in retired NFL players? Neuroradiology, neuropsychology, and neurology examinations of 45 retired players. Sports Health 2014;6(5):384–95.

61. Faul M, Coronado V. Epidemiology of traumatic brain injury. Handb Clin Neurol 2015;127:3–13.

62. Denst J, Sinton DW, Neuberger KT. Chronic encephalopathy following minor head injury. AMA Arch Pathol 1959;67(2):134–9.

63. Mez J, Solomon TM, Daneshvar DH, et al. Pathologically confirmed chronic traumatic encephalopathy in a 25-year-old former college football player. JAMA Neurol 2016;73(3):353–5.

64. DeKosky ST, Blennow K, Ikonomovic MD, et al. Acute and chronic traumatic encephalopathies: pathogenesis and biomarkers. Nature reviews. Neurology 2013;9(4):192–200.

65. Turner RC, Lucke-Wold BP, Logsdon AF, et al. Modeling chronic traumatic encephalopathy: the way forward for future discovery. Front Neurol 2015;6:223.

66. Neubuerger KT, Sinton DW, Denst J. Cerebral atrophy associated with boxing. AMA Arch Neurol Psychiatry 1959;81(4):403–8.

67. Mawdsley C, Ferguson FR. Neurological disease in boxers. Lancet 1963; 2(7312):795–801.

68. Payne EE. Brains of boxers. Neurochirurgia 1968;11(5):173–88.

69. Corsellis JA, Bruton CJ, Freeman-Browne D. The aftermath of boxing. Psychol Med 1973;3(3):270–303.

70. Roberts GW, Allsop D, Bruton C. The occult aftermath of boxing. J Neurol Neurosurg Psychiatry 1990;53(5):373–8.

71. McKee AC, Cantu RC, Nowinski CJ, et al. Chronic traumatic encephalopathy in athletes: progressive tauopathy after repetitive head injury. J Neuropathol Exp Neurol 2009;68(7):709–35.

72. Kovacs GG, Ferrer I, Grinberg LT, et al. Aging-related tau astrogliopathy (ARTAG): harmonized evaluation strategy. Acta Neuropathol 2016;131(1):87–102.

73. Kurland D, Hong C, Aarabi B, et al. Hemorrhagic progression of a contusion after traumatic brain injury: a review. J neurotrauma 2012;29(1):19–31.

74. Johnson VE, Stewart W, Smith DH. Widespread tau and amyloid-beta pathology many years after a single traumatic brain injury in humans. Brain Pathol 2012; 22(2):142–9.

75. Johnson VE, Stewart JE, Begbie FD, et al. Inflammation and white matter degeneration persist for years after a single traumatic brain injury. Brain 2013; 136(Pt 1):28–42.

76. Oppenheimer DR. Microscopic lesions in the brain following head injury. J Neurol Neurosurg Psychiatry 1968;31(4):299–306.

77. Ryan GA, McLean AJ, Vilenius AT, et al. Brain injury patterns in fatally injured pedestrians. J Trauma 1994;36(4):469–76.

78. Blumbergs PC, Scott G, Manavis J, et al. Staining of amyloid precursor protein to study axonal damage in mild head injury. Lancet 1994;344(8929):1055–6.

79. Sherriff FE, Bridges LR, Sivaloganathan S. Early detection of axonal injury after human head trauma using immunocytochemistry for beta-amyloid precursor protein. Acta Neuropathol 1994;87(1):55–62.

80. Bieniek KF, Ross OA, Cormier KA, et al. Chronic traumatic encephalopathy pathology in a neurodegenerative disorders brain bank. Acta Neuropathol 2015; 130(6):877–89.

81. Finkbeiner NW, Max JE, Longman S, et al. Knowing what we don't know: long-term psychiatric outcomes following adult concussion in sports. Can J Psychiatry 2016;61(5):270–6.

82. Spillane JD. Five boxers. Br Med J 1962;2(5314):1205–10.

83. Geddes JF, Vowles GH, Robinson SF, et al. Neurofibrillary tangles, but not Alzheimer-type pathology, in a young boxer. Neuropathol Appl Neurobiol 1996;22(1):12–6.

84. Geddes JF, Vowles GH, Nicoll JA, et al. Neuronal cytoskeletal changes are an early consequence of repetitive head injury. Acta Neuropathol 1999;98(2): 171–8.

85. McKee AC, Stern RA, Nowinski CJ, et al. The spectrum of disease in chronic traumatic encephalopathy. Brain 2013;136(Pt 1):43–64.

86. Reams N, Eckner JT, Almeida AA, et al. A clinical approach to the diagnosis of traumatic encephalopathy syndrome: a review. JAMA Neurol 2016;73(6):743–9.

87. Rafaels KA, Bass CR, Panzer MB, et al. Brain injury risk from primary blast. J Trauma 2012;73(4):895–901.

88. Gennarelli TA, Thibault LE, Adams JH, et al. Diffuse axonal injury and traumatic coma in the primate. Ann Neurol 1982;12(6):564–74.

89. Johnson VE, Stewart W, Smith DH. Axonal pathology in traumatic brain injury. Exp Neurol 2013;246:35–43.

90. Byrnes KR, Wilson CM, Brabazon F, et al. FDG-PET imaging in mild traumatic brain injury: a critical review. Front Neuroenergetics 2014;5:13.

91. Altmeyer W, Steven A, Gutierrez J. Use of magnetic resonance in the evaluation of cranial trauma. Magn Reson Imaging Clin N Am 2016;24(2):305–23.

92. Oehmichen M, Meissner C, Schmidt V, et al. Axonal injury–a diagnostic tool in forensic neuropathology? A review. Forensic Sci Int 1998;95(1):67–83.

93. Reichard RR, Smith C, Graham DI. The significance of beta-APP immunoreactivity in forensic practice. Neuropathol Appl Neurobiol 2005;31(3):304–13.

94. Kaur B, Rutty GN, Timperley WR. The possible role of hypoxia in the formation of axonal bulbs. J Clin Pathol 1999;52(3):203–9.

95. Selkoe DJ, Hardy J. The amyloid hypothesis of Alzheimer's disease at 25 years. EMBO Mol Med 2016;8(6):595–608.

96. Neve RL, McPhie DL, Chen Y. Alzheimer's disease: a dysfunction of the amyloid precursor protein. Brain Res 2000;886(1–2):54–66.

97. Lambri M, Djurovic V, Kibble M, et al. Specificity and sensitivity of betaAPP in head injury. Clin Neuropathol 2001;20(6):263–71.

98. Niess C, Grauel U, Toennes SW, et al. Incidence of axonal injury in human brain tissue. Acta Neuropathol 2002;104(1):79–84.

99. Lazarus C, Soheilypour M, Mofrad MR. Torsional behavior of axonal microtubule bundles. Biophys J 2015;109(2):231–9.

100. Bogoslovsky T, Wilson D, Chen Y, et al. Increases of plasma levels of glial fibrillary acidic protein, tau, and amyloid β up to 90 days after traumatic brain injury. J Neurotrauma 2017;34(1):66–73.

101. Plummer S, Van den Heuvel C, Thornton E, et al. The neuroprotective properties of the amyloid precursor protein following traumatic brain injury. Aging Dis 2016; 7(2):163–79.

102. Smith DH, Chen XH, Iwata A, et al. Amyloid beta accumulation in axons after traumatic brain injury in humans. J Neurosurg 2003;98(5):1072–7.

103. Scott G, Ramlackhansingh AF, Edison P, et al. Amyloid pathology and axonal injury after brain trauma. Neurology 2016;86(9):821–8.

104. King A, Sweeney F, Bodi I, et al. Abnormal TDP-43 expression is identified in the neocortex in cases of dementia pugilistica, but is mainly confined to the limbic system when identified in high and moderate stages of Alzheimer's disease. Neuropathology 2010;30(4):408–19.

105. McKee AC, Gavett BE, Stern RA, et al. TDP-43 proteinopathy and motor neuron disease in chronic traumatic encephalopathy. J Neuropathol Exp Neurol 2010; 69(9):918–29.

106. Johnson VE, Stewart W, Trojanowski JQ, et al. Acute and chronically increased immunoreactivity to phosphorylation-independent but not pathological TDP-43 after a single traumatic brain injury in humans. Acta Neuropathol 2011;122(6): 715–26.

107. Chio A, Calvo A, Dossena M, et al. ALS in Italian professional soccer players: the risk is still present and could be soccer-specific. Amyotroph Lateral Scler 2009; 10(4):205–9.

108. Spillantini MG, Schmidt ML, Lee VM, et al. Alpha-synuclein in Lewy bodies. Nature 1997;388(6645):839–40.

109. Lepreux S, Auriacombe S, Vital C, et al. Dementia pugilistica: a severe tribute to a career. Clin Neuropathol 2015;34(4):193–8.

110. Iacono D, Geraci-Erck M, Rabin ML, et al. Parkinson disease and incidental Lewy body disease: just a question of time? Neurology 2015;85(19):1670–9.

111. Hutson CB, Lazo CR, Mortazavi F, et al. Traumatic brain injury in adult rats causes progressive nigrostriatal dopaminergic cell loss and enhanced vulnerability to the pesticide paraquat. J neurotrauma 2011;28(9):1783–801.

112. Acosta SA, Tajiri N, de la Pena I, et al. Alpha-synuclein as a pathological link between chronic traumatic brain injury and Parkinson's disease. J Cell Physiol 2015;230(5):1024–32.

113. Mortimer JA, Snowdon DA, Markesbery WR. The effect of APOE-epsilon4 on dementia is mediated by Alzheimer neuropathology. Alzheimer Dis Assoc Disord 2009;23(2):152–7.

114. Michaelson DM. APOE epsilon4: the most prevalent yet understudied risk factor for Alzheimer's disease. Alzheimer's Dement 2014;10(6):861–8.

115. Diaz-Arrastia R, Gong Y, Fair S, et al. Increased risk of late posttraumatic seizures associated with inheritance of APOE epsilon4 allele. Arch Neurol 2003; 60(6):818–22.

116. Li L, Bao Y, He S, et al. The association between apolipoprotein e and functional outcome after traumatic brain injury: a meta-analysis. Medicine 2015;94(46): e2028.

117. Friedman G, Froom P, Sazbon L, et al. Apolipoprotein E-epsilon4 genotype predicts a poor outcome in survivors of traumatic brain injury. Neurology 1999; 52(2):244–8.

118. Chuang PY, Conley YP, Poloyac SM, et al. Neuroglobin genetic polymorphisms and their relationship to functional outcomes after traumatic brain injury. J Neurotrauma 2010;27(6):999–1006.

119. Osier ND, Bales JW, Pugh B, et al. Variation in PPP3CC genotype is associated with long-term recovery after severe brain injury. J Neurotrauma 2017;34(1): 86–96.

120. Myrga JM, Juengst SB, Failla MD, et al. COMT and ANKK1 genetics interact with depression to influence behavior following severe TBI: an initial assessment. Neurorehabil Neural Repair 2016;30(10):920–30.

121. Ritter AC, Kammerer CM, Brooks MM, et al. Genetic variation in neuronal glutamate transport genes and associations with posttraumatic seizure. Epilepsia 2016;57(6):984–93.

122. Sofroniew MV, Vinters HV. Astrocytes: biology and pathology. Acta Neuropathol 2010;119(1):7–35.

123. Bouzier-Sore AK, Pellerin L. Unraveling the complex metabolic nature of astrocytes. Front Cell Neurosci 2013;7:179.

124. Diaz-Arrastia R, Wang KK, Papa L, et al. Acute biomarkers of traumatic brain injury: relationship between plasma levels of ubiquitin C-terminal hydrolase-L1 and glial fibrillary acidic protein. J neurotrauma 2014;31(1):19–25.

125. Carron SF, Yan EB, Alwis DS, et al. Differential susceptibility of cortical and subcortical inhibitory neurons and astrocytes in the long term following diffuse traumatic brain injury. J Comp Neurol 2016;524(17):3530–60.

126. Tay TL, Savage J, Hui CW, et al. Microglia across the lifespan: from origin to function in brain development, plasticity and cognition. J Physiol 2016. [Epub ahead of print].

127. Perry VH, Nicoll JA, Holmes C. Microglia in neurodegenerative disease. Nat Rev Neurol 2010;6(4):193–201.

128. Smith C. Review: the long-term consequences of microglial activation following acute traumatic brain injury. Neuropathol Appl Neurobiol 2013;39(1):35–44.

129. Jungner M, Siemund R, Venturoli D, et al. Blood-brain barrier permeability following traumatic brain injury. Minerva Anestesiol 2015;82(5):525–33.

130. Doherty CP, O'Keefe E, Wallace E, et al. Blood-brain barrier dysfunction as a hallmark pathology in chronic traumatic encephalopathy. J Neuropathol Exp Neurol 2016;75(7):656–62.

131. Glass CK, Saijo K, Winner B, et al. Mechanisms underlying inflammation in neurodegeneration. Cell 2010;140(6):918–34.

132. Corps KN, Roth TL, McGavern DB. Inflammation and neuroprotection in traumatic brain injury. JAMA Neurol 2015;72(3):355–62.

133. Karve IP, Taylor JM, Crack PJ. The contribution of astrocytes and microglia to traumatic brain injury. Br J Pharmacol 2016;173(4):692–702.

134. Stein TD, Montenigro PH, Alvarez VE, et al. Beta-amyloid deposition in chronic traumatic encephalopathy. Acta Neuropathol 2015;130(1):21–34.

135. Costanza A, Weber K, Gandy S, et al. Review: contact sport-related chronic traumatic encephalopathy in the elderly: clinical expression and structural substrates. Neuropathol Appl Neurobiol 2011;37(6):570–84.

136. Washington PM, Villapol S, Burns MP. Polypathology and dementia after brain trauma: does brain injury trigger distinct neurodegenerative diseases, or should they be classified together as traumatic encephalopathy? Exp Neurol 2016;275 Pt 3:381–8.

137. Jellinger KA, Attems J. Challenges of multimorbidity of the aging brain: a critical update. J Neural Transm 2015;122(4):505–21.

138. Kovacs GG, Milenkovic I, Wohrer A, et al. Non-Alzheimer neurodegenerative pathologies and their combinations are more frequent than commonly believed in the elderly brain: a community-based autopsy series. Acta Neuropathol 2013; 126(3):365–84.

139. Southborough L. Report of the War Office committee of enquiry into "shell shock". London: HMSO; 1922.

140. American Psychiatric Association. Diagnostic and statistical manual of mental disorders. 5th edition. 2015. p. 271–80.

141. Jones E, Wessely S. Shell shock to PTSD. Military psychiatry from 1900 to the Gulf War. IN; Maudsley monographs 47. Hove (United Kingdom): Psychology Press; Taylor & Francis Group; 2005.

142. Mott FW. The microscopic examination of the brains of two men dead of commotio cerebri (shell shock) without visible external injury. BMJ 1917;2(2967):612–5.

143. Fulton JF. Blast and concussion in the present war. N Engl J Med 1942;226:1–8.

144. Alexander E Jr. The blasted pheasant. Br J Neurosurg 1991;5(2):183–5.

145. Shively SB, Horkayne-Szakaly I, Jones RV, et al. Characterization of interface astroglial scarring in the human brain after blast exposure: a post-mortem case series. Lancet 2016;15(9):944–53.

146. Shively SB, Perl DP. Traumatic brain injury, shell shock, and posttraumatic stress disorder in the military–past, present, and future. J Head Trauma Rehabil 2012; 27(3):234–9.

147. Peskind ER, Brody D, Cernak I, et al. Military- and sports-related mild traumatic brain injury: clinical presentation, management, and long-term consequences. J Clin Psychiatry 2013;74(2):180–8 [quiz: 188].

148. Edlow BL, Wu O. Advanced neuroimaging in traumatic brain injury. Semin Neurol 2012;32(4):374–400.

149. McNab JA, Edlow BL, Witzel T, et al. The Human Connectome Project and beyond: initial applications of 300 mT/m gradients. Neuroimage 2013;80: 234–45.

150. Pandit AS, Expert P, Lambiotte R, et al. Traumatic brain injury impairs small-world topology. Neurology 2013;80(20):1826–33.

151. Barrio JR, Small GW, Wong KP, et al. In vivo characterization of chronic traumatic encephalopathy using [F-18]FDDNP PET brain imaging. Proc Natl Acad Sci U S A 2015;112(16):E2039–47.

152. Trotter BB, Robinson ME, Milberg WP, et al. Military blast exposure, ageing and white matter integrity. Brain 2015;138(Pt 8):2278–92.

153. Riedy G, Senseney JS, Liu W, et al. Findings from structural MR imaging in military traumatic brain injury. Radiology 2016;279(1):207–15.

154. Absinta M, Nair G, Filippi M, et al. Postmortem magnetic resonance imaging to guide the pathologic cut: individualized, 3-dimensionally printed cutting boxes for fixed brains. J Neuropathol Exp Neurol 2014;73(8):780–8.

155. Sharp DJ, Ham TE. Investigating white matter injury after mild traumatic brain injury. Curr Opin Neurol 2011;24(6):558–63.

156. Mac Donald CL, Dikranian K, Bayly P, et al. Diffusion tensor imaging reliably detects experimental traumatic axonal injury and indicates approximate time of injury. J Neurosci 2007;27(44):11869–76.

157. Pierpaoli C, Jezzard P, Basser PJ, et al. Diffusion tensor MR imaging of the human brain. Radiology 1996;201(3):637–48.

158. Kondo A, Shahpasand K, Mannix R, et al. Antibody against early driver of neurodegeneration cis P-tau blocks brain injury and tauopathy. Nature 2015; 523(7561):431–6.

Unique Aspects of Traumatic Brain Injury in Military and Veteran Populations

CrossMark

Patrick Armistead-Jehle, PhD, ABPP-CN[a],*,
Jason R. Soble, PhD, ABPP-CN[b], Douglas B. Cooper, PhD, ABPP-CN[c,d],
Heather G. Belanger, PhD, ABPP-CN[e,f,g,h]

KEYWORDS

- Blast injury • Military • Veteran • Concussion • Posttraumatic stress disorder
- Polytrauma • Postconcussive syndrome

KEY POINTS

- Traumatic brain injury (TBI), in particular mild TBI, is a relatively common injury experienced by service members across both deployed and nondeployed environments.
- Several unique aspects of the military environment render the identification and treatment of service members and Veterans who experience a TBI dissimilar from their civilian counterparts.
- The Departments of Defense and Veterans Affairs have developed specific protocols and systems of care for addressing TBI-related care in deployed and nondeployed environments.
- Comorbidities are a frequent occurrence with service members and Veterans with history of TBI that represent for care and must be considered in treatment planning.

Disclosure Statement: The views, opinions, and/or findings contained in this article are those of the authors and should not be construed as an official Department of the Army, Department of Veterans Affairs, Defense and Veterans Brain Injury Center, or US Government position, policy, or decision unless so designated by other official documentation.
[a] Concussion Clinic, Munson Army Health Center, 550 Pope Avenue, Fort Leavenworth, KS 66027, USA; [b] Psychology Service, South Texas Veterans Healthcare System, 7400 Merton Minter, San Antonio, TX 78229, USA; [c] Defense and Veterans Brain Injury Center, Department of Neurology, San Antonio Military Medical Center, Joint Base San Antonio, MCHE-ZDM-N, 3551 Roger Brooke Drive, Fort Sam Houston, TX 78234-4504, USA; [d] Department of Psychiatry, University of Texas Health Science Center, 7703 Floyd Curl Drive, San Antonio, TX 78229-3900, USA; [e] HSR&D, Tampa VA TBI/Polytrauma Rehabilitation Center, Center of Innovation on Disability and Rehabilitation Research (CINDRR), James A. Haley Veterans' Hospital, 13000 Bruce B. Downs Boulevard - 116A, Tampa, FL 33612, USA; [f] Department of Mental Health and Behavioral Sciences, James A. Haley Veterans' Hospital, 13000 Bruce B Downs Boulevard (116B), Tampa, FL 33612, USA; [g] Department of Psychiatry and Behavioral Neurosciences, University of South Florida, 4202 E Fowler Avenue, Tampa, FL 33612, USA; [h] Defense and Veterans Brain Injury Center, 13000 Bruce B Downs Boulevard (116B), Tampa, FL 33612, USA
* Corresponding author.
E-mail address: Patrick.j.armistead-jehle.civ@mail.mil

Phys Med Rehabil Clin N Am 28 (2017) 323–337
http://dx.doi.org/10.1016/j.pmr.2016.12.008
1047-9651/17/Published by Elsevier Inc.

pmr.theclinics.com

INTRODUCTION/EPIDEMIOLOGY OF TRAUMATIC BRAIN INJURY IN THE MILITARY

Prompted by the protracted nature of the conflicts in Afghanistan and Iraq and by enemy combatants' frequent use of explosive devices, traumatic brain injuries (TBI) have become the focus of notable clinical and research attention in the military and Veteran health care environments. Although many of the medical principles and treatment protocols used in the civilian sector to evaluate and treat TBI are applicable to care in the military, there are several unique factors specific to this injury in military and Veteran populations. These factors, which include sustainment of injuries within combat zones, distinct mechanisms of TBI, psychiatric comorbidities, and influences of the military culture on health care utilization, are the focus of this review.

According to the Defense and Veterans Brain Injury Center, between 2000 and the first quarter of 2016, there have been approximately 348,000 active duty military service members (SMs) who have experienced a TBI.[1] These injuries increased from 10,958 in 2000 to a peak of 32,907 in 2011. The annual number of SMs diagnosed with a TBI then steadily declined to 22,594 in 2015. The vast majority of these injuries (82%) have been categorized as mild in severity, and as such, mild traumatic brain injury (mTBI) is the primary focus of this review.[1] As SMs separate from active duty status, their treatment transitions to the Veterans Health Administration (VHA), which also tracks epidemiologic data. In fiscal year 2014, 7% of Iraq and Afghanistan War Veterans seen in the VHA system carried a diagnosis of TBI.[2] According to Taylor and colleagues,[2] in 2014 the average cost of health care services in those with a diagnosis of TBI (mean = $15,161 [SD = $33,460]) was consistently higher than those without such a diagnosis (mean = $5058 [SD = $12,368]); this difference represents a moderate effect size (Cohen's d = .40). Moreover, in 2014, 6% of Veterans were service connected for TBIs.[2]

Despite the attention given to injuries sustained in the combat theater, most recorded concussions occur in garrison (nondeployed) environments.[1] Outside of deployment to a combat zone, SMs routinely engage in operational and training activities that are physically demanding and can increase the risk for TBIs. Furthermore, as most SMs are men between 18 and 24 years of age, there is a higher demographic risk for concussion via events like motor vehicle crashes and sporting and recreational activities. Consequently, even with the relatively recent reduction of SMs deployed in support of direct combat operations, TBI will continue to be a condition of interest in the military and Veteran populations. Several factors reviewed in later discussion are unique to the military and Veteran populations and should be considered in evaluating and treating TBI within these populations.

MILITARY CULTURE

Over the past 25 years, there has been a growing appreciation that individual factors, such as one's cultural identification, can influence medical treatment, development of a therapeutic alliance, and health care outcomes. Although cultural competence in modern health care has frequently focused on the influence of various ethnic and religious backgrounds, individuals who have served in the US military identify with a military culture that has its own set of unique values, traditions, language, and customs.[3] Military values such as selfless service, mission focus, and decreased focus on personal needs over the good of the group are entrenched through military service and training. High levels of acculturation often remain following the end of a military career, as can be exemplified by the clothing and hats worn by Veterans in the community. Although some military personnel and Veterans receive their care in the Military Healthcare System and Veterans Healthcare System, nearly 66% of Veterans access their health care entirely in civilian settings.[4] Accordingly, health care providers treating individuals with TBI need to have an understanding of and sensitivity to military culture to optimize health care outcomes.

For clinicians working with SMs and Veterans with TBI, military cultural competence is important in optimizing communication and developing skills to promote a strong therapeutic alliance and provide effective clinical care. Core values of military service that may serve as motivation and inspiration during the course of rehabilitation include (1) personal courage, (2) not accepting failure, (3) self-sacrificing, and (4) a commitment to the mission. The physical and psychological strength required to accomplish a mission can be recruited to persevere through challenges and reach treatment goals. Group-based treatment within a rehabilitation milieu can be adapted to align with military values of teamwork and comradery. Inclusion of family members, where applicable, can enhance compliance in Veterans and SMs.

In addition to fostering those military values that may enhance rehabilitation treatment, it is important to be sensitive to cultural issues that can represent a barrier to treatment or compliance with treatment recommendations. As discussed in other sections of this article, psychological comorbidities occur at a higher rate in those with deployment-related TBI than in the civilian population.[5–7] In addition, there remains a stigma attached to behavioral health treatment for many individuals who served in the military, related to a perceived negative impact on one's military career, self-sacrifice as a core military value, and the belief that accessing mental health care may indicate failure. For those who served in battle, exposure to life-threatening danger and death may alter life perspectives and expectations. Wounds may be not only physical or mental, but also moral, from participating in or witnessing traumatic events. Particularly in the context of moral injuries, clinicians need to be sensitive to the role of spirituality as it relates to resilience, healing, and recovery from the patient's perspective. Fostering resilience through social supports, such as family and spirituality, as well as integration of behavioral health treatment into TBI care can help enhance this process and protect the individual from feeling alienated or becoming noncompliant with treatment recommendations.

In a recent RAND report on capacity to provide culturally competent care to military personnel and their families, cultural competence was operationalized through 3 general areas: (1) familiarity and awareness of military and Veteran culture; (2) comfort level in working with military/Veterans and their families; and (3) skills/training in serving this population.[8] General principles to enhance cultural competence in one's practice should include asking about military experience (including family members) when taking a clinical history, clarifying unfamiliar acronyms or military language, and considering military cultural factors when developing treatment plans and recommendations.[9] Although there is a growing movement to integrate formal training about military culture into medical school curricula on a more systematic basis,[10] many tools/training resources are currently available to enhance military/Veteran cultural competence in serving individuals with TBI and their families. For example, Ross and colleagues[11] provide a listing of specific resources reproduced in **Table 1**.

IDENTIFYING AND TREATING CONCUSSION IN THE WAR ZONE

The theater of combat provides unique challenges to the identification and treatment of concussion that are distinct from injuries sustained in civilian settings. Historically, SMs in a combat zone have been unlikely to come forward with or be recognized for injuries that are not easily visible. That is, for injuries involving external indications of damage (eg, compound fractures, external bleeding, inability to breathe, extended

Table 1
Suggested topics for Veteran-centered curriculum for Veterans Affairs and civilian-based trainees

Topic	Instruction Focus	Teaching Methods	Teaching Resources (Ref.)
VHA utilization	Share patterns of Veteran usage of VHA health care facilities	Focus didactics/lecture Self-paced learning	68 69
Military cultural competence/ consciousness	Provide trainees with an overview of the structure of the US military and military conflicts, and demographic background of US Veterans, as well as military socialization processes, traditions, values, and behavioral norms	Focus didactics/lecture Self-paced learning	70 71 72
Military health history	Demonstrate how to obtain a focused military history, elicit service-related health concerns, and assess life stressors	Vignettes/trigger tapes Medical encounter videos	73 74 75
Health care disparities	Identify causes of health disparities for US Veterans, highlighting the social determinants of health and the ways in which social location creates challenges in optimal health care	Problem-based learning cases Individual care-based discussion	76
Empathetic communication	Instruct trainees to provide care that is concordant with the patient's values and preferences that promotes active participation in decision making regarding their health and health care	Faculty role models/ mentors Medical encounter video	77 78
Common diagnoses in Veterans	Summarize conditions particularly prevalent in Veterans (eg, PTSD, TBI, anxiety, depression) and instruct trainees on how to identify these conditions within this population	Individual case-based discussion Workshops Problem-based learning cases	79 80 81 82

loss of consciousness), the need for medical care is accepted. However, for injuries that are not readily evidenced by external signs, many SMs will seek to avoid medical care in an effort to continue mission engagements with their units. mTBI is such an injury whereby the pursuit of subsequent medical care has been limited, particularly within the first several years of the conflicts in Iraq and Afghanistan. Beyond the point of injury, when SMs return from deployment, there are mandated postdeployment screening measures that include evaluation for concussion-related symptoms. However, once injuries are reported, medically related appointments can be scheduled and delay the SM's postdeployment leave and family reunification. Consequently, injuries and symptoms may be minimized at this time, which could conceivably forestall treatment and potentially complicate care. As the effects of mTBI on the war fighter have become better understood, policy has been instituted to more effectively identify and manage these injuries. Clinical and educational efforts have been aimed at improving early identification of mTBI as well as standardizing guidelines for return to duty.

In regards to clinical care in the deployed environment, a concussion management algorithm was established by the Department of Defense (DoD).[12] This policy, instituted in 2012 and in effect through 2022, mandates use of the most recent DoD clinical practice guidelines and management algorithms in the deployed environment. At present, this states that SMs involved in a potentially concussive event are required to have at least 24 hours of rest and symptom resolution before returning to duty. If an SM experiences 2 concussions in a 12-month period, he or she is mandated an additional 7 days of rest following symptom resolution. With 3 diagnosed concussions within the past 12 months, a recurrent concussion evaluation is to be engaged. This comprehensive evaluation includes neurologic, neuropsychological, and functional assessments, with appropriate neuroimaging as indicated. In addition, all concussion evaluations require the administration of the Military Acute Concussion Evaluation (MACE).[13,14] This mTBI screening and mental status evaluation have standardized the examination of acute and subacute concussion care across DoD medical providers and paraprofessionals. Next, since 2007, the DoD has mandated that each deploying SM complete baseline neurocognitive testing within 12 months of scheduled deployment. The Automated Neuropsychological Assessment Metrics (ANAM) was chosen as the neurocognitive assessment tool for the vast majority of SMs across the DoD. This measure can also be administered postinjury in theater, so that providers can use comparison scores to assist in return to duty decisions. These policies and related clinical tools have positively impacted TBI-related care in the combat theater. In Afghanistan, regional Concussion Care Centers (CCCs) staffed by specialty providers with expertise in concussion and rehabilitation were established so that SMs could obtain necessary services in theater. The CCCs allowed for 7 to 10 days of structured return to duty programs that reduce the need to medically evacuate SMs from the war zone.[15] Of note, given the high incidence of concussion in nondeployed environments, the Army mandated nearly identical management algorithms for Soldiers experiencing an mTBI in garrison.[16]

In regards to education, the DoD has implemented mandatory training sessions for all personnel that address the nature of mTBI, the mandated requirements for care, and the likely short-term impacts on unit readiness. The overarching message of such training is that SMs who experience an mTBI are expected to return to duty in a relatively short period of time; however, management of symptoms in the acute and subacute phases of recovery are essential to ensure optimal outcomes. Training is also required for all credentialed health care providers regardless of specialty, including primary care providers (PCP), medics, and non-PCPs. Given that most acute or subacute mTBIs can be successfully managed in primary care, the most intense of these trainings is for the PCP. Of note, as most of mTBIs occur in nondeployed settings, concussion-related training is mandated not only for those SMs that deploy but also for all civilian and active duty providers in garrison.

Mechanism of Injury

Mechanism of injury, and more specifically, high rates of blast-related injuries, further differentiates military TBI from TBI in the civilian sector. Briefly, blast-related injuries can be primary (ie, injury due to rapid atmospheric pressure changes), secondary (ie, impact injury resulting from propelled debris), tertiary (ie, injury from being thrown by the blast), or quaternary (eg, burns, toxic exposure following the blast).[17] Moreover, the frequent occurrence of blast exposure in combat has resulted in a significant population of military personnel who sustained injuries to multiple body regions and/or systems (eg, amputations, visual damage, burns) in addition to TBI, which is classified as a "polytrauma injury" within the DoD and VHA systems of care (discussed later). Despite the complex medical and mental health comorbidities often associated with blast-related polytrauma, to date, studies have generally revealed few differences between blast- and non-blast-related TBIs for postconcussion symptom endorsement, neuropsychological test performance, or psychological symptoms, suggesting that the mechanism of injury may not be as critical as the actual TBI with regard to these functional outcomes.[18–21]

VETERANS HEALTH ADMINISTRATION AND DEPARTMENT OF DEFENSE SYSTEMS OF CARE FOR IDENTIFICATION AND TREATMENT OF TRAUMATIC BRAIN INJURY AFTER DEPLOYMENT
Traumatic Brain Injury Screening

Because of the increase in polytrauma injuries and concomitant increase in TBI seen in returning active duty personnel, the VHA and DoD developed a comprehensive and integrated system of care to treat TBI, particularly those with associated physical and emotional comorbidities. Because mTBI is so common in those injured, and because it is not always an obvious or visible injury, a system was needed to identify these patients and triage them accordingly. The DoD instituted Post-Deployment Health Assessment (PDHA) and Reassessment (PDHRA) programs. The PDHA is scheduled with trained health care providers within 30 days from deployment return. The purpose is to review each service member's current health, mental health, psychosocial issues commonly associated with deployments, possible deployment-related occupational and environmental exposures (including TBI), and to discuss deployment-related health concerns. Positive responses require supplemental assessment and/or referrals for medical consultation. Similarly, the PDHRA, which is completed within 3 to 6 months after return from deployment, is designed to identify and address health concerns, with specific emphasis on mental health, that have emerged over time since deployment.

Similarly, VHA implemented a series of Operation Enduring Freedom/Operation Iraqi Freedom/Operation New Dawn clinical reminders (ie, mandated clinical questions to ask the Veteran, prompted by the electronic medical record), including a TBI clinical reminder protocol. Clinical reminders are completed by any provider within the VHA system of care who first encounters that patient following deployment. In addition to first asking about deployment location, the TBI screen asks the Veteran whether they have already been diagnosed with TBI related to deployment. Those who confirm deployment and report no prior TBI diagnosis are asked additional questions about: (1) injury event, (2) immediate loss or alteration of consciousness,

(3) immediate/acute postconcussive symptoms, and (4) current (past week) postconcussive symptoms. A positive response to all 4 sections constitutes a positive screen. The screen is to be repeated if a Veteran is redeployed. Positive screens automatically generate a consult to a TBI specialist or specialty clinic if the Veteran agrees to further assessment or care. This mandated follow-up evaluation, called the Comprehensive TBI Evaluation, consists of further evaluation of blast exposures and TBI events, targeted review of systems, and a physical examination. The purposes of the follow-up evaluation are to (1) confirm the diagnosis of TBI, even if the present symptoms are thought to be secondary to other factors such as posttraumatic stress disorder (PTSD), stress, depression, or chronic pain; and (2) institute an appropriate plan for follow-up care (eg, other evaluations or diagnosis-based or symptom-based treatment). A VA/DoD evidence-based mild TBI treatment guideline was developed (http://www.healthquality.va.gov/management_of_concussion_mtbi.asp) to help the clinician develop a plan of care and treat the symptom complex identified through the comprehensive evaluation. So, for instance, if concentration problems are endorsed, a review of sleep hygiene is one of many recommended assessments, along with possible treatments.

Traumatic Brain Injury Rehabilitation

Stateside, the rehabilitation process for those returning from combat theater begins at acute medical settings, such as Military Treatment Facilities with the initiation of individual physical, occupational, and speech therapy. Collaboration via video teleconferences has allowed earlier physiatric input into the care of these complex patients and helped to coordinate a smooth transition from acute care facilities to rehabilitation units.

In response to the complexity inherent in those returning from war for rehabilitation, VHA set up a Polytrauma System of Care housed at its existing TBI Centers. This entire system of care is described in detail elsewhere.[22,23] Briefly, the Polytrauma System of Care has the 4 following components:

1. Polytrauma Rehabilitation Centers (located in Tampa, FL; Minneapolis, MN; Palo Alto, CA; Richmond, VA; San Antonio, TX) provide acute medical and rehabilitation care, research, and education related to polytrauma/TBI within the context of accreditation by the Commission on Accreditation of Rehabilitation Facilities for both acute TBI and Comprehensive Rehabilitation.
2. Polytrauma Network Sites (located within each of VHA's regional Veterans Integrated Service Networks) provide postacute rehabilitation care for individuals with polytrauma/TBI, including inpatient and outpatient rehabilitation and vocational rehabilitation programs. They are responsible for coordinating access to services to meet the needs of patients recovering from polytrauma.
3. Polytrauma Support Clinic Teams are geographically distributed across VHA to facilitate access to specialized rehabilitation services close to the Veterans' and active duty SM's home communities. These interdisciplinary teams of rehabilitation specialists are responsible for managing the care of patients by providing treatment plans, regular follow-up, and any care needs as they arise.
4. Polytrauma Points of Contact in remaining facilities are responsible for managing consultations for patients with polytrauma and referring these patients to appropriate programs.

Disability Process

Patients who participate in rehabilitation frequently are involved in disability proceedings. When SMs develop a medical condition that may render them unable to continue their military service, they are entered into the Integrated Disability Evaluation System (IDES), which combines the DoD Disability Process with the Veterans Affairs (VA) Disability Process.[24] The first half of the IDES is known as the Medical Evaluation board (MEB) process. Eventually, a VA disability claim is filed and a Compensation and Pension evaluation is scheduled. The purpose of these processes is to ascertain the history and severity of the SM's medical conditions and their impact on his/her ability to perform job duties. As noted above, disability for mTBI is not uncommon with an estimated 6% of Veterans carrying a service connection for mTBI. Of note, within the context of mTBI, validity of data obtained in various evaluations must be considered. For example, in cognitive testing of mTBI patients in Veteran settings, questionable validity is obtained in 29% to 59%[25–28] of cases. In active duty patients, the rate varies from 38%[29] to 59%,[30] depending on which performance validity measure is used and whether the sample exclusively consisted of those involved in an MEB. In military samples with a history of mild TBI, performance validity test results account for the most variance in cognitive test scores, above demographic, concussion history, symptom validity, and psychological distress variables.[25,31] Although much of the research on validity testing uses professional or paraprofessional administered instruments specific to cognition, a few self-report measures designed to assess respondent validity and possible overreporting have been developed. The mild Traumatic Brain Injury Atypical Symptoms scale[32] and Validity-10 of the Neurobehavioral Symptom Inventory (NSI)[33] can be administered across a variety of medical disciplines, to include primary care and physiatry. Although these measures are not as sensitive to invalid test performance and symptom exaggeration as traditional neuropsychological measures of performance and symptom validity, they can serve to alert the evaluating provider of gross levels symptom exaggeration.[34–37]

PSYCHIATRIC COMORBIDITIES IN MILITARY AND VETERANS HEALTH ADMINISTRATION SAMPLES WITH TRAUMATIC BRAIN INJURY

Another unique aspect of TBI in the military population is the high occurrence of psychiatric comorbidity. Among Operation Enduring Freedom/Operation Iraqi Freedom/Operation New Dawn Veterans, prevalence rates of 23% for PTSD,[38] 17% to 21% for depression,[39,40] and 7% to 15% for alcohol-related problems and disorders have been reported[39,41] with multiple psychiatric diagnoses being common.[42] For instance, 24% of Veterans receiving VHA care in 2008 to 2010 had a mental health issue and comorbid substance abuse.[41] Among Veterans with TBI, 89% had a comorbid psychiatric diagnosis, most commonly with PTSD with rates of 44% to 54%[5,6,43] Seventy percent also had pain diagnoses, which along with persisting postconcussive symptoms and PTSD constitute the Polytrauma Clinical Triad.[5,44] The high psychiatric comorbidity among military personnel presents several clinical challenges related to accurate diagnosis and treatment of TBI. First, TBI is a historical diagnosis, one often dependent on self-report. Diagnosis is further complicated among military personnel because exposure to psychologically traumatic events is common in active combat zones and can have strikingly similar sequelae. For instance, traumatic events (eg, surprise improvised explosive device attack) can result in acute nervous system activation, anxiety, and alterations in attention and awareness, which can closely resemble TBI-related confusion and disorientation despite the absence of actual insult to the brain.[45] This diagnostic complexity is further complicated by the fact that clinicians are often tasked with rendering a TBI diagnosis based on retrospective, self-reported symptoms long after an event, frequently without additional corroborating information.[46]

Second, many of the core emotional, behavioral, and cognitive symptoms associated with these psychiatric comorbidities overlap considerably with TBI symptoms, especially mTBI and postconcussion symptoms.[21] Accordingly, many of the Postconcussive Syndrome diagnostic criteria, such as sleep disturbance, cognitive difficulties, and mood/behavior changes (eg, irritability), are nonspecific and mirror symptoms included in the formal diagnostic criteria for PTSD and Major Depressive Disorder.[47,48] In fact, prior studies found that postconcussion symptoms were more strongly correlated with measures of PTSD and depression than TBI, and Veterans with psychiatric disorders more frequently met diagnostic criteria for Postconcussive Syndrome compared with those with mTBI.[49–51] The issue of psychiatric co-morbidities is perhaps best illustrated in **Fig. 1**, which shows that National Guard members with PTSD, but no history of TBI, endorsed substantially greater symptoms across all 4 subscales of the NSI,[52] a self-report measure of postconcussion symptoms, compared with those with a history of mTBI, but no psychiatric disturbance as well as nondeployed and deployed nonclinical controls.[50] Thus, it is critical to maintain awareness of the role that psychiatric comorbidities have in maintaining persisting postconcussion symptoms, especially because many of these disorders are amenable to evidenced-based mental health intervention.

Effective treatment of these psychiatric comorbidities also poses a distinctive challenge for clinicians working with military personnel due to a combination of historically low levels of TBI education in the military, high rates of TBI misinformation among Veterans and behavioral health professionals, a greater reluctance to attribute difficulties to a mental health problem as opposed to a physical one (ie, TBI), and stigma/negative beliefs about mental health treatment as barriers to care.[45,53–56] The myriad of obstacles impacting veteran's engagement in treatment is particularly problematic given prior meta-analytic findings have consistently indicated that individuals with mTBI generally recover quickly from acute neuropsychological sequelae, although residual impairment often remains for moderate-severe TBI.[57–59] Furthermore, persisting

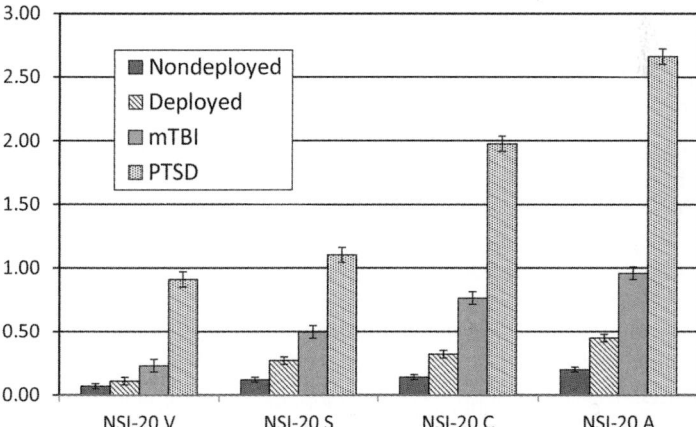

Fig. 1. Mean NSI subscale scores for nondeployed nonclinical group (n = 1453), deployed nonclinical group (n = 1064), deployed mTBI group (n = 108), and deployed PTSD group (n = 52). A, affective subscale; C, cognitive subscale; S, somatic subscale; V, vestibular subscale. NSI-20 subscale averages are reported due to differences in number of items per subscale. (*From* Soble JR, Silva MA, Vanderploeg RD, et al. Normative data for the Neurobehavioral Symptom Inventory (NSI) and post-concussion symptom profiles among TBI, PTSD, and nonclinical samples. Clin Neuropsychol 2014;28:614–32; with permission.)

symptoms often are more related to psychiatric conditions and emotional distress, especially PTSD, rather than mTBI.[42,60,61] Nevertheless, despite the evidence implicating psychiatric disturbances in maintaining postconcussive symptoms, stigma and negative beliefs associated with mental health conditions often result in greater non/underutilization of mental health care and premature treatment dropout among Veterans and military SMs, such that a subsection of this population does not receive adequate mental health services.[40,54,62] For example, a recent study found that among a cohort of soldiers diagnosed with PTSD following combat deployment, 22% had only one mental health visit and 24% dropped out of treatment.[63]

For those that do pursue mental health treatment, findings have shown that Veterans with mTBI are able to tolerate evidence-based Cognitive Processing Therapy (CPT) for PTSD.[64] Furthermore, prolonged exposure therapy for PTSD has been found to be effective among those with TBI, with some studies documenting treatment effectiveness across varying levels of TBI severity.[64–66] In addition to traditional PTSD treatments, several novel, integrative mental health interventions for those with comorbid PTSD and TBI, including mindfulness-based stress reduction and a hybrid program that integrates standard CPT with compensatory cognitive rehabilitation training, have been recently proposed to address both PTSD symptoms and cognitive difficulties often found in this population, although future randomized clinical trials are needed to further assess their effectiveness.[63,67]

SUMMARY/FUTURE DIRECTIONS

As reviewed above, several factors specific to the military and Veteran environments differentiate identification and care of TBI from the civilian sector. Since the inception of the conflicts in Afghanistan and Iraq, the DoD and VHA have initiated various policies and systems of care to address the specific needs of these populations. Future work will likely need to focus on the potential long-term consequences of repeated mTBIs via impact and blast injuries, in terms of both neuropathology and any related functional deficits. Furthermore, efforts to more quickly identify and care for acute and subacute mTBI may expedite return to duty in active duty SMs. Finally, future research to efficiently identify and treat comorbidities of mTBI will likely be of benefit to SMs and Veterans.

REFERENCES

1. Defense and Veterans Brain Injury Center. DoD Worldwide Numbers for TBI. Available at: http://dvbic.dcoe.mil/dod-worldwide-numbers-tbi. Accessed July 5, 2016.
2. Taylor BC, Campbell E, Nugent S, et al. Fiscal Year 2014 VA Utilization Report for Iraq and Afghanistan War Veterans Diagnosed with TBI. Prepared for the VA Polytrauma and Blast-Related Injuries QUERI #PLY 05-2010-2. November 2015. Available at: http://www.polytrauma.va.gov/TBIReports/FY14-TBI-Diagnosis-HCU-Report.pdf. Accessed June 7, 2016.
3. Meyer EG. The importance of understanding military culture. Acad Psychiatry 2015;39:416–8.
4. The Healthcare System for Veterans: An Interim Report. Congressional budget office. 2007. Available at: https://www.cbo.gov/sites/default/files/110th-congress-2007-2008/reports/12-21-va_healthcare.pdf. Accessed June 6, 2016.
5. Cifu DX, Taylor BC, Carne WF, et al. Traumatic brain injury, posttraumatic stress disorder, and pain diagnoses in OIF/OEF/OND veterans. J Rehabil Res Dev 2013;50:1169–76.

6. Taylor BC, Hagel EM, Carlson KF, et al. Prevalence and costs of co-occurring traumatic brain injury with and without psychiatric disturbance and pain among Afghanistan and Iraq War Veteran V.A. users. Med Care 2012;50:342–6.

7. Cooper DB, Kennedy JE, Cullen MA, et al. Association between combat stress and post-concussive symptom reporting in OEF/OIF service members with mild traumatic brain injuries. Brain Inj 2011;25:1–7.

8. Tanielian T, Farris C, Batka C, et al. Ready to serve: community-based provider capacity to deliver culturally competent, quality mental health care to veterans and their families. Santa Monica (CA): RAND Corporation; 2014. Available at: http://www.rand.org/pubs/research_reports/RR806.html. Accessed June 7, 2016.

9. Meyer EG, Writer BW, Brim W. The importance of military cultural competence. Curr Psychiatry Rep 2016;18:26–32.

10. Gleeson TD, Hemmer PA. Providing care to military personnel and their families: how we can all contribute. Acad Med 2014;89:1201–3.

11. Ross PT, Ravindranath D, Clay M, et al. A greater mission: understanding military culture as a tool for serving those who have served. J Grad Med Educ 2015;7: 519–22.

12. Department of Defense Instruction 6490.11. Available at: http://www.usaisr. amedd.army.mil/cpgs/DODI_6490.11_Policy_Guidance_for_Mgmt_of_Mild_Trau matic_Brain_Injury_or_Concussion_in_the_Deployed_Setting.pdf. Accessed June 7, 2016.

13. French L, McCrea M, Baggett M. The military acute concussion evaluation. (MACE). J Spec Oper Med 2008;8:68–77.

14. Defense and Veterans Brain Injury Center. The Military Acute Concussion Evaluation. Available at: http://dvbic.dcoe.mil/research/military-acute-concussion-evaluation-mace. Accessed June 7th, 2016.

15. Helmick KM, Spells CA, Malik SZ, et al. Traumatic brain injury in the US military: epidemiology and key clinical and research programs. Brain Imaging Behav 2015;9:358–66.

16. HQDA Executive Order 165-13: Department of the Army Guidance for Management of Concussion/Mild Traumatic Brain Injury in the Garrison Setting.

17. Depalma RG, Burris DG, Champion HR, et al. Blast injuries. N Engl J Med 2005; 352:1335–42.

18. Belanger HG, Proctor-Weber Z, Kretzmer T, et al. Symptom complaints following reports of blast versus non-blast mild TBI: does mechanism of injury matter? Clin Neuropsychol 2011;25:702–15.

19. Lange RT, Pancholi S, Brickell TA, et al. Neuropsychological outcome from blast versus non-blast: mild traumatic brain injury in U.S. military service members. J Int Neuropsychol Soc 2012;18:595–605.

20. Macdonald CL, Johnson AM, Nelson EC, et al. Functional status after blast-plus-impact complex concussive traumatic brain injury in evacuated United States military personnel. J Neurotrauma 2014;31:889–98.

21. Cooper DB, Chau P, Armistead-Jehle P, et al. Relationship between mechanism of injury and neurocognitive functioning in OEF/OIF Service Members with mild traumatic brain injuries. Mil Med 2012;177:1157–60.

22. Belanger HG, Uomoto JM, Vanderploeg RD. The Veterans Health Administration's (VHA's) Polytrauma System of Care for mild traumatic brain injury: costs, benefits, and controversies. J Head Trauma Rehabil 2009;24:4–13.

23. Sigford BJ. "To care for him who shall have borne the battle and for his widow and his orphan" (Abraham Lincoln): the Department of Veterans Affairs polytrauma system of care. Arch Phys Med Rehabil 2008;89:160–2.

24. Department of Defense Manual Number 1332.18, Volume 2, August 2014. Available at: http://warriorcare.dodlive.mil/files/2016/03/DoDM_1332.18_Vol2.pdf. Accessed June 21, 2016.

25. Cooper DB, Vanderploeg RD, Armistead-Jehle P, et al. Factors associated with neurocognitive performance in OIF/OEF service members with postconcussive complaints in postdeployment clinical settings. J Rehabil Res Dev 2014;51: 1023–34.

26. Reslan S, Axelrod BN. Evaluating the Medical Symptom Validity Test (MSVT) in a sample of veterans between the ages of 18 to 64. Appl Neuropsychol Adult 2017; 24:132–9. Available at: http://dx.doi.org/10.1080/23279095.2015.1107565. Accessed June 7, 2016.

27. Armistead-Jehle P. Symptom validity test performance in U.S. veterans referred for evaluation of mild TBI. Appl Neuropsychol 2010;17:52–9.

28. Nelson NW, Hoelzle JB, McGuire KA, et al. Evaluation context impacts neuropsychological performance of OEF/OIF veterans with reported combat-related concussion. Arch Clin Neuropsychol 2010;25:713–23.

29. Armistead-Jehle P, Buican B. Comparison of select Advanced Clinical Solutions embedded Effort measures to the Word Memory Test in the detection of suboptimal effort. Arch Clin Neuropsychol 2013;28:297–301.

30. Grills CE, Armistead-Jehle PJ. Performance validity test and neuropsychological assessment battery screening module performances in an active-duty sample with a history of concussion. Appl Neuropsychol Adult 2016;23:295–301.

31. Armistead-Jehle P, Cooper DB, Vanderploeg RD. The role of performance validity tests in the assessment of cognitive functioning after military concussion: a replication and extension. Appl Neuropsychol Adult 2015;23:264–73.

32. Cooper DB, Nelson L, Armistead-Jehle P, et al. Utility of the mild brain injury atypical symptoms scale as a screening measure for symptom over-reporting in Operation Enduring Freedom/Operation Iraqi Freedom service members with postconcussive symptoms. Arch Clin Neuropsychol 2011;26:718–27.

33. Vanderploeg RD, Cooper DB, Belanger HG, et al. Screening for postdeployment conditions: development and cross-validation of an embedded validity scale in the neurobehavioral symptom inventory. J Head Trauma Rehabil 2014;29:1–10.

34. Lange RT, Brickell TA, Lippa SM, et al. Clinical utility of the Neurobehavioral Symptom Inventory validity scales for symptom exaggeration following traumatic brain injury. J Clin Exp Neuropsychol 2015;37:853–62.

35. Lange RT, Brickell TA, French LM. Examination of the Mild Brain Injury Atypical Symptom Scale and the Validity-10 Scale to detect symptom exaggeration in US military service members. J Clin Exp Neuropsychol 2015;37:325–37.

36. Lange RT, Edmed SL, Sullivan KA, et al. Utility of the Mild Brain Injury Atypical Symptoms Scale to detect symptom exaggeration: an analogue simulation study. J Clin Exp Neuropsychol 2013;35:192–209.

37. Sullivan KA, Lange RT, Edmed SL. Utility of the neurobehavioral symptom inventory validity-10 index to detect symptom exaggeration: an analogue simulation study. Appl Neuropsychol Adult 2016;23(5):353–62.

38. Fulton JJ, Calhoun PS, Wagner HR, et al. The prevalence of posttraumatic stress disorder in Operation Enduring Freedom/Operation Iraqi Freedom (OEF/OIF) Veterans: a meta-analysis. J Anxiety Disord 2015;31:98–107.

39. Seal KH, Metzler TJ, Gima KS, et al. Trends and risk factors for mental health diagnoses among Iraq and Afghanistan veterans using Department of Veterans Affairs health care, 2002-2008. Am J Public Health 2009;99:1651–8.

40. Vaughan CA, Schell TL, Tanielian T, et al. Prevalence of mental health problems among Iraq and Afghanistan veterans who have and have not received VA services. Psychiatr Serv 2014;65:833–5.

41. Jacobson IG, Ryan MA, Hooper TI, et al. Alcohol use and alcohol-related problems before and after military combat deployment. JAMA 2008;300:663–75.

42. Seal KH, Bertenthal D, Miner CR, et al. Bringing the war back home: mental health disorders among 103,788 US veterans returning from Iraq and Afghanistan seen at Department of Veterans Affairs facilities. Arch Intern Med 2007;167:476–82.

43. Hoge CW, Mcgurk D, Thomas JL, et al. Mild traumatic brain injury in U.S. Soldiers returning from Iraq. N Engl J Med 2008;358:453–63.

44. Pugh MJ, Finley EP, Copeland LA, et al. Complex comorbidity clusters in OEF/OIF veterans: the polytrauma clinical triad and beyond. Med Care 2014;52:172–81.

45. Lew HL, Otis JD, Tun C, et al. Prevalence of chronic pain, posttraumatic stress disorder, and persistent postconcussive symptoms in OIF/OEF veterans: polytrauma clinical triad. J Rehabil Res Dev 2009;46:697–702.

46. Brenner LA, Vanderploeg RD, Terrio H. Assessment and diagnosis of mild traumatic brain injury, posttraumatic stress disorder, and other polytrauma conditions: burden of adversity hypothesis. Rehabil Psychol 2009;54:239–46.

47. Word Health Organization. The ICD-10 classification of mental and behavioural disorders, clinical descriptions and diagnostic guidelines. Geneva: World Health Organization; 1992.

48. American Psychiatric Association. Diagnostic and statistical manual of mental disorders. 5th edition. Washington, DC: American Psychiatric Association; 2013.

49. Lippa SM, Pastorek NJ, Benge JF, et al. Postconcussive symptoms after blast and nonblast-related mild traumatic brain injuries in Afghanistan and Iraq war veterans. J Int Neuropsychol Soc 2010;16:856–66.

50. Soble JR, Silva MA, Vanderploeg RD, et al. Normative data for the Neurobehavioral Symptom Inventory (NSI) and post-concussion symptom profiles among TBI, PTSD, and nonclinical samples. Clin Neuropsychol 2014;28:614–32.

51. Donnell AJ, Kim MS, Silva MA, et al. Incidence of postconcussion symptoms in psychiatric diagnostic groups, mild traumatic brain injury, and comorbid conditions. Clin Neuropsychol 2012;26:1092–101.

52. King PR, Donnelly KT, Donnelly JP, et al. Psychometric study of the neurobehavioral symptom inventory. J Rehabil Res Dev 2012;49:879–88.

53. Block C, Fabrizio K, Bagley B, et al. Assessment of veteran and caregiver knowledge about mild traumatic brain injury in a VA medical center. J Head Trauma Rehabil 2014;29:76–88.

54. Bradford LS. Misconceptions about traumatic brain injury among U.S. Army behavioral health professionals. Rehabil Psychol 2015;60:344–52.

55. Pietrzak RH, Johnson DC, Goldstein MB, et al. Perceived stigma and barriers to mental health care utilization among OEF-OIF veterans. Psychiatr Serv 2009;60:1118–22.

56. Hoge CW, Castro CA, Messer SC, et al. Combat duty in Iraq and Afghanistan, mental health problems and barriers to care. N Engl J Med 2004;351:13–22.

57. Schretlen DJ, Shapiro AM. A quantitative review of the effects of traumatic brain injury on cognitive functioning. Int Rev Psychiatry 2003;15:341–9.

58. Belanger HG, Vanderploeg RD. The neuropsychological impact of sports-related concussion: a meta-analysis. J Int Neuropsychol Soc 2005;11:345–57.

59. Rohling ML, Binder LM, Demakis GJ, et al. A meta-analysis of neuropsychological outcome after mild traumatic brain injury: re-analyses and reconsiderations of

Binder, et al. (1997), Frencham et al. (2005), and Pertab et al. (2009). Clin Neuropsychol 2011;25:608–23.

60. Meares S, Shores EA, Taylor AJ, et al. The prospective course of postconcussion syndrome: the role of mild traumatic brain injury. Neuropsychology 2011;25: 454–65.

61. Belanger HG, Kretzmer T, Vanderploeg RD, et al. Symptom complaints following combat-related traumatic brain injury: relationship to traumatic brain injury severity and posttraumatic stress disorder. J Int Neuropsychol Soc 2010;16:194–9.

62. Hoge CW, Grossman SH, Auchterlonie JL, et al. PTSD treatment for soldiers after combat deployment: low utilization of mental health care and reasons for dropout. Psychiatr Serv 2014;65:997–1004.

63. Davis JJ, Walter KH, Chard KM, et al. Treatment adherence in cognitive processing therapy for combat-related PTSD with history of mild TBI. Rehabil Psychol 2013;58:36–42.

64. Wolf GK, Kretzmer T, Crawford E, et al. Prolonged exposure therapy with veterans and active duty personnel diagnosed with PTSD and traumatic brain injury. J Trauma Stress 2015;28:339–47.

65. Sripada RK, Rauch SA, Tuerk PW, et al. Mild traumatic brain injury and treatment response in prolonged exposure for PTSD. J Trauma Stress 2013;26:369–75.

66. Cole MA, Muir JJ, Gans JJ, et al. Simultaneous treatment of neurocognitive and psychiatric symptoms in veterans with post-traumatic stress disorder and history of mild traumatic brain injury: a pilot study of mindfulness-based stress reduction. Mil Med 2015;180:956–63.

67. Jak AJ, Aupperle R, Rodgers CS, et al. Evaluation of a hybrid treatment for Veterans with comorbid traumatic brain injury and posttraumatic stress disorder: study protocol for a randomized controlled trial. Contemp Clin Trials 2015; 45(Pt B):210–6.

68. US Department of Veterans Affairs. VA Health. Care Utilization by Recent Veterans. Available at: http://www.publichealth.va.gov/epidemiology/reports/oefoifond/health-care-utilization. Accessed January 30, 2017.

69. US Department of Veterans Affairs. National Center for Veterans Analysis and Statistics. Available at: http://www.va.gov/vetdata/index.asp. Accessed January 30, 2017.

70. Goldenberg MN, Hamaoka D, Santiago P, et al. Basic training: a primer on military life and culture for health care providers and trainees. MedEdPORTAL. 2012. Available at: https://www.mededportal.org/icollaborative/resource/192. Accessed January 30, 2017.

71. Reger MA, Etherage JR, Reger GM, et al. Civilian psychologists in the Army culture: the ethnical challenge of cultural competence. Mil Psychol 2008;20:21–35.

72. Center for Deployment Psychology. Learn About Military Culture Course. Available at: http://deploymentpsych.org/military-culture. Accessed January 30, 2017.

73. Association of American Medical Colleges.Taking a military health history: four critical questions. 2013. Available at: https://www.aamc.org/advocacy/campaigns_and_coalitions/360908/takingamilitaryhealthhistory.html. Accessed January 30, 2017.

74. Brown JL. A piece of my mind: the unasked question. JAMA 2012;308(18): 1869–70.

75. Pankow SH, Dill MJ, Navarro AM, et al. Health care provider awareness of the military status of patients: asking the question. Analysis in Brief. Association of American Medical Colleges. 2013;13(5). Available at: https://www.aamc.org/download/

358546/data/oct2013analysisinbrief-awarenessofmilitarystatusofpatients.pdf. Accessed January 30, 2017.

76. National Ethics Committee of the Veterans. Health Administration. An ethical analysis of ethnic disparities in health care. National Center for Ethics, Veterans Health Administration, Department of Veterans Affairs. 2001. Available at: www.ethics.va.gov/docs/net/net_topic_20021218_ethnic_disparities_in_health_care.doc. Accessed January 30, 2017.

77. Lypson ML, Page A, Bernat CK, et al. Patient-doctor communication: the fundamental skill of medical practice. iCollaborative. 2012. Available at: https://www.mededportal.org/icollaborative/resource/595. Accessed January 30, 2017.

78. Bellet PS, Maloney MJ. The importance of empathy as an interviewing skill in medicine. JAMA 1991;266(13):1831–2.

79. Lypson ML, Ravindranath D, Ross PT. Developing skills in veteran-centered care: understanding where soldiers really come from. MedEdPORTAL. 2014. Available at: http://www.mededportal.org/publication/9818. Accessed January 30, 2017.

80. PTSD: National Center for PTSD. Available at: http://www.ptsd.va.gov/index.asp. Accessed January 30, 2017.

81. Krakower J, Navarro AM, Prescott JE. Training for the treatment of PTSD and TBI in US medical schools. In: Analysis in Brief. Association of American Medical Colleges. 2012;12(5). Available at: https://www.aamc.org/download/313126/data/november2012anaysisinbrief-trainingforthetreatmentofptsdandtbii.pdf. Accessed January 30, 2017.

82. Spelman JF, Hunt SC, Seal KH, et al. Post deployment care for returning combat veterans. J Gen Intern Med 2012;27(9):1200–9.

Neuropsychological Evaluation in Traumatic Brain Injury

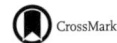 CrossMark

Jason R. Soble, PhD, ABPP*, Edan A. Critchfield, PsyD, ABPP,
Justin J.F. O'Rourke, PhD, ABPP

KEYWORDS

- Neuropsychology • Assessment • Cognition • Brain-behavior relationships
- Psychometrics • Outcome • Rehabilitation

KEY POINTS

- Neuropsychology is a subspecialty of professional psychology that involves the scientific study and clinical application of brain-behavior relationships.
- Neuropsychological evaluation integrates objective psychometric tests with other clinical data to comprehensively characterize the cognitive, behavioral, and emotional effects secondary to traumatic brain injury (TBI).
- Neuropsychological evaluation can help delineate normal individual differences from the neurologic effects of injury. Neuropsychological testing is also useful for identifying if psychological conditions (eg, depression) or other non-neurologic factors are affecting symptom presentation.
- Neuropsychological evaluation can further contribute to evidence-based TBI patient care through serial assessment of cognitive and functional status over time, informing TBI rehabilitation, and evaluating the effectiveness of interventions.

AN OVERVIEW OF NEUROPSYCHOLOGY

Neuropsychology involves the scientific study and clinical application of brain-behavior relationships.[1] It is a specialty of professional psychology that "applies principles of assessment and intervention based upon the scientific study of human behavior as it relates to normal and abnormal functioning of the central nervous system."[2] A clinical neuropsychologist has advanced doctoral education as well as

Disclosure Statement: The views, opinions, and/or findings expressed herein are those of the authors and do not necessarily reflect the views or the official policy of the Department of Veterans Affairs or US Government.
Psychology Service (116B), South Texas Veterans Healthcare System, 7400 Merton Minter, San Antonio, TX 78229, USA
* Corresponding author.
E-mail address: jason.soble@va.gov

Phys Med Rehabil Clin N Am 28 (2017) 339–350
http://dx.doi.org/10.1016/j.pmr.2016.12.009
1047-9651/17/Published by Elsevier Inc.

internship and specialty postdoctoral residency/fellowship training in the foundations of brain-behavior relationships (eg, functional neuroanatomy, neurologic disease, and psychopharmacology) in addition to clinical (eg, psychopathology and personality assessment) and general (eg, learning, development, and statistics and psychometrics) psychology.[3] Specialty board certification in clinical neuropsychology is also available.

Professionally, clinical neuropsychologists engage in evaluation/assessment, intervention, consultation, and research related to the cognitive, behavioral, and emotional manifestation(s) of known or suspected brain dysfunction with an extensive array of clinical populations, such as TBI and other acquired brain injury (eg, anoxia and stroke), neurodegenerative/dementing and neurologic conditions (eg, Alzheimer disease, Parkinson disease, multiple sclerosis, and epilepsy), learning disorders, neurodevelopmental conditions, and psychiatric disorders.[2] Among the varied professional activities performed by clinical neuropsychologists, evaluation through the use of objective, psychometric tests is most predominant and serves as the main focus of this review, with emphasis on its relevance to moderate to severe TBI.

CLINICAL UTILITY OF NEUROPSYCHOLOGICAL EVALUATION

Although modern neuroimaging techniques have greatly reduced the historical role of the neuropsychologist in localizing lesions of the central nervous system based on psychometric testing, neuropsychological evaluation continues to meaningfully contribute to patient care by elucidating the functional sequelae secondary to central nervous system pathology/dysfunction. From a clinical and patient care standpoint, this is particularly valuable given that similar structural neuroanatomic lesions can have striking diverse cognitive and behavioral symptom presentations among individual patients.[4,5] Consequently, there are 6 broad clinical questions that commonly generate a referral for a neuropsychological evaluation[5]:

Referral Question	Examples
1. Differential diagnosis	Are the patient's reported cognitive difficulties due to TBI or is some other condition, such as a psychiatric disorder, sleep disturbance, chronic pain, or substance misuse, or are other non-neurologic factors contributing?
2. Characterization of cognitive, behavioral, and emotional abilities/limitations	What cognitive and behavioral deficits does a patient with a moderate TBI have? How may these affect daily functioning?
	How have a patient's cognitive deficits resulting from a penetrating TBI and subsequent posttraumatic epilepsy changed over the past year since initial evaluation?
	Is a treatable psychiatric condition that can have an adverse impact on engagement in TBI rehabilitation (eg, depression) present?
3. Treatment planning	What specific cognitive impairments should be targeted for rehabilitation for a patient with a subarachnoid hemorrhage?
	What behavioral interventions would be effective for a patient with disinhibited and hypersexual behavior after TBI?
	What academic accommodations does a patient with a TBI and residual cognitive deficits need if he/she wishes to pursue college coursework?

(continued on next page)

(continued)	
Referral Question	**Examples**
4. Treatment evaluation	Has there been an improvement in mental status and cognition after surgical evacuation of a subdural hematoma? Has the patient's attention improved after initiation of medication X? Has a cognitive remediation protocol resulted in an improvement in the patient's memory?
5. Research	Is a newly developed test able to accurately predict cognitive and functional outcomes after TBI? Has an investigational medication resulted in objective improvements in cognition among patients with TBI?
6. Forensic	Does this person have cognitive deficits from a TBI sustained during a workplace injury that prevents him/her from holding employment?

DECONSTRUCTING THE NEUROPSYCHOLOGICAL EVALUATION

The interpretation of neuropsychological test results is central to the role of clinical neuropsychologists and their unique expertise in the neuroanatomic correlates of cognition, neurologic disease processes, statistical analysis, and measurement. A vast majority of non-neuropsychologists, however, understandably view test selection and interpretation as the most enigmatic aspect of the neuropsychological evaluation. The seemingly endless test descriptions, standard scores, and percentiles in reports can seem overwhelming and unintelligible to other health care providers. The forthcoming sections attempt to explain approaches to neuropsychological test interpretation and highlight the importance of evidence-based neuropsychological measurement principles to avoid underpathologizing or overpathologizing patients.

It is also essential for consumers of neuropsychological services to understand that test scores represent only 1 component of an evaluation. Additional data sources might include a patient's medical record (eg, history and physical, neuroimaging findings, and active medications), behavioral observations both during testing and in the clinical milieu, a neurobehavioral examination, assessment of psychological symptoms, including personality idiosyncrasies and/or personality disorders, and often most importantly, an interview with collateral sources. As such, although other clinical disciplines may have familiarity with individual aspects of functioning (cognition, mental health, and so forth), a unique contribution of neuropsychological evaluation is that it integrates the totality of this information to establish a comprehensive conceptualization of a patient's cognitive, emotional, and behavioral functioning after TBI.

Test Selection

Counterintuitively, the first step of neuropsychological test interpretation begins before any tests are administered, with the selection of appropriate measures. Proper test selection depends on several variables, including consistency over time (ie, reliability), susceptibility to measurement error, association with theoretically similar/dissimilar tests (ie, validity), and lesion analysis research demonstrating tests' relationships with neural structures and systems. Several other factors that affect baseline expectations for neuropsychological test performance need to be considered, including age, level and type of education, occupational achievement, primary language, ethnicity, reading level, and physical disability.[6] A patient's expected level of cognitive impairment also needs to be anticipated to avoid ceiling or floor effects in the selected tests. Failing to consider any of these factors compromises the accuracy of neuropsychological test interpretation before an evaluation begins.

Once psychometrically sound measures are selected, neuropsychologists often take 1 of 2 approaches to neuropsychological evaluation: the fixed battery approach or the flexible battery approach.[7] The fixed battery approach involves administration of the same tests to every patient in a standardized manner. Examples of fixed batteries are the Halstead-Reitan Neuropsychological Battery[8] and the Meyers Neuropsychological Battery.[9] This approach allows for the comprehensive and systematic assessment of multiple cognitive domains, which allows neuropsychologists to make direct comparisons between patients' performance over time to assess decline or monitor recovery. Disadvantages of the fixed batteries include their length (ie, up to 8 hours of testing) that can lead to higher health care costs and poor patient tolerance for such a long session. Additionally, fixed battery assessments may include the administration of superfluous measures that are not be required to answer the referral question.

In response to the limitations of the fixed-battery approach, most neuropsychologists use a hypothesis-driven or flexible battery approach toward test selection. Flexible batteries are tailored to the needs of individual patients based on the referral question, medical history, and information gathered during the clinical interview. A brief set of probing tests is initially administered, and additional in-depth tests of more specific abilities are completed if a patient exhibits deficits on any initial measures. A popular flexible approach to testing is the Iowa-Benton method,[10] which requires that clinicians administer a core battery that is followed-up with tests that assess suspected impairments in more detail.

Test Validity Versus Assessment Validity

Whether or not a fixed or flexible battery approach is used, neuropsychological evaluations are only useful if a patient's personal performance and symptom report are an accurate reflection of cognitive abilities. Outright malingering, adoption of the sick role, somatization, chronic pain, and a litany of other secondary influences on cognitive functioning often can lead to artificially low test scores that may result in misdiagnosis and treatments that harm the patient. A complete neuropsychological evaluation includes objective measures of assessment validity, which Larrabee[11] succinctly defines as the ability to determine if an individual patient is producing valid test results during the evaluation. Assessment validity differs from test validity, which is related to the psychometric properties of individual neuropsychological tests (eg, construct and criterion validity) regardless of patient performance.

Assessment validity can refer to either symptom validity or performance validity.[12] Symptom validity refers to patients' self-reported symptoms and complaints. Symptom validity tests are often found in personality inventories and other questionnaires that require patients to describe their subjective experience of physical, cognitive, and emotional problems. Examinees' reported symptoms are compared with the reports of various patient groups to determine if their responses are consistent with known conditions. In contrast to symptom validity tests, performance validity tests (PVTs) identify whether or not a patient's objective cognitive test results are a valid reflection of neuropsychological functioning. Stand-alone tests dedicated to assessing performance validity, measures embedded with genuine tests of ability, and atypical patterns of results are all used to establish performance validity. Multiple PVTs throughout the battery are necessary to minimize false-positive errors and avoid labeling genuine impairment as noncredible. Furthermore, it is recommended that each PVT have a specificity of at least 90%.[13] Sensitivity and specificity are often established through known-groups studies, which compare PVT results of a genuine patient group with that of healthy individuals instructed to feign symptoms of the genuine patient group.

A substantial amount of research on PVTs has been conducted in patients with brain injury, in particular mild TBI (mTBI) (ie, concussions), simulators, and patients with moderate to severe TBI. Using various statistical methodologies, such as chained likelihood ratios,[13–15] this research has consistently established that if a patient with a history of mTBI in the context of substantial external incentive (eg, military benefits, litigation, and criminal prosecution) fails 2, 3, or more PVTs during an evaluation, then the false-positive rate is practically zero and it can be safely concluded that non-neurologic factors (eg, feigning) are artificially lowering scores. If malingering is suspected, criteria for malingered neurocognitive dysfunction[16] have been established to meaningfully integrate results from validity measures, clinical history and context (benefits, prosecution, and so forth), and testing behavior to provide a rationale for discerning whether a patient is purposefully underperforming. These criteria are particularly helpful in cases of mTBI where persistent cognitive impairments are not expected.[17]

Neuropsychological Domains and Tests

The table below outlines the domains often assessed in an evaluation as well as some common tests that may be encountered in an evaluation report. Before proceeding, however, 3 important caveats are in order. First, this list is by no means inclusive. Readers are referred to other authoritative references for a complete compendium of neuropsychological tests[5,18] as well as the Center for Outcome Measurement in Brain Injury for additional TBI-specific measures.[19] Second, the specific domains assessed/tests administered in any single evaluation vary based on the referral question and clinical presentation. For example, it is unlikely that full academic achievement testing is indicated in a 75-year-old patient with a subdural hematoma secondary to a fall. Likewise, assessment of a patient with acute posttraumatic amnesia (PTA) and agitation may initially involve bedside serial monitoring with orientation and behavioral measures followed by comprehensive evaluation after resolution of PTA. Third, although each test is listed under the domain it is primarily intended to measure, it is essential to understand that few tests are pure measures of a specific cognitive ability. For instance, a patient with severe visuospatial impairments may perform poorly on a confrontation naming test due to difficulty with accurately perceiving test stimuli rather than a frank language deficit.

Domain of Functioning	Neuropsychological Tests
Serial monitoring after acute TBI	JFK Coma Recovery Scale-Revised Orientation Log Galveston Orientation and Amnesia Test Agitated Behavior Scale
General cognitive functioning and full neuropsychological batteries	Wechsler Adult Intelligence Scale–Fourth Edition Halstead-Reitan Neuropsychological Test Battery Repeatable Battery for the Assessment of Neuropsychological Status Neuropsychological Assessment Battery

(continued on next page)

(continued)	
Domain of Functioning	**Neuropsychological Tests**
Academic achievement	Woodcock-Johnson Tests of Achievement–Fourth Edition Wide-Range Achievement Test 4
Sensory-motor functions	Grooved Pegboard Test Finger Tapping Test
Language	Multilingual Aphasia Examination Boston Diagnostic Aphasia Examination Boston Naming Test Verbal Fluency Tests
Visuospatial/constructional	Judgment of Line Orientation Hooper Visual Organization Test Clock Drawing Test
Learning and memory	Rey Auditory Verbal Learning Test Rey Complex Figure Test California Verbal Learning Test–Second Edition Wechsler Memory Scale–Fourth Edition
Attention	Ruff 2 and 7 Selective Attention Test Trail Making Test Paced Serial Addition Test Continuous performance tests Symbol Digit Modalities Test
Executive functions	Wisconsin Card Sorting Test Delis-Kaplan Executive Function System Booklet Category Test Stroop Test
Functional abilities	Independent Living Scales Texas Functional Living Scale
Emotional functioning/personality	Minnesota Multiphasic Personality Inventory-2 Personality Assessment Inventory Beck Depression Inventory–Second Edition

Test Interpretation

Assuming that the evaluation is valid, the neuropsychologist can proceed with clinical interpretation of the test scores. A test score does not indicate the presence or absence of cognitive impairment. Rather, a patient's overall performance across a test battery is what indicates the presence or absence of impairment. One cannot simply look at the total score on a screening measure such as the Montreal Cognitive Assessment (MoCA) or Mini Mental Status Exam (MMSE) and confidently assume that the entirety of a patient's cognitive functioning has been captured. No neuropsychological measure captures an isolated aspect of cognitive functioning, because each test depends on patients' simultaneous use of multiple cognitive abilities. For instance, measures of declarative verbal memory (eg, word list memory tasks) are used to objectively measure learning, encoding, storage, and retrieval; however, performance on these tasks is also dependent on attention, processing speed, and executive functioning and the neural correlates of those abilities. Therefore, an impaired score on a verbal memory task does not necessarily indicate amnesia but could be a reflection of a problem in other cognitive functions. It is the neuropsychologist's task to determine which cognitive deficits are causing impaired performances by looking for a pattern of deficits across the overall the battery and by comparing the neuropsychological profile with known patterns of disease.

Test interpretation also involves normative comparisons to both population and individual data. For instance, stating that a patient recalled 7 words (raw score) after a delay on a verbal memory task has, in and of itself, limited clinical value because this score may be within normal limits for a 65-year-old patient but abnormal for a 45-year-old. Given that certain demographic variables (eg, age and education) have been consistently found to account for significant variance across a majority of tests, comparing raw test performance to relevant demographically corrected normative benchmarks allows a neuropsychologist to more accurately determine the degree to which an individual patient's score deviates from normality for a selected population.[1,5,8,18,20] Interpretation is further contingent on individual comparison of a patient's scores to his or her own premorbid abilities. For example, language scores at the 16th percentile may be within normal limits for a patient with 9 years of education but may reflect a significant decline in functioning for one with a college degree (ie, 16 years of education). Although premorbid neuropsychological data are ideal for determining individual premorbid ability, such information is rarely available; as such, methods for estimating an individual's premorbid baseline, such as performance on tasks that are more resistant to brain dysfunction (eg, word reading tasks), have been developed.[1,5] Finally, quantitative test scores are integrated with qualitative information related to a patient's observable test-taking behavior (eg, how a patient approaches tests, types of errors, and behavioral abnormalities, such as perseveration, stimulus-boundedness, and so forth) to provide essential context and enhance the utility of the test scores.[5]

Given the nuances of interpretation, evidence-based neuropsychological evaluation attempts to improve the accuracy of cognitive test interpretation by accounting for the complexities of human cognition and normal intraindividual differences that can have a substantial impact on cognitive presentation. Much as neuroradiologists want to minimize motion artifacts to obtain a clear picture of the brain's structural integrity, evidence-based neuropsychological evaluation attempts to minimize statistical artifacts and patients' normal idiosyncrasies to obtain a clear picture of neurocognitive functioning. To do this, neuropsychologists use well-defined neuropsychological outcomes, account for base rates of low scores, and use a combination of inferential statistics and bayesian analyses (eg, sensitivity, specificity, positive and negative predictive values, and likelihood ratios) that minimize measurement error and diagnostic misclassification.[21] For example, base rate studies indicate that a certain number of low test scores is common among the general population. Healthy people of average intelligence are expected to have 30% of their test scores fall below the 16th percentile (1 SD), 15% below the 10th percentile, and 10% below the 5th percentile.[22] Without a working knowledge of normal test performances, there is a risk of overdiagnosing patients. Other extracognitive factors that need to be considered include the number of tests administered, statistical distribution of scores (ie, normal vs skewed distributions), demographic characteristics of the patient, the choice of cut scores chosen to indicate impairment, and secondary factors, such as pain or mood problems.[23]

NEUROPSYCHOLOGICAL EVALUATION AND TRAUMATIC BRAIN INJURY OUTCOMES

During the acute period after a moderate to severe TBI, there is often a great deal of uncertainty regarding the extent of cognitive and physical recovery and long-term functional outcome. Much of this uncertainty is due to variability in the recovery course that takes place primarily in the first year after TBI.[24] Although accurate prognostication during the acute period is not always straightforward, having a general awareness of likely outcomes is often helpful for families to plan for supervision needs and changes in family roles and to remain hopeful for recovery. Even when the outlook is bleak, having an accurate idea of what to expect allows the grieving process to begin and adjustments to be made. Among interdisciplinary teams, neuropsychologists' expertise in the neuroanatomic correlates of cognition and behavior, neuroimaging, and skills of a clinical psychologist often make them apt medical liaisons for communicating with patients and their family members regarding prognostic predictions.

There are several factors to consider when evaluating prognosis post–moderate to severe TBI. Research has consistently indicated that during the acute period, the most reliable prognostic indicators are the length of loss of consciousness, duration of PTA, the highest Glasgow Coma Scale score during the first 24 hours, and lesion size and location on neuroimaging.[25–27] Concurrently, the use of postacute neuropsychological evaluations has also proved useful in adding to prognostic models of functional outcome. Specifically, global neuropsychological functioning and performance within specific domains, such as working memory, memory, and cognitive flexibility, have been useful in predicting long-term productivity, level of supervision, and employment.[28–30] Aside from cognitive functioning, most neuropsychological evaluations also assess comorbid psychopathology, which has been found to predict vocational outcomes and overall quality of life.[31,32]

MEASURING CHANGE OVER TIME

During the acute period after moderate to severe TBI, patients are at an increased risk for secondary injury due to hydrocephalus, hypoxia, edema, and/or hemorrhage. Having a neuropsychological baseline level of attention and processing speed can help to objectively assess for a decline in cognitive functioning, which would warrant escalation to a higher level of care for neuroimaging and possibly surgical intervention.[33,34]

Acutely, serial cognitive assessment is also used to assess orientation and memory to determine emergence from PTA. Generally, a patient who has obtained a score of greater than or equal to 76 on the Galveston Orientation and Amnesia Test or greater than or equal to 25 on the Orientation Log across 2 consecutive days is considered to have emerged from PTA. Thus, the neuropsychologist may initially contribute to acute TBI care by evaluating orientation and situational awareness over time to monitor for resolution of PTA. Once a patient has emerged from PTA, then a more thorough neuropsychological evaluation and cognitive rehabilitation can be implemented.[35,36]

Finally, neuropsychological evaluation can be used to objectively measure cognitive recovery and provide a guide for updating rehabilitative interventions and limits to functional independence. This might include specific evaluations to assess decision-making capacity, driving evaluations, or supervision needs. There also may be a comprehensive follow-up neuropsychological evaluation completed 1 year post-injury because this milestone generally marks the period where the majority of natural recovery has occurred and rehabilitation often shifts to a more compensatory nature.[37] It is critical that any repeat evaluations take into account a patient's familiarity with testing procedures/items and can account for true cognitive changes versus change in scores that might be due to practice effects or measurement error.[38]

USE OF NEUROPSYCHOLOGICAL EVALUATION TO INFORM INTERVENTIONS

One of the most basic yet critical interventions after TBI is providing patients and their families with accurate education. This is true for both mTBI (ie, concussion)[39] and moderate to severe TBI.[40] Important educational topics to cover include the recovery course after TBI as well as factors that promote a positive recovery, such as sleep, exercise, and avoiding secondary injury. It is also critical for family members to be educated on the topic of managing problematic behavior that might appear after TBI (irritability, disinhibition, perseveration, and so forth). Finally, and possibly most importantly, the neuropsychologist can provide the patient and family with a comprehensive understanding of the specific injury. Often patients and their families remark that there are numerous evaluations and tests completed during the acute period with little to no feedback provided. It is also understandable that if results were provided during the acute stages that the recipients were not at a cognitive or emotional point where they could appreciate the information. As a result, neuropsychologists are often used to meet with patients and family members to review the outcome and implications of acute events, evaluations, or reports from neuroimaging.[40]

NEUROPSYCHOLOGICAL EVALUATION IN REHABILITATION

Given the substantial variability in cognitive profiles after TBI, once a patient has cleared PTA, a comprehensive neuropsychological evaluation is critical to determine the approach to cognitive rehabilitation, including a determination of the type and severity of cognitive impairments to address in rehabilitation and the identification of cognitive strengths, which can be used to offset areas of cognitive weakness. Neuropsychological evaluation can also be used to identify the cause of functional cognitive deficits and ensure that the correct cognitive deficit is addressed. For example, patients might present with memory complaints; however, their memory itself might be intact but seem impaired due to upstream deficits in attention or verbal comprehension.[41]

Once a patient's neuropsychological profile of strengths and weaknesses has been established, specific cognitive rehabilitation interventions can be initiated. Although there is often much overlap, cognitive rehabilitation interventions typically can be categorized as restorative, compensatory, or metacognitive. In theory, restorative interventions are used during the acute phase of rehabilitation by means of drills and specific cognitive exercises, which are meant to stimulate brain plasticity.[42] Compensatory cognitive strategies have been described as the utilization of either internal or external strategies to complete functional tasks. With internal compensatory strategies, patients might rely on preserved strengths to offset weaknesses. For example, a patient might rely on visual memory rather than verbal memory to recall instructions. In contrast, a patient's use of external compensatory strategies focuses on environmental manipulation or external devices to offset cognitive weaknesses. This might include the use of a notebook or calendar to remember upcoming appointments. Finally, metacognitive rehabilitation strategies focus on patients' awareness of their cognitive strengths and weaknesses and their implication for daily functioning. Ideally, the goal of metacognitive rehabilitation is to have a patient able to recognize the need either to use cognitive compensatory strategies in the moment or to anticipate the use of strategies at a future setting.[43,44]

SUMMARY

In sum, neuropsychological evaluation is a valuable clinical tool that involves integration of psychometric test data along with other pertinent clinical information to objectively (and flexibly) assess the range of cognitive, behavioral, and emotional sequelae that may emerge after TBI. Neuropsychology can further contribute to TBI patient care through delineation of normal individual differences from the neurologic effects of injury, determining the effect that psychological factors may have on symptom presentation, and serial assessment after acute TBI to monitor for resolution of PTA. Data derived from a neuropsychological evaluation can also be used to identify individual patient strengths, inform cognitive and behavioral rehabilitation targets, and objectively evaluate the effectiveness of TBI-related interventions.

REFERENCES

1. Schoenberg MR, Scott JG. The little black book of neuropsychology: a syndrome-based approach. New York: Springer; 2011.
2. American Psychological Association. Clinical neuropsychology. Available at: http://www.apa.org/ed/graduate/specialize/neuro.aspx. Accessed May 15, 2016.
3. Hannay J, Bieliauskas L, Crosson B, et al. Proceedings of the Houston Conference on Specialty Education and Training in Clinical Neuropsychology. Arch Clin Neuropsychol 1998;13:157–250.
4. Heilman KM, Valenstein E. Clinical neuropsychology. New York: Oxford University Press; 2003.
5. Lezak MD, Howieson DB, Bigler ED, et al. Neuropsychological assessment. 5th edition. New York: Oxford University Press; 2012.
6. Smith GE, Ivnik RJ, Lucas J. Assessment techniques: tests, test batteries, norms, and methodological approaches. In: Morgan JE, Ricker JH, editors. Textbook of clinical neuropsychology. New York: Taylor & Francis; 2008. p. 38–57.
7. Barr WB. Historical development of the neuropsychological test battery. In: Morgan JE, Ricker JH, editors. Textbook of clinical neuropsychology. New York: Taylor & Francis; 2008. p. 3–17.
8. Heaton RK, Miller SW, Taylor MJ, et al. Revised comprehensive norms for an expanded halstead-reitan battery: demographically adjusted neuropsychological norms for African American and caucasian adults. Odessa (FL): Psychological Assessment Resources; 2004.
9. Bush SS. Meyers neuropsychological battery. In: Kreutzer JS, Deluca J, Caplan B, editors. Encyclopedia of clinical neuropsychology. New York: Springer; 2011. p. 1589–90.
10. Tranel D. Theories of clinical neuropsychology and brain-behavior relationships. In: Morgan JE, Ricker JH, editors. Textbook of clinical neuropsychology. New York: Taylor & Francis; 2008. p. 25–37.
11. Larrabee GJ. The multiple validities of neuropsychological assessment. Am Psychol 2015;70(8):779–88.
12. Larrabee GJ. Performance validity and symptom validity in neuropsychological assessment. J Int Neuropsychol Soc 2012;18(4):625–30.
13. Boone KB, Lu P. Noncredible cognitive performance in the context of severe brain injury. Clin Neuropsychol 2003;17(2):244–54.
14. Grimes DA, Schulz KF. Refining clinical diagnosis with likelihood ratios. Lancet 2005;365(9469):1500–5.
15. Larrabee GJ. Aggregation across multiple indicators improves the detection of malingering: relationship to likelihood ratios. Clin Neuropsychol 2008;22(4):666–79.
16. Slick DJ, Sherman EM, Iverson GL. Diagnostic criteria for malingered neurocognitive dysfunction: proposed standards for clinical practice and research. Clin Neuropsychol 1999;13(4):545–61.

17. McCrea M. Mild traumatic brain injury and postconcussion syndrome: the new evidence base for diagnosis and treatment. New York: Oxford University Press; 2008.
18. Strauss E, Sherman EM, Spreen O. A compendium of neuropsychological tests, administration, norms, and commentary. 3rd edition. New York: Oxford University Process; 2006.
19. The Center for Outcome Measurement in Brain Injury. COMBI: Featured Scales. Available at: http://www.tbims.org/combi/list.html. Accessed June 9, 2016.
20. Mitrushina M, Boone KB, Razani J, et al. Handbook of normative data for neuropsychological assessment. 2nd edition. New York: Oxford University Process; 2005.
21. Chelune GJ. Evidence-based research and practice in clinical neuropsychology. Clin Neuropsychol 2010;24(3):454–67.
22. Iverson GL, Brooks BL, Holdnack JA. Evidence-based neuropsychological assessment following work-related injury. In: Bush SS, Iverson GL, editors. Neuropsychological assessment of work-related injuries. New York: Guildford; 2012. p. 360–400.
23. Iverson GL, Brooks BL. Improving accuracy for identifying cognitive impairment. In: Schoenberg MR, Scott JG, editors. Little black book of neuropsychology: a syndrome based approach. New York: Springer; 2011. p. 923–50.
24. Sandhaug M, Andelic N, Bernsten SA, et al. Functional level during the first year after moderate and severe traumatic brain injury: Course and predictors of outcome. J Neurol Res 2011;1(2):48–58.
25. Lingsma HF, Roozenbeek B, Steyerberg EW, et al. Early prognosis in traumatic brain injury: from prophecies to predictions. Lancet Neurol 2010;9(5):543–54.
26. Dikmen SS, Corrigan JD, Levin HS, et al. Cognitive outcome following traumatic brain injury. J Head Trauma Rehabil 2009;24(6):430–8.
27. Maas AI, Steyerberg EW, Butcher I, et al. Prognostic value of computerized tomography scan characteristics in traumatic brain injury: results from the IMPACT study. J Neurotrauma 2007;24(2):303–14.
28. Dikmen SS, Machamer JE, Winn HR, et al. Neuropsychological outcome at 1-year post head injury. Neuropsychology 1995;9(1):80–90.
29. Spitz G, Ponsford JL, Rudzki D, et al. Association between cognitive performance and functional outcome following traumatic brain injury: a longitudinal multilevel examination. Neuropsychology 2012;26(5):604–12.
30. Hanks RA, Millis SR, Ricker JH, et al. The predictive validity of a brief inpatient neuropsychologic battery for persons with traumatic brain injury. Arch Phys Med Rehabil 2008;89(5):950–7.
31. Van der horn HJ, Spikman JM, Jacobs B, et al. Postconcussive complaints, anxiety, and depression related to vocational outcome in minor to severe traumatic brain injury. Arch Phys Med Rehabil 2013;94(5):867–74.
32. Bombardier CH, Fann J, Temkin NR, et al. Rates of major depressive disorder and clinical outcomes following traumatic brain injury. JAMA 2010;303(19):1938–45.
33. Vanneste JA. Diagnosis and management of normal-pressure hydrocephalus. J Neurol 2000;247(1):5–14.
34. Hellstrom P, Edsbagge M, Archer T, et al. The neuropsychology of patients with clinically diagnosed idiopathic normal pressure hydrocephalus. Neurosurgery 2007;61:1219–26.
35. Levin HS, O'donnell VM, Grossman RG. The Galveston Orientation and Amnesia Test. A practical scale to assess cognition after head injury. J Nerv Ment Dis 1979; 167(11):675–84.

36. Frey KL, Rojas DC, Anderson CA, et al. Comparison of the O-Log and GOAT as measures of posttraumatic amnesia. Brain Inj 2007;21(5):513–20.
37. Sherer M, Novack TA, Sander AM, et al. Neuropsychological assessment and employment outcome after traumatic brain injury: a review. Clin Neuropsychol 2002;16(2):157–78.
38. Maassen GH, Bossema E, Brand N. Reliable change and practice effects: outcomes of various indices compared. J Clin Exp Neuropsychol 2009;31(3): 339–52.
39. Mittenberg W, Canyock EM, Condit D, et al. Treatment of post-concussion syndrome following mild head injury. J Clin Exp Neuropsychol 2001;23(6):829–36.
40. Mateer CA, Sira C. Practical rehabilitation strategies in the context of clinical neuropsychological feedback. In: Morgan JE, Ricker JH, editors. Textbook of clinical neuropsychology. New York: Taylor & Francis; 2008. p. 996–1007.
41. Eapen BC, Allred DB, O'rourke J, et al. Rehabilitation of moderate-to-severe traumatic brain injury. Semin Neurol 2015;35(1):e1–3.
42. Sohlberg MM, Turkstra LS. Optimizing cognitive rehabilitation: effective instructional methods. New York: Guilford; 2011.
43. Cicerone KD, Langenbahn DM, Braden C, et al. Evidence-based cognitive rehabilitation: updated review of the literature from 2003 through 2008. Arch Phys Med Rehabil 2011;92(4):519–30.
44. Prigatano GP. Principles of neuropsychological rehabilitation. New York: Oxford University Press; 1999.

Educational and Vocational Issues in Traumatic Brain Injury

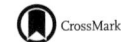

Paul Howard Wehman, PhD[a], Pamela Sherron Targett, MEd[b],
Lauren Elizabeth Avellone, PhD[b],*

KEYWORDS

- Traumatic brain injury • Special education • Employment • Rehabilitation

KEY POINTS

- Communication and collaboration between health care providers who treat children with traumatic brain injury (TBI) and school personnel increase the likelihood that a student with a TBI receives appropriate and timely educational supports and services to maximize success at school.
- Training school personnel about TBI and educating health care providers about a student's rights in the educational process and possible services and supports that schools can provide enhance a child's return to school postinjury.
- Communication and collaboration between health care providers and disability employment service providers increase the likelihood that an individual with TBI receives appropriate services and supports to gain and maintain work.
- Supported employment (SE) is a vocational service option that can assist an individual with a severe TBI with gaining and maintaining employment.

TBI can have a serious impact on functional life activities, including the ability to succeed in school or perform on the job. Along with balancing the demands of returning to work or school with receipt of continued medical care, an individual with a TBI may face a difficult adjustment period learning how to function with physical or cognitive impairments resulting from the TBI. Coping with the symptoms of TBI or learning

Disclosure Statement: Research reported in this article was supported by the US Department of Health and Human Services (USDHS), National Institute on Disability, Independent Living, and Rehabilitation Research (NIDILRR) grant # 90DP0033-02-01. The content is solely the responsibility of the authors and does not necessarily represent the official views of USDHS NIDILRR.
[a] Division of Rehabilitation Research, Medical College of Virginia, Virginia Commonwealth University, 1314 West Main Street, Box 842011, Richmond, VA 23284-2011, USA; [b] VCU-RRTC, Virginia Commonwealth University, 1314 West Main Street, Box 842011, Richmond, VA 23284-2011, USA
* Corresponding author.
E-mail address: leavellone@vcu.edu

alternative methods to perform activities previously executed with ease can also be emotionally difficult for some patients. The added pressures of having to find proper supports to successfully transition back to life activities can hinder school and employment outcomes for individuals with TBI. Therefore, it is important for communication and collaboration to occur between health care providers (eg, physicians, nurses, and medical staff) and school personnel (eg, teachers, paraprofessionals, and school representatives) or employment service providers (eg, job coaches and case managers).

INTRODUCTION TO EDUCATIONAL ISSUES IN TRAUMATIC BRAIN INJURY

Each year approximately 700,000 children aged 0 to 19 sustain TBI and survive.[1] Therefore, more children with TBI are returning to school. Changes in physical,[2] cognitive,[3] and social behavior skills[4] postinjury often result in students needing educational interventions, supports, and services.[5] During the 2009 to 2010 academic year, approximately 25,000 students (0.38% of all special education students) received services under the classification of TBI.[6] Variables that may influence student outcomes include age at injury,[7] developmental status, nature and extent of injury,[8] preinjury psychological status or cognitive status,[9] history of prior injury,[10] postinjury pain or stress,[11] family functioning,[12] socioeconomic resources, and parenting behavior.[12] Several common factors found to mediate and moderate the effects of TBI on school performance have also been identified.[12] For example, earlier age at injury and more severe injuries are associated with poorer school outcomes. Predicting the impact of these changes on school performance is difficult, however, because no 2 injuries are alike. In addition, the same etiologic factor can lead to different outcomes, depending on the student and the context.

In a 2013 review of current issues in education for students with TBI, Glangand colleagues[12] reported that although the impact of TBI on school performance is unique, the most reported sequelae postinjury are lag in academic achievement due to cognitive deficits and disruptions in executive functioning along with social behavior problems. Glang and colleagues[12] also indicated perceptual skills deficits, physical impairments, fatigue, diminished stamina, and the effects of medications on a student's behavior, attention, mood, and learning can also have an impact on academic performance. Reduced federal funding has led to shorter inpatient rehabilitation and limited access to long-term rehabilitation. Consequently, many students with TBI do not receive the long-term rehabilitation treatment needed. This exacerbates difficulties with adaptive skills, academics, and the development of unwanted behaviors in the classroom. To combat these concerns, Glang and colleagues[12] suggested increased training for school personnel on effective strategies for teaching students with TBI and strengthening links between schools and hospitals treating children with TBI.

After a TBI, health care providers and school personnel should consider the long-term educational challenges a student faces. In 2016, Prasad and colleagues[13] found that although children with complicated mild/moderate TBI were less likely to receive educational services at 2 years postinjury than children with severe TBI, those assessed at 6 years postinjury had comparable services. The researchers concluded that children with complicated mild/moderate TBI are often left vulnerable to the sequential effects of poor academic outcomes for too long. Long-term monitoring of educational performance and service delivery is needed for all students with TBI regardless of severity of injury. Acquiring proper supports requires a movement of information through the correct channels, which does not always seem to happen.

Prasad and colleagues[13] stated that schools primarily rely on parent information and often do not get advice or recommendations from health care providers.

Effective planning for returning to school requires a collaborative approach between health care providers and school personnel.[12] Several states have implemented models that require collaboration between parents, the school, and medical rehabilitation professionals. These allow students to return to the classroom with strategies in place and an ongoing plan for communication to make adjustments as needed based on performance. This type of approach prevents students from returning to school with no or only written recommendations from health care providers that parents and the school may find difficult to implement. The likelihood that school reentry is successful is increased if a child receives adequate support to prevent unnecessary adjustment problems when academic and social activities are resumed.[12] Health care providers are uniquely positioned to promote a child's transition back to school. They can influence outcomes and help children, their families, and school staff meet various challenges associated with this process by

- Collaborating to increase educators' and other school personnel's knowledge about pediatric TBI[14–16]
- Understanding students' rights, their state's educational system, and the requirements related to students accessing various types of interventions, supports, and services
- Determining and assigning interdisciplinary roles, functions, and responsibilities that promote successful return to school[12]

COLLABORATION AND INFORMATION DISSEMINATION

Health care providers need to know how to support a child's return to school. Communication between health care providers and school personnel ensures that the school supports and interventions a student requires are put into place in a timely manner. Health care providers need to provide specific information to the school system, such as diagnosis, medical reports stating why the child is under a physician's care, and length of time the child is expected to be absent. Guidelines that need to be followed on return to school should also be communicated to school personnel, including partial-day versus full-time attendance, plan to transition to full day, need for rest breaks, need to attend medical and therapy appointments, and participation in certain classes or sports. Information from health care providers regarding type or severity of impairment may also be needed for a student to meet eligibility for educational supports and services. In addition, educators and other school staff need to understand how to translate medical findings into meaningful individualized interventions, supports, and services for a particular student. A list of questions health care providers need to answer is presented in **Box 1**.

Providing patient-specific information increases the likelihood that a student has access to what is needed.

EDUCATIONAL SERVICES FOR STUDENTS WITH DISABILITIES

Health care providers need to be familiar with basic special education laws, including the referral process and eligibility requirements for their state.[12] They also need to understand the various types of educational supports schools can offer students, such as interventions and accommodations available as a general education student, with a Section 504 accommodation plan or with special education supports and services under the Individuals with Disabilities Education Act (IDEA)[17] through an

> **Box 1**
> **Questions for health care providers concerning return to school**
>
> Health care providers are likely to receive questions from school personnel regarding the following information:
>
> - What are the student's strengths?
> - How has the student's ability to learn been impacted?
> - How have the student's ability to plan and carry out activities, initiative to start and finish things, and ability to self-evaluate been impacted?
> - How have the student's social skills been impacted with respect to emotional status, sensitivity, and ability to handle stress?
> - What events or settings may trigger inappropriate behavior?
> - How have the student's physical abilities been impacted, such as strength, balance, and endurance?
> - What are some strategies that can be used in the classroom and/or outside the classroom setting to help the student with changes cited as well as academics (eg, attention and concentration, memory, and learning new things), participation in extracurricular activities, peer relations, and relationships with school personnel?

Individualized Education Program (IEP). An IEP specifies a student's academic goals and states how these goals will be obtained through specially designed instruction and related services. A Section 504 accommodation plan is provided under federal law, of the Rehabilitation Act of 1973.[18] The Act is designed to protect the rights (ie, prevent discrimination) of individuals with disabilities in programs and activities that receive federal financial assistance from the US Department of Education (ie, public schools and private schools receiving federal funding). A child must have "a physical or mental impairment that substantially limits one or more major life activities (eg, walking, learning, thinking or concentrating) have a record of such impairment or is regarded as having such impairment" to be covered under this law.[18] Special education provides specialized academic instruction, supports, and services as stated within an IEP. As stated previously, an IEP is a requirement under the IDEA, because public schools are mandated to provide a free and appropriate education to eligible children with disabilities.

Assessment of a student's current level of academic and functional performance is necessary to determine if the child is eligible for special education services.[19] The request should be made in writing to school administration (eg, principal) with a copy sent to the school district's special education office. An authorization to release medical and or therapy records to the schools also is required. Most states require a medical doctor to make a diagnosis of TBI and use that report as evidence. An assessment plan (which includes reviewing information provided by parents and the medical staff) is made by the school district, signed off on by a parent, and performed within a specified timeframe. Once assessments are completed, an IEP meeting is held. The time frame to complete assessments and an IEP meeting varies state to state but is typically 60 days. With information in hand, appropriate school personnel (ie, school nurse or school psychologist), parents, student (to the degree possible), and treating medical team should come together to discuss services and establish a timeline for the student to return to school. Health care providers and parents may need to be informed about the special education process, services, and the student's rights under the law. For example, the parents need to know that if they do not agree with the school's assessment findings, they can follow procedures to request an Individual Education Evaluation at the district's expense by a qualified professional with expertise in evaluating students with TBI. In addition, some students, with obvious disability, may require less information to qualify for special education.

Additional evaluations may be held after the initial assessment or after a child is found eligible to determine if related services can help the student benefit from special education.[19] Services can vary from state to state. Some examples of related services include medical services for diagnostic or evaluation purposes, physical therapy, occupational therapy, assistive technology assessments, parent counseling and training, and transportation. Schools are obligated to provide educationally relevant opposed to medically relevant therapies. A student who receives medical therapy outside of school may also be eligible for school-based therapy. The approach to school therapies is different from what is found in a medical setting. To receive school-based therapy, a student is assessed by the school-based therapist. If eligible, goals are written and implemented in group or individual therapy sessions. For example, in the school setting, a physical therapist might focus on improving a child's posture or mobility or enhancing functional life skills, such as eating or drinking. Knowledge of available educational services can help health care providers be involved in planning and referral in the most beneficial manner possible.

ROLES AND RESPONSIBILITIES

The link between the health care facility and the school has been found the most important factor associated with a student's transition back to school.[20] Both health care providers and school personnel, however, may be confused about what type of information needs to be communicated to the other party to facilitate successful return to school for a child with moderate to severe TBI. Suggestions regarding general knowledge to be distributed among parties are presented in **Table 1**.

Roles and responsibilities for completing various tasks during return-to-school activities can be confusing when multiple parties are involved. Collaboration should include a thorough discussion designed to determine who is responsible for communication, identify important deadlines, and confirm what information is needed or not needed with respect to patient needs and confidentiality rights. **Table 2** outlines suggested activities to be assumed by parties involved in the return-to-school process, namely school personnel, health care providers, and the student or family.[12,21–23]

VOCATIONAL ISSUES IN TRAUMATIC BRAIN INJURY

Employment is an important life activity with recognized benefits, including monetary independence, access to socialization, daily structure through routines, and improved mental health.[24] TBI can have a serious impact on competitive employment outcomes for both youth entering the workforce for the first time and adults attempting to return to work (RTW) after an injury. Employment rates for individuals with disabilities are disparagingly low, at 17.5%, according to the Bureau of Labor Statistics in 2015.[25] Although estimates of RTW rates among individuals with TBI vary widely, typically 30% to 40% is reported across studies.[26] An individual with a TBI may experience challenges in physical mobility, cognition, or psychosocial functioning that have a direct impact on employment. Advancements in legislation, vocational services, and funding, however, have made positive employment outcomes attainable of all individuals, including those with the most significant disabilities.

Table 1
Suggested information needed by relevant parties during return-to-school process

Information Needed by School Personnel	Information Needed by Health Care Providers
• Basic brain anatomy	• Referral process for educational services
• Head injury and level classifications	• Basic information about special education services eligibility
• Multidimensional assessments	• Suitable documentation for proof of disabling condition
• Training or explanations of clinical reports	• Applicable legislation, such as the IDEA
• Suggested accommodations and supports	• Types of educational plan, such as an IEP and a Section 504 accommodation plan
• Symptoms or behavior change that issue concern	• Types of accommodations available (eg, seating at the front of the class, extended time completing assignments or tests, alternate settings to take tests, audio recording or Braille)
• Medical restrictions or considerations	• Progress meeting IEP or other educational objectives
• Path to recovery	• Pertinent academic assessments or evaluations
• Suspected impact of symptoms on learning	• School-based therapy, such as occupational therapy or speech language therapy
• Considerations regarding changing needs	• Natural breaks in school calendar that could be used for additional treatment
• Referral to didactic resources	• Effective procedures for collaboration and proper paperwork for release of information
• Demand of treatment regimen on a student's time or emotional energy	
• Effective procedures for collaboration and proper paperwork for release of information with respect to confidentiality	

PREDICTORS OF EMPLOYMENT

Research investigating predictors of employment outcomes for individuals with TBI have yielded widely different results. Comparisons across studies are difficult, largely due to vastly different methodology, patient characteristics, definitions of injury severity, and sampling sizes.[27,28] Generally, research findings suggest that better employment outcomes are associated with the following unmodifiable variables: younger age at injury, higher educational attainment preinjury, and employment prior to injury.[29] Importantly, many modifiable factors have a positive impact on employment outcomes as well, including supportive work cultures[30] and receipt of appropriate vocational services.[31]

WORKPLACE SUPPORTS

Employment is a multistep process involving seeking, securing, and then maintaining a job long term. Individuals with TBI may require assistance with some or all of the employment process, depending on individual need. Workplace supports refers to services, accommodations, or modifications used to assist an individual with a disability successfully obtain and retain a job. Workplace supports are provided by trained professionals (eg, job coaches), which are often acquired through an employment service agency, such as vocational rehabilitation (VR). Supports are tailored to meet individual needs but may include

- Assistance identifying employment opportunities
- Assistance developing a job within a business that matches a job seeker's abilities

Party	Roles and Responsibilities
Table 2 **Roles and responsibilities for return to school**	
School personnel	• Observe the student in the hospital. • Attend the hospital predischarge meeting. • Request and obtain information from the hospital prior to a student's discharge. • Plan ways to disseminate information learned from hospital staff with appropriate parties. • On receipt of the letter from the family about the student's medical and functional status, determine the student's need for intervention by holding a Student Study Team meeting and gathering and reviewing facts on diagnosis and impact on education. • Make recommendations for interventions (ie, 504 accommodation plan or evaluation for special education). • Educate parents and medical personnel about accessing school services.
Health care providers	• Communicate with the school as early as possible. • Develop and distribute training materials to be sent to the school about TBI. • Assist parent in writing a letter notifying the school of a child's diagnosis, treatment, or need for educational supports. • Communicate the status and needs of the student, along with ideas on how to support the student to help set up a successful return to school. • Offer specific functional information about interventions to parents, educators, and others in the school setting who will be supporting the student. • If receiving inpatient services, coordinate lessons with the child's teachers • Translate the student's challenges into academic and social supports and accommodations.
Parents	• Request that school personnel and hospital staff get involved and begin communicating early on, very soon after the time of injury. • Sign necessary release forms for medical and educational institutions to exchange information. • Ask hospital staff to assist in writing a letter notifying the school of the child's diagnosis, treatment, and need to set up an initial meeting.
All	• Understand the guidelines for referral, evaluation, eligibility determination, parent involvement in decision making, IEPs, delivery of specially designed instruction, and related services for students with TBI.

- On-the-job training
- Social skills training related to work culture
- Personal assistant services
- Facilitation using natural supports within the workplace
- Provision of follow-up services, including frequent contact with the employer, the individual with a disability, family or guardians, or advocates to promote job retention

Determination of proper supports is derived using multiple information-gathering techniques, such as interviewing the job seeker and conducting vocational assessments. For example, with permission, job coaches may review relevant records from the job seeker, such as a document of employment experience or medical records, to determine restrictions or health concerns pertinent to work. A job coach may also observe the job seeker performing actual work tasks in an applied setting to determine existing skills. Assessment results provide information regarding a job seeker's strengths, preferences, interest, and needs, which can be used to match individuals with TBI to a job they like with the supports they need to be successful. Suggested workplace supports available for individuals with TBI-related cognitive, physical, or psychosocial impairments are presented in **Table 3**.

EMPLOYMENT AVENUES

There are multiple ways individuals with TBI can become competitively employed. The Rehabilitation Act of 1973 created federal funding for VR services to operate in all 50 states.[32] Individuals with TBI must meet eligibility criteria to receive services. VR assists individuals with TBI in creating an Individualized Plan for Employment, which identifies workplace supports and action steps necessary for achieving employment goals. Funding through VR may be applied toward the receipt of many beneficial services, including assessments and evaluations, vocational counseling, physical or mental restoration, rehabilitation technology, and collaboration with transition services.[33,34] VR also provides funding for recognized pathways to employment, including SE, customized employment (CE), internships, apprenticeships, and advanced educational training pertinent to employment.

Supported Employment

SE is an evidenced-based practice that uses a combination of personalized supports to assist individuals who have the most significant disabilities achieve competitive and integrated work in community settings. Vocational assessments are used to determine a job seeker's strengths. A job matching an individual's strengths and preferences is

Table 3
Suggested workplace supports

Traumatic Brain Injury Impairment	Workplace Support
Cognition	• Job-seeking services • Job development capitalizing on job seeker strengths • Compensatory strategies (checklists, charts, and manuals) • On-the-job training support • Assistive technology • Facilitation of discussion with business to modify processes or procedures • Follow-along services to promote job stability • With permission, training for the employer regarding how to support the individual with the disability
Physical mobility	• Job development targeting strengths rather than impairments • Modify work environment • Modify work schedule to combat fatigue • Assistive technology • Adaptive equipment • Transportation to work site
Psychosocial	• Social skills training and support • Rearranging environment to avoid triggers • Counseling services • Cognitive behavior therapy

developed through discussions with a business. Proper supports to assist with job training and follow-along services are provided.[35] VR often funds SE services for eligible individuals.

Customized Employment

CE is a natural extension of SE and was added to the definition of SE under the Workforce Innovation and Opportunity Act of 2014. CE uses a qualitative approach to gaining information about a job seeker via a process called *discovery*. Collected information is used to develop a job by means of job carving, job negotiation, job creation, self-employment, or resource ownership. Job-site training and follow-along services are provided.[36] VR funding can be applied to CE services.

Internships

Youth with disabilities who have little or no work experience can benefit from work opportunities in a supervised setting. Internships provide an opportunity for individualized supports to be identified and put in place to help individuals with TBI learn work skills. VR collaborates with transition teams to assist youth with disabilities interested in participating in internship programs.

Apprenticeships

Apprenticeship opportunities help prepare individuals for jobs in specific disciplines (construction trade, medical field, and so forth). Businesses offering apprenticeships typically intend to hire the individual after completion of an extensive training period. Therefore, time invested in education and training is rewarding to both the individual with a disability who receives a permanent job and the business that acquires a well-trained employee. VR services may apply toward work-related supports in apprenticeship settings.

Postsecondary Education

Individuals who are returning to work after TBI may need advanced training to change fields. Youth with TBI may also need supports to be successful in postsecondary settings. Technical schools, community colleges, and universities house disability support services offices, where approved accommodations and modifications related to postsecondary education may be obtained. Proper documentation of disability is required. Support through VR, for services like transportation or a personal assistant, may be applied toward postsecondary training.

PROMOTING SUCCESSFUL RETURN TO WORK

A variety of supports and services are available to help individuals with TBI obtain meaningful work for competitive wages in integrated settings and in a variety of professional fields. Antiquated models of work that waste valuable time preparing individuals with disabilities to work have been replaced by successful strategies that place individuals in a work environment immediately and then train them in the applied setting. Furthermore, work models that segregate individuals with TBI and other disabilities from nondisabled peers and offer subminimum compensation for work are not acceptable employment outcomes. Individuals with even the most significant disabilities can, and have, a right to work.

Several measures can be taken to enhance employment outcomes after TBI. Referrals to VR or other service provider agencies should occur in a timely manner after injury. Conducting and sharing results of important neuropsychological and vocational assessments among relevant parties can aid in proper job development procedures.[37] Ensuring that individuals with TBI receive individualized supports is essential. Providing comprehensive services is also necessary, such as emotional support, in addition to vocational support, to address the psychological difficulties of adjusting to the impact of TBI in a work setting. Finally, continued collaboration long term among relevant parties, including health care providers, employment service providers, and the business, helps alleviate any emerging concerns and bolsters job security.[37]

ROLE OF CLINICIANS RELATED TO EMPLOYMENT

Clinicians play integral role in helping individuals with TBI in work settings. Students entering work for the first time might need doctors to indicate what is and is not reasonable concerning types of job duties (physical restrictions). Individuals returning to work may need documentation of when and in what capacity they are able to return. Adjustments, such as removal of a restriction at follow-ups, may also be needed in writing for individuals to present to their job coach or other employment service providers as they consider job opportunities. Individuals with TBI enrolled in postsecondary settings need documentation of their disability to receive accommodations and modifications. It may be that individuals with TBI are unaware of what they might need in work and school settings. Therefore, it may be helpful for health care providers to probe about an individual's employment or postsecondary plans, explain the type of assistance a health care provider can offer, and set up a plan for how and when the individual with TBI can communicate what is needed.

SUMMARY AND RECOMMENDATIONS

The purpose of this is article is to describe some of the current issues related to return to school and employment for individuals with TBI. A smooth reentry to school or work after TBI is critically important. A strong, collaborative partnership between an individual's health care team and stakeholders is essential. This article concludes with some recommendations on areas for future research.

More research is needed to help bridge the gap between the health care and education fields to facilitate a more seamless transition back to school for students post-TBI. Future research should investigate ways to improve communication and collaboration between health care providers and school personnel.[12,21–23] Ways to clarify the roles and responsibilities of health care providers and school personnel[14,15,19] in the transition process should be examined. Continued research into effective classroom interventions for students with TBI is needed.[5,19] Finally, steps states can take to create infrastructure and begin addressing gaps in educational services for children with TBI are essential.[12,16,19]

More research is also needed to improve employment outcomes for youth and adults with TBI. Research investigating the types of work experience, including paid employment, that promote a successful transition from school to work for students with TBI should be examined.[31,32] The types of support employers need to employ individuals with TBI is needed.[31,35] Finally, fidelity in implementation of employment services that successfully assist individuals with TBI with gaining and maintaining employment should be researched. Until more research is conducted, key stake holders should follow best practices, which should assist individuals with TBI with becoming as successful as possible whether they are in school or at work.

REFERENCES

1. Faul M, Xu L, Wald MM, et al. Traumatic brain injury in the United States. Atlanta (GA): National Center for Injury Prevention and Control; Centers for Disease Control and Prevention; 2010.
2. Zonfrillo MR, Durbin DR, Winston FK, et al. Physical disability after injury-related inpatient rehabilitation in children. Pediatrics 2013;131(1):206–13.
3. Vu J, Babikian T, Asarnow RF. Academic and language outcomes in children after traumatic brain injury: a meta-analysis. Except Child 2011;3:263–81.
4. Greenham M, Spencer-Smith MM, Anderson PJ, et al. Social functioning in children with brain insult. Front Hum Neurosci 2010;4:22.
5. Wehman P, West M, Targett P, et al. Applications for youth with traumatic brain injury and other health impairments. In: Life beyond the classroom. 5th edition. Baltimore (MD): Paul H. Brookes; 2013. p. 473–500.
6. Snyder TD, de Brey C, Dillow SA. Digest of Education Statistics 2014 (NCES 2016-006). Washington, DC: National Center for Education Statistics, Institute of Education Sciences, U.S. Department of Education; 2016.
7. McKinlay A, Dalrymple-Alford JC, Horwood LJ, et al. Long term psychosocial outcomes after mild head injury in early childhood. J Neurol Neurosurg Psychiatry 2002;73(3):281–8.
8. Hessen E, Nestvold K, Sundet K. Neuropsychological function in group of patients 25 years after sustaining minor head injuries as children and adolescents. Scand J Psychol 2006;47(4):245–51.
9. Massagli TL, Fann JR, Burington BE, et al. Psychiatric illness after mild traumatic brain injury in children. Arch Phys Med Rehabil 2004;85:1428–34.
10. Swaine BR, Tremblay C, Platt RW, et al. Previous head injury is a risk factor for subsequent head injury in children: a longitudinal cohort study. Pediatrics 2007;119(4):749–58.
11. Luis CA, Mittenberg W. Mood and anxiety disorders following pediatric traumatic brain injury: a prospective study. J Clin Exp Neuropsychol 2002;24(3):270–9.
12. Glang A, Ettel D, Tyler JS, et al. Educational issues and school reentry for students with traumatic brain injury. In: Zasler ND, Katz DI, Zafonte RD, editors. Brain injury medicine: principles and practice. 2nd edition. New York: Demos Medical Publishing; 2013. p. 602–20.
13. Prasad MR, Swank PR, Ewing-Cobbs L. Long-term school outcomes of children and adolescents with traumatic brain injury. J Head Trauma Rehabil 2017;32(1): E24–32.
14. Glang A, Dise-Lewis J, Tyler J. Identification and appropriate service delivery for children who have TBI in schools. J Head Trauma Rehabil 2006;21(5):411–2.
15. Ettel D, Glang AE, Todis B, et al. Traumatic brain injury: persistent misconceptions and knowledge gaps among educators. Exceptionality Education Int 2016;26:1–18.
16. Glang A, Ettel D, Todis B, et al. Services and supports for students with traumatic brain injury: Survey of state educational agencies. Exceptionality 2015;23(4): 211–24.
17. Individuals with Disabilities Education Act, 20 U.S.C. 1400 et seq.; 34 CFR Part 300.
18. Section 504 of the Rehabilitation Act of 1973, 29 U.S.C. 794; 35 CFR Part 104.
19. Brown J, Grandinette S, Kang K. Pediatrics and adolescents. The essential brain injury guide. 5th edition. Brain Injury Association of America; 2016. p. 286–317.
20. Glang A, Todis B, Thomas CW, et al. Return to school following childhood TBI: who gets services? NeuroRehabilitation 2008;23:477–86.

21. Ylvisaker M, Hartwick P, Stevens MB. School reentry following head injury: managing the transition from hospital to school. J Head Trauma Rehabil 1991;6(1): 10–22.

22. Savage RC. Identification, classification, and placement issues for students with traumatic brain injuries. J Head Trauma Rehabil 1991;6(1):1–9.

23. Savage RC, DePompei R, Tyler J, et al. Pediatric traumatic brain injury: a review of pertinent issues. Pediatr Rehabil 2005;8(2):92–103.

24. Hoare PN, Machin MA. The impact of reemployment on access to the latent and manifest benefits of employment and mental health. J Occup Organ Psy 2010;83: 759–70.

25. The United States Bureau of Labor Statistics. Persons with a disability: labor force characteristics - 2014. 2015. Available at: http://www.bls.gov/news.release/pdf/ disabl.pdf.

26. Malec J, Moessner A. Replicated positive results for the VCC model of vocational intervention after ABI within the social model of disability. Brain 2006;20:227–36.

27. Cancelliere C, Kristman VL, Cassidy JD, et al. Systematic review of return to work after mild traumatic brain injury: results of the international collaboration on mild traumatic brain injury prognosis. Arch Phys Med Rehabil 2014;95:S201–9.

28. Saltychev M, Eskola M, Tenovuo O, et al. Return to work after traumatic brain injury: systematic review. Brain 2013;27:1516–27.

29. Dahm J, Ponsford J. Predictors of global functioning and employment 10 years following traumatic brain injury compared with orthopaedic injury. Brain Inj 2015;29(13–14):1539–46.

30. Stergiou-Kita M, Mansfield E, Sokoloff S, et al. Gender influences on return to work after mild traumatic brain injury. Arch Phys Med Rehabil 2016;97:S40–5.

31. Rumrill P, Wehman P, Cimera R, et al. Vocational rehabilitation services and outcomes for transition-age youth with traumatic brain injuries. J Head Trauma Rehabil 2016;31:159–232.

32. Wehman P, Chan F, Ditchman N, et al. Effect of supported employment on vocational rehabilitation outcomes of transition-age youth with intellectual and developmental disabilities: a case control study. Intellect Dev Disabil 2014;52: 296–310.

33. Huang I, Holzbauer JJ, Lee EJ, et al. Vocational rehabilitation services and employment outcomes for adults with cerebral palsy in the United States. Dev Med Child Neurol 2013;55:1000–8.

34. Sung C, Sánchez J, Kuo HJ, et al. Gender differences in vocational rehabilitation service predictors of successful competitive employment for transition-aged individuals with autism. J Autism Dev Disord 2015;45:3204–18.

35. West M, Targett P, Wehman P, et al. Separation from supported employment: a retrospective chart review study. Disabil Rehabil 2015;37:1055–9.

36. Smith JT, Dillahunt-Aspillaga C, Kenney C. Integrating customized employment practices within the vocational rehabilitation system. J Vocat Rehabil 2015;42:201–8.

37. Wehman P, Goodwin M, McNamee SD, et al. Return to work following traumatic brain injury. In: Zollman FS, editor. Manual of traumatic brain injury management. New York: Demos Medical Publishing, LLC; 2011. p. 451–6.

Integrative Medicine in Traumatic Brain Injury

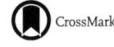

David F. Drake, MD[a,b,]*, Anne M. Hudak, MD[a,b], William Robbins, MD[a,b]

KEYWORDS

- Integrative medicine • Traumatic brain injury • Complementary and integrative health

KEY POINTS

- Integrative medicine combines complementary and alternative medicine (CAM) practices in which there is some high-quality evidence of safety and effectiveness in addition to conventional medicine for patient care.
- The scope of CAM includes mind-body practices, manipulative therapies, traditional Chinese medicine, and natural products among others.
- There is growing evidence to support CAM techniques in the treatment of common comorbidities, recovery, and symptom management in the traumatic brain injury population.
- Acupuncture, tai chi, qigong, yoga, and mindfulness are all CAM techniques that have been researched in treatment of patients with a traumatic brain injury.
- Nutraceutical use in the treatment of traumatic brain injury is based on physiologic properties of specific substances but has yet to be proven in high-quality clinical trials.

INTRODUCTION
Integrative Medicine

Complementary and Integrative medicine (CIM) is a holistic, interdisciplinary approach, designed to treat the person, not just the disease. It is a partnership between the patient and his or her providers, where the goal is to treat the mind, body, and spirit, all at the same time. CIM combines treatments of conventional medicine and elements of complementary and alternative medicine (CAM) where there is strong evidence of safety and effectiveness.

The Osher Center for Integrative Medicine at the University of California, San Francisco, says on its Web site: "Our Center strives to successfully integrate modern medicine,

Disclosure Statement: The authors have nothing to disclose.
[a] Department of Physical Medicine and Rehabilitation, Richmond VAMC, 1201 Broad Rock Boulevard, Richmond, VA 23249, USA; [b] Department of Physical Medicine and Rehabilitation, Virginia Commonwealth University, 1223 East Marshall Street, 4th Floor, P.O. Box 980677, Richmond, VA 23298-0677, USA
* Corresponding author. Department of Physical Medicine and Rehabilitation, Interventional Pain and Integrative Medicine, Richmond VAMC, 1201 Broad Rock Boulevard, Richmond, VA 23249.
E-mail address: David.drake4@va.gov

Phys Med Rehabil Clin N Am 28 (2017) 363–378
http://dx.doi.org/10.1016/j.pmr.2016.12.011
1047-9651/17/Published by Elsevier Inc.

healthy lifestyle practices, and established healing approaches from around the globe, in an effort to meet the need for a new model of care and daily living that promotes healing and well-being of the whole person—mind, body and spirit."[1] CIM encompasses east and west, mind and body, individual and family. Most importantly, CIM is patient centered. It transforms the current medical model to a personalized, proactive, patient-driven approach that enables engagement with life in accordance with how an individual wants to live. CIM focuses on empowering the consumer through comprehensive education regarding their health and wellness, thereby encouraging active participation in one's own well-being.

Complementary and Integrative Health

The National Center for Complementary and Integrative Health uses the term "complementary health approaches" and defines 2 specific subgroups: natural products and mind-body practices; and offers a third: other complementary health approaches.

Natural products are herbs and supplements, such as probiotics, and vitamins and minerals. Mind-body practices include a very diverse large group of techniques or procedures that include acupuncture, massage, meditation, mindfulness, movement therapies, relaxation techniques, spinal manipulation, traditional Chinese medicine (to include tai chi and qigong), yoga, and others not specifically listed. Ayurvedic medicine, traditional Chinese medicine, homeopathy, and naturopathy are examples of approaches that fall into the other complementary health subgroup.[2]

Complementary medicine involves the use of non-mainstream techniques or treatments in conjunction with conventional medicine. Alternative medicine, on the other hand, is the use of CAM in place of conventional medicine.

Although limited specific research has been directed toward the use of integrative medicine for individuals with traumatic brain injury (TBI), the overall principles and specific techniques are appropriate for TBI rehabilitation and should be applied based on the individual's specific needs and progress.

ACUPUNCTURE

Acupuncture is a form of energy medicine and is one of the more common and more researched of the CAM modalities; however, it shares with the others a similar treatment setting. Acupuncture also shares a conceptual framework similar to tai chi or qigong, in that life energy, called Qi (pronounced chee), is thought to be circulating though all parts of the body via energy channels, called meridians. These meridians connect the exterior to the interior, the organs to each other and the exterior.

The classical Chinese explanation is that channels of energy run in regular patterns through the body and over its surface in channels, called meridians. Much like blood flow may cause infarction, an obstruction in the movement of these energy rivers will cause the flow of Qi to become blocked or unbalanced, thus causing abnormality. Acupuncture is one of the treatments used to re-establish the flow of Qi by placing needles at points along the meridians, thus allowing the body to return to a homeostasis, easing the ailment for which it was prescribed.

The modern scientific explanation is that needling the acupuncture points stimulates the nervous system to release chemicals in the muscles, spinal cord, and brain. These chemicals will either change the experience of pain or they will trigger the release of other chemicals and hormones that influence the body's own internal regulating system.

The physiology of acupuncture effects is beginning to emerge. Stimulation of acupuncture points has been shown to create signal change in the amygdala, anterior hippocampus, and subgenual cingulate cortex on functional MRI (fMRI).[2] Other studies confirm these findings, defining the role of the amygdala in affect, fear, and defensive behavior as well as the processing of pain[3–5] and motivation.[6] The hippocampus is thought to link affective states with memory processing. The signal decrease within the amygdala and anterior hippocampus is consistent with past acupuncture fMRI studies at acupoints LI-4 and GB-34 as well as ST-36.[7–11]

Ahsin and colleagues[12] linked electroacupuncture to functional improvement they thought was related to the measured increase in endorphins and a decrease in cortisol, in subjects given electroacupuncture.

The improved energy and biochemical balance produced by acupuncture results in stimulating the body's natural healing abilities, and in promoting physical and emotional well-being. The anatomy of acupuncture points is not clear; however, a theory proposed by Langevin and Yandow[13] suggests that the meridians are located within tissues planes, that acupuncture points occur at a convergence of these, that meridian qi is the connective tissue biochemical and bioelectrical signaling, and that a blockage of qi may lead to an altered connective tissue matrix composition leading to altered signal transduction and therefore pain or other symptoms.

Clinically, acupuncture does appear to be of benefit in some patients; however, there is no good evidence for the use of acupuncture in TBI. According to a *Cochrane Review* in 2013, "The small number of studies together with their low methodological quality means that they are inadequate to allow any conclusion to be drawn about the efficacy and safety of acupuncture in the treatment of TBI."[14] Acupuncture has, however, been found helpful for some often seen comorbid conditions such as headache, pain, spasticity, and posttraumatic stress disorder (PTSD). For example, one *Cochrane Review* concluded that acupuncture was effective for treating frequent episodic or chronic tension–type headaches,[15] and another stated, "Available studies suggest that acupuncture is at least as effective as, or possibly more effective than, prophylactic drug treatment, and has fewer adverse effects. Acupuncture should be considered a treatment option for patients willing to undergo this treatment."[16,17] According to the *Journal of Rheumatology*, there is sufficient evidence to warrant positive recommendations for osteoarthritis, low back pain, and lateral epicondylitis in routine care of rheumatic patients.[18] Acupuncture has shown to be effective in low back pain,[19] lateral epicondylitis,[20] shoulder pain due to subacromial impingement,[21] and headache pain.[22] Nausea and vomiting has also shown to be effectively managed by acupuncture.[23–25] A meta-analysis showed that acupuncture significantly decreased spasticity after stroke, noting most significant decreases in the wrist, knee, and elbow.[26] Finally, a systematic review and meta-analysis by Kim and colleagues[27] in 2013 suggested that the evidence of effectiveness of acupuncture for PTSD is encouraging but further qualified trials are needed to prove its effectiveness. Acupuncture is an ancient medical modality, with physiologic changes that seem to suggest neurologic and neurochemical effects that can lead to clinical improvement in patients with TBI.

NUTRACEUTICALS

In recent years, much attention has been paid to TBI. This attention has not yet yielded a successful pharmaceutical clinical trial. The reasons for this are likely multifactorial because TBI is a varied and complex injury that scientists are just beginning to understand. Although many of today's treatments focus on maximizing residual function, minimizing damage via interruption of the cellular pathologic mechanisms may be more effective. Given its heterogeneous nature, TBI may not be well suited for the typical pharmacologic approach to intervention testing, that is, aiming for an isolated target within the currently known biochemical pathways.[28] Nutritional supplements often have influence in more than one pathway and have the potential of a multitargeted approach.

Survivors of trauma need proper nutrition to counter the catabolic metabolism that occurs after injury. The Brain Trauma Foundation Guidelines recommend initiation of nutritional support by day 7.[28] They do not, however, provide specific guidelines. Further exploration is needed to establish recommended nutritional components that can not only provide the required calories, but foster recovery from TBI. Many of the current nutrition-based research targets have deficiency states with known neurologic deficits (eg, zinc [Zn], vitamin B3). Some of the more promising nutritional supplements for TBI are addressed in later discussion.

OMEGA-3 FATTY ACIDS

Omega-3 fatty acids (FA) are polyunsaturated fats unable to be synthesized in the human body, and therefore, must come from dietary sources.[29] The important omega-3 FA are docosahexaenoic acid (DHA), eicosapentaenoic acid, and alpha-linolenic acid. Omega-3 FA are found in significant concentrations in cold water marine food sources (eg, oily fish, krill). Non-marine animal and plant-based sources exist.[30] Omega-3 FAs are key factors in membrane organization, function, and plasticity, thereby influencing cell adhesion, synapse maintenance, and neurotransmission speed.[31,32] A major structural component of the mammalian cerebral cortex,[32] DHA supplementation has been showed to enhance learning during aging.[31] A body of animal studies on omega-3 FAs has shown the potential benefits of these compounds after TBI.

Consumption of omega-3 FAs reduces reactive oxygen species (ROS) production.[32] DHA pretreatment for 30 days before TBI leads to decreased axonal injury, apoptotic marker, and improved memory in rodents.[33] Postinjury treatment with omega-3 FA for 30 days demonstrated decreased β-APP-positive neurons when compared with controls in rodents.[33] An array of studies supports the role of omega-3 FA in ameliorating TBI-related injury in areas such as mitochondrial malfunction, apoptotic cell death, oxidative stress, inflammation, and excitotoxicity.[32] To date, no human studies involving omega-3 FA on TBI have been published, but several clinical trials are underway (NCT01814527, recruiting, mild TBI; NCT01903525, recruiting, mild, adolescents; NCT02762539, not yet recruiting). Use of omega-3 FA in TBI is a promising area of effort.

ZINC

Zn is an essential trace element, which has been linked to a variety of neurologic disorders. Occurring in both protein-bound and free forms, the balance between the 2 is critical for normal brain performance.[34] Zn participates in neurotransmitter activity, cell signaling, DNA binding of transcription factors, enzymatic activity, and adult neurogenesis.[34,35] Zn is required for normal central nervous system development. Mild gestational Zn deficiency has been shown to have learning and memory abnormalities in animals.[34] Free Zn is postulated to be responsible for developmental programmed neuronal pruning.[36] Free Zn is stored in neuronal synaptic vesicles and is released into the synaptic cleft triggering post–synaptic neuronal death, and excessive Zn has been associated with neuronal morbidity and mortality.[37] After TBI, Zn serum levels decline and urinary levels are elevated.[34] Research has demonstrated that Zn deficiencies after TBI are more problematic than elevated levels.[34] Choi and colleagues[38] demonstrated in animals that removal of Zn reduced TBI-induced progenitor cell proliferation and neurogenesis. A human randomized controlled trial (RCT) involving 68 severe TBI patients reported lower mortality at 1 month after injury when compared with controls. Mean Glasgow Coma Scale (GCS) of the Zn-supplemented group was higher at day 28, and mean motor GCS was higher on days 15, 21, and 28; however, the control group had a greater number of craniotomies for hematoma evacuation. Although Zn appears to have some promise, more work needs to be done for a better understanding of its impact on TBI.

VITAMIN D

Vitamin D is a fat-soluble vitamin that is synthesized by human skin upon exposure to sunlight, specifically UV-B rays, or gained through dietary sources such as fatty fish, cod liver oil, mushrooms, and eggs. Vitamin D gained through dietary sources, light exposure, and supplements must undergo transformation of 2 hydroxylations to be biologically useful.[28] Vitamin D deficiency has been linked with neurodegenerative processes and cognitive impairment.[39]

A human study from Iran compared 3 groups (control, progesterone, vitamin D and progesterone) of 20 severe TBI patients. At 3 months, 35% of the progesterone and vitamin D had good recovery on Glasgow Outcome Scale (GOS); progesterone alone had 25% had good recovery, and 15% of placebo had good recovery.[40] Jamall and colleagues[39] performed a retrospective chart review on patients that attended a TBI clinic. They examined the relationship between vitamin D and outcome measures such as cognitive testing, while controlling for confounding variables such as time from injury and injury severity. Vitamin D levels were correlated with cognition; depression was correlated between the vitamin D–depleted and –insufficient groups. Currently, no listing for an RTC was found on ClinicalTrials.gov.

VITAMIN B3

Nicotinamide in the body originates from dietary intake or primarily plant sources or can be synthesized.[41] Current clinical usage is treatment of the deficiency state, pellagra, and to decrease cholesterol (high doses) and atherosclerosis. Nicotinamide serves as a source of energy supplementation by functioning as the precursor for β-nicotinamide adenine dinucleotide (NAD+) and nicotinamide adenine dinucleotide phosphate (NADP+).[41] It has been shown to inhibit both poly(adenine dinucleotide phosphate [ADP]-ribose) polymerase-1 and sirtuins that balance the repair of DNA damage. Inhibition of these has been shown to improve outcomes after TBI in rodent models. Histologically, nicotinamide reduced degenerating neurons, edema, and apoptosis, and decreased lesion size in the acute period.[42–44] In the more chronic phase, reduced lesion size and active astrocytes were found.[45] Examination of downstream markers substantiated these findings.[45] Use of nicotinamide in TBI animal models has improved sensory, motor, and cognitive function and reduced lesion volume.[42,43,46] Of concern, a study in middle-aged rats demonstrated no improvement, and higher doses trended toward impairment for a variety of measures, including vestibulomotor and lesion size[47,48] compared with high- and low-dose nicotinamide across 3 different TBI animal models. Low-dose administration provided no benefit. At high-dose level, the controlled cortical impact model had significant tissue sparing. Concern has been expressed about converting the high doses used in animal studies for human consumption.

VITAMIN E

Vitamin E is a group of fat-soluble compounds that includes tocopherols (α, β, γ, δ) and tocotrienols. Of these, α-tocopherol is the most widely studied. Vitamin E inhibits ROS formation during fat oxidation. Wu and colleagues[49] found vitamin E–pretreated rats performed better on the Morris water maze; neurotrophic factors were restored, and there was evidence of less oxidative stress. Ishaq and colleagues[50] studied vitamin C and vitamin E at 2 dosing levels as well as a combination of vitamins. The intervention drug started before injury and continued after injury. The combination of C and E group had significantly reduced mortalities that were not dose dependent.

A randomized clinical trial on severe TBI patients (N = 100) divided subjects into 1 of 4 groups: placebo, vitamin E, high-dose vitamin C, and low-dose vitamin C. At discharge, the vitamin E group had lower mortality and better GOS (P = .04). Of note, both vitamin C groups had higher rates of unfavorable outcome at discharge. Perilesional edema was measured by imaging and found to be decreased by 68% in the high-dose vitamin C group. The small sample size is a noteworthy limitation of this study.[51]

CREATINE

Humans synthesize creatine in the liver, kidneys, pancreas,[52] and brain,[53] and the primary dietary source of creatine is meat. Intracellular creatine exists in 2 forms: free creatine and phosphocreatine.[54] Creatine kinase (CK) metabolizes creatine and catalyzes the reversible transfer of a phosphate group between ATP and creatine. Creatine/phosphocreatine (Cr/PCr) serves as a temporal and spatial energy buffer[52] (connecting energy production with utilization sites). Although CK is functionally coupled to ATP-consuming processes, creatine maintains local ATP/ADP ratios.[52,55,56] Cr/PCr prevents inactivation of cellular ATPases by limiting elevations of intracellular ADP.[56]

In addition to energy metabolism, creatine inhibits opening of mitochondrial permeability transition pore (MPTP), thereby assisting in Ca^{2+} homeostasis,[57] decreasing ROS production (Mazzeo A) and inhibiting apoptosis.[58] Creatine can serve as an antioxidant by scavenging ROS[59] and by decreasing production of ROS by mitochondria.[60,61] Creatine inhibits many of the processes associated with TBI-related secondary injury, including providing an alternative energy source, inhibiting MPTP, decreasing apoptosis, and acting as an antioxidant.

Creatine-specific genetic anomalies reveal the importance of creatine for normal brain function. The three known genetic errors of creatine transport and production exist,[62] each of which is associated with decreased to absent creatine levels in the brain. Each deficiency clinical picture includes cognitive impairment and developmental delay, highlighting the relationship between cognition and Cre.[55] In non-TBI humans, creatine supplementation has demonstrated reduced mental fatigue,[63] improved working memory,[64–66] increased intelligence test scores,[65] and in the face of sleep deprivation, improved central executive function tasks.[64] In summary, it appears that creatine-deficient and physically stressed but otherwise healthy humans have a positive response to creatine supplementation.

Creatine–Traumatic Brain Injury Studies

After mild TBI, rats[67] and cats[68] were found to have a decrease in cerebral concentration of creatine. Pretreatment with creatine in both mice[57] and rats[57,69] decreased lesion size after cortical contusion, reduced activation of MPTP, and lowered production of reactive oxygen intermediates.[57] Creatine did not reverse Na/K ATPase inhibition in a severe TBI model, but did reduce oxidative damage.[70]

There is one published report on administration of creatine to post-TBI humans. Children, ages 1 to 18 years, with severe TBI were supplemented for 6 months in an open-label design. At 3 months, participants had better outcomes than controls ($P = .004$), with 65% having Glasgow Outcome Scale-Extended (GOS-E) of 8 (good recovery) compared with 0% in controls. At 6 months, the creatine group continued to do better on GOS-E ($P<.001$), with "good recovery" found for 88.9% of creatine group compared with 5.9% of controls. Participants demonstrated decreased duration of posttraumatic amnesia ($P = .019$), decreased length of intubation ($P = .051$), and decreased intensive care unit stay ($P = .056$).[71] In a follow-up publication, decreased rates of headaches, dizziness, and fatigue were reported at 6 months.[72] Although creatine appears to have promise, much work needs to be done before any recommendations can be made.

CURCUMIN

Curcumin is a yellow pigment that comes from the *Curcuma longa* rhizome and is typically used as a flavoring in curries. Prior work supports the wide variety of biological actions of curcumin (anti-inflammatory, antioxidant, inhibitor of proinflammatory cytokine interleukin-1β]).[73] Curcumin crosses the blood-brain barrier.[73] Animal studies have demonstrated an energy regulatory control function when pretreatment with curcumin is used in a TBI fluid percussion model.[74] Post-TBI use of curcumin in fluid percussion TBI animal models showed normalized brain-derived neurotrophic factor, and a transcription factor involved in learning and memory (CREB).[75] Zhu and colleagues[73] demonstrated reduced cerebral edema, neurologic deficit, and cytokine release in mice after weight drop TBI model. Using a hypoxia model of injury on rats, Yu and colleagues[76] found reduced apoptosis and cerebral edema using pretreatment with curcumin. No human studies of curcumin in the TBI population were located.

QIGONG

Qigong (pronounced chee-gung) is a "moving" mindfulness practice that uses slow graceful movements often with coordinated breathing to promote the circulation of Qi ("energy flow" or "life force") within the human body to enhance overall health, relaxation, and mental focus. There are several forms of qigong, which allow for it to be practiced in standing, sitting, and lying positions, some with little or no movement at all.

Qigong is often confused with the Chinese martial art of tai chi. This misunderstanding can be attributed to the fact that most Chinese martial arts practitioners will usually also practice some form of qigong. It is best to think of qigong as the roots and trunk of the tree whose branches form much of the eastern martial arts.

Qigong's great appeal is that anyone can practice it, regardless of their fitness level, age, belief system, income, or life circumstances. Qigong may benefit anyone, from the most physically challenged to the superathlete.

Most Western medical practitioners view qigong as a set of breathing and movement exercises, with benefits to health through stress reduction and exercise. One of the more important long-term effects is that qigong is said to re-establish the body/mind/spirit connection. When these 3 aspects of our being are integrated, it is thought to encourage a positive outlook on life and help eliminate harmful attitudes and behaviors.

Research supports these thoughts in many areas. Meta-analysis and systematic reviews support the use of qigong to improve stress and anxiety as well as depression.[77]

A RCT indicated that medical qigong can improve overall quality of life mood status of patients with cancer and reduce fatigue.[78] Evidence also supports the use of qigong in patients with fibromyalgia, showing significant improvements in pain, sleep, as well as physical and mental function when compared with the wait-list/usual care control group. Although this was an 8-week study, the benefits extended well beyond this time, indicating significant changes for 6 months.[79,80]

TAI CHI

Tai chi (TIE-chee) involves performing a series of postures or movements in a slow, graceful manner. It is often referred to as "meditation in motion." Each posture flows into the next without pause, ensuring that the body is in constant motion. Forms of tai chi include rhythmic patterns of movement, synchronized with breathing.

Similar to qigong, most forms of tai chi are gentle and suitable for everyone regardless of age or physical ability as technique is emphasized over speed or strength. It is inexpensive, requires no special equipment, and can be done indoors or out, alone or in a group, so it is accessible to many.

Beyond the study mentioned above, further evidence supports the benefits of tai chi. It has been used in patients with Parkinson disease for years, because studies have shown that tai chi training reduces balance impairments in patients with mild to moderate Parkinson disease.[81] Additional benefits include improved functional capacity and reduced falls.[82,83]

A study looking at patients aroused from prolonged coma after severe TBI determined that a goal-oriented rehabilitation program supplemented with elements of tai chi was more effective than the standard rehabilitation program in improving the performance of activities of daily living.[84]

Tai chi practice may exert its effects by changing brain morphology. A controlled study compared tai chi practitioners with controls and showed significantly thicker cortex in precentral gyrus, insula sulcus and middle frontal sulcus in the right hemisphere, and superior temporal gyrus and medial occipitotemporal sulcus and lingual sulcus in the left hemisphere. Greater intensity of tai chi practice was associated with a thicker cortex in the left medial occipitotemporal sulcus and lingual sulcus. These findings suggest that committed long-term practice may induce regional structural change, suggesting tai chi might share similar patterns of neural correlates with meditation and aerobic exercise.[85]

A National Institute's of Health comprehensive review of health benefits of qigong and tai chi concluded that research has demonstrated consistent, significant results for several health benefits in RCTs and suggested a similarity and equivalence of qigong and tai chi.[86]

Tai chi is simply a safe and effective form of physical exercise. As noted, it enhances cardiovascular fitness, muscular strength, balance, and physical function. It also appears to be associated with reduced stress, anxiety, and depression and improved quality of life. Tai chi can be safely recommended to patients with osteoarthritis, rheumatoid arthritis, and fibromyalgia as a complementary and alternative medical approach to affect patient health and wellness.[87]

A review of scientific literature published in the *American Journal of Health Promotion* suggests that there is strong evidence of beneficial health effects of both tai chi and qigong, to include bone health, cardiopulmonary fitness, balance, and quality of life. Because of the apparent similarities between tai chi and qigong, the researchers reviewed the literature on both practices together. The review, conducted by the Institute of Integral Qigong and Tai Chi (Santa Barbara, California), Arizona State

University, and the University of North Carolina, included 77 articles reporting on 66 RCTs that included 6410 participants of tai chi and qigong. Most of the studies used a non–exercise control group, but some included a control group that practiced other forms of exercise, whereas others included both exercise and nonexercise groups as controls. They concluded that the strongest and most consistent evidence of health benefits for tai chi or qigong is for bone health, cardiopulmonary fitness, balance, and factors associated with preventing falls, quality of life, and self-efficacy (the confidence in and perceived ability to perform a behavior). They went on to suggest that tai chi and qigong are viable forms of exercise with health benefits. Because of the similarities in philosophy and critical elements between tai chi and qigong, they thought the outcomes could be analyzed across both types of studies.[86]

YOGA

With many different types of yoga being practiced today, it may be difficult for a patient to figure out which style fits them best. It is important for them to discover which type of yoga meets their needs.[88]

Research has shown a benefit to yoga practice. In one study, the yoga group significantly improved their standing balance, sit-to-stand test, 4-m walk, and one-legged stand with eyes closed, compared with control group.[89]

In another study, the post–yoga testing showed a significant decrease in the heart rate and respiratory rate. Maximum changes were seen in autonomic variables and breathing rate during the state of effortless meditation (dhyana). The changes were all suggestive of reduced sympathetic activity and/or increased vagal modulation.[90]

In a population with TBI, one study revealed that the yoga group demonstrated significant longitudinal change on measures of observed respiratory functioning as well as self-reported physical and psychological well-being over a 40-week period. The control group, on the other hand, showed marginal improvement on 2 of the 6 measures of respiratory health, physical and social functioning, emotional well-being, and general health. The small sample sizes precluded the analysis of between-group differences. This study suggests that breath-focused yoga may improve respiratory functioning and self-perceived physical and psychological well-being of adults with severe TBI.[91]

One study of yoga on poststroke patients did not find significant changes in depression or anxiety in those practicing yoga; however, they did report that comparison of individual case results was clinically relevant. Participants reported no adverse events, and the study experienced high retention of participants and high compliance in the yoga program. They concluded that yoga after stroke is a feasible, safe, and acceptable intervention, but that additional investigations with a larger sample sizes are needed.[92]

MEDITATION/MINDFULNESS

Meditation has been practiced for thousands of years and, today, is commonly used for relaxation and stress reduction. Attention is focused to help control the stream of stressful thoughts, which may result in enhanced physical and emotional well-being. Anyone can practice meditation. It is simple, does not require special equipment, and can be practiced anywhere.

Although meditation and mindfulness have been a significant part of the human experience for millennia, modern medicine has recently shown an increased interest in meditation and mindfulness, primarily due to Jon Kabat-Zinn's work on stress reduction. In a 1982 article, he described a 10-week stress reduction and relaxation program to train chronic pain patients in self-regulation. He reported on 51 chronic pain patients who had not improved despite given modern medical interventions. At the end of the 10 weeks, he noted 65% showed a reduction of $\geq$33% in mean total pain rating, whereas 50% showed a reduction of $\geq$50%. He also reported improvement in mood and psychiatric symptoms.[93]

One study used fMRI to assess the neural mechanisms by which mindfulness meditation influences pain in healthy human participants. Each participant underwent a 4-day training period where they learned mindfulness meditation techniques. A painful stimulus was applied at rest, to establish a baseline, and then was applied again while they were practicing the mindfulness meditation they were taught. The study found a reduction in the pain unpleasantness by 57% and pain intensity ratings by 40% when the participants were practicing mindfulness meditation. The fMRI was then reviewed, and they found that meditation reduced pain-related activation of the contralateral primary somatosensory cortex. In addition, meditation-induced reductions in pain intensity ratings were associated with increased activity in the anterior cingulate cortex and anterior insula, areas involved in the cognitive regulation of nociceptive processing. Reductions in pain unpleasantness ratings were associated with orbitofrontal cortex activation, an area implicated in reframing the contextual evaluation of sensory events. The drop in pain unpleasantness seemed to be associated with thalamic deactivation. They thought this might reflect a limbic gating mechanism involved in modifying interactions between afferent input and executive-order brain areas. This study seemed to show that meditation engages multiple brain mechanisms that may alter the pain experience from the afferent information.[94]

Mindfulness practice in individuals with a TBI history has been shown to improve quality of life in both 10- and 12-week pilot programs; the latter study showed improvements were maintained at a 1-year follow-up.[95,96] Furthermore, other relaxation techniques reduced the number of symptoms and improved performance on cognitive tests among college students with mild TBI.[97]

Veterans enrolled in the Mindfulness Based Stress Reduction program who were diagnosed with PTSD showed a reduction in PTSD symptoms and specifically showed increases in Acting With Awareness and Non-Reactivity. They also noted increases in mindfulness were strongly related to decreases in Hyperarousal and Emotional Numbing.[98]

Mantram repetition has been shown in 2 RCTs to assist in managing psychological distress in HIV patients and to reduce symptoms in self-reported and clinician-rated posttraumatic stress syndrome symptom severity.[99,100]

In RCTs on the efficacy of mantram repetition in Veterans with PTSD, findings have shown significant and clinically meaningful reductions in PTSD symptom severity and hyperarousal as well as reported improvements in interpersonal relationships, mindful attention awareness, and spiritual well-being.[101–103]

SUMMARY

Integrative medicine is more accurately described as an approach to the delivery of health care, not as a separate entity in and of itself. In fact, many think that Integrative Medicine is the way all medical care, not just rehabilitation, will be in the future. Although it often incorporates many complementary practices, the key is a patient-centered integrative approach that includes all health and wellness practices that best serve each individual.

REFERENCES

1. Osher Center for Integrative Medicine. 2012. Available at: http://www.osher.ucsf.edu/. Accessed June 18, 2016.
2. Gahche J, Bailey R, Burt V, et al. Dietary supplement use among U.S. adults has increased since NHANES III (1988–1994). NCHS Data Brief 2011;(61):1–8.
3. Bornhord K, Quante M, Blauche V, et al. Painful stimuli evoke different stimulus-response functions in the amygdala, prefrontal, insula and somatosensory cortex: a single-trial fMRI study. Brain 2002;125:1326–36.
4. Jasmin L, Rabkin SD, Granato A, et al. Analgesia and hyperalgesia from GABA-mediated modulation of the cerebral cortex. Nature 2003;424:316–20.
5. Bingel U, Quante M, Knab R, et al. Subcortical structures involved in pain processing: evidence from single-trail fMRI. Pain 2002;99(1-2):313–21.
6. Zald DH. The human amygdala and the emotional evaluation of sensory stimuli. Brain Res Rev 2003;41:88–123.
7. Hui K, Liu J, Chen A. Effects of acupuncture on human limbic system and basal ganglia measured by fMRI. Neuroimage 1997;5:226.
8. Hui KK, Liu J, Makris N, et al. Acupuncture modulates the limbic system and subcortical gray structures of the human brain: evidence from fMRI studies in normal subjects. Hum Bran Mapp 2000;9:13–25.
9. Wu MT, Hsieh JC, Xiong J, et al. Central nervous pathway for acupuncture stimulation: localization of processing with functional MR imaging of the brain—preliminary experience. Radiology 1999;212:133–41.
10. Wu MT, Sheen JM, Chuang KH, et al. Neuronal specificity of acupuncture response: a fMRI study with electroacupuncture. Neuroimage 2002;16:1028–37.
11. Zhang WT, Jin Z, Cui GH, et al. Relations between brain network activation and analgesic effect induced by low vs. high frequency electrical acupoint stimulation in different subjects: a functional magnetic resonance imaging study. Brain Res 2003;982:168–78.
12. Ahsin S, Saleem S, Bhatti AM, et al. Clinical and endocrinological changes after electro-acupuncture treatment in patients with osteoarthritis of the knee. Pain 2009;147:60–6.
13. Langevin HM, Yandow JA. Relationship of acupuncture points and meridians to connective tissue planes. Anat Rec 2002;269:257–65.
14. Wong V, Cheuk DK, Lee S, et al. Acupuncture for acute management and rehabilitation of traumatic brain injury. Cochrane Database Syst Rev 2011;(5):CD007700.
15. Linde K, Allais G, Brinkhaus B, et al. Acupuncture for the prevention of tension-type headaches. Cochrane Database Syst Rev 2016;4:CD007587.
16. Linde K, Allais G, Brinkhaus B, et al. Acupuncture for migraine prophylaxis. Cochrane Database Syst Rev 2009;(1):CD001218.
17. Bingel U, Quante M, Knab R, et al. Subcortical structures involved in pain processing: evidence from single-trail fMRI. Pain 2002;99:313–21.
18. Ernst E, Lee MS. Acupuncture for rheumatic conditions: an overview of systematic reviews. Rheumatology 2010;49(10):1957–61.
19. Haake M, Muller HH, Schade-Brittinger C, et al. German acupuncture trials (GERAC) for chronic low back pain: randomized, multicenter, blinded, parallel-group trial 3 groups. Arch Intern Med 2007;167(17):1892–8.
20. Fink M, Wolkenstein E, Karst M, et al. Acupuncture in chronic epicondylitis: a randomized controlled trial. Rheumatology 2002;41(2):205–9.
21. Johansson K, Bergstrom A, Schroder K, et al. Subacromial corticosteroid injection or acupuncture with home exercises when treating patients with

subacromial impingement in primary care—a randomized clinical trial. Fam Pract 2011;28(4):355–65.

22. Linde K, Allais G, Brinkhaus B, et al. Acupuncture for migraine prophylaxis. Cochrane Database Syst Rev 2009;(1):CD001218.

23. Carlsson CP, Axemo P, Bodin A, et al. Manual acupuncture reduces hyperemesis gravidarum: a placebo-controlled, randomized, single-blind, crossover study. J Pain Symptom Manage 2000;20(4):273–9.

24. Lee A, Done ML. The use of nonpharmacologic techniques to prevent postoperative nausea and vomiting: a meta-analysis. Anesth Analg 1999;88(6):1362–9.

25. Lim SM, Yoo J, Lee E, et al. Acupuncture for spasticity after stroke: a systematic review and meta-analysis of randomized controlled trials. Evid Based Complement Alternat Med 2015;2015:870398.

26. Lim SM, Yoo J, Lee E, et al. Acupuncture for spasticity after stroke: a systematic review and meta-analysis of randomized controlled trials. Evid Based Complement Alternat Med 2015;2015:870398.

27. Kim YD, Heo I, Shin BC, et al. Acupuncture for posttraumatic stress disorder: a systematic review of randomized controlled trials and prospective clinical trials. Evid Based Complement Alternat Med 2013;2013:615857.

28. Scrimgeour AG, Condlin ML. Nutritional treatment for traumatic brain injury. J Neurotrauma 2014;31:989–99.

29. Wang T, Van KC, Gavitt BJ, et al. Effect of fish oil supplementation in a rat model of multiple mild traumatic brain injuries. Restor Neurol Neurosci 2013;31(5):647–59.

30. Tur JA, Bibiloni MM, Sureda A, et al. Dietary sources of omega 3 fatty acids: public health risks and benefits. Br J Nutr 2012;107(Suppl 2):S23–52.

31. Bazan NG, Molina MF, Gordon WC. Docosahexaenoic acid signalolipidomics in nutrition: significance in aging, neuroinflammation, macular degeneration, Alzheimer's, and other neurodegenerative diseases. Annu Rev Nutr 2011;31:321–51.

32. Hasadsri L, Wang BH, Lee JV, et al. Omega-3 fatty acids as a putative treatment for traumatic brain injury. J Neurotrauma 2013;30(11):897–906.

33. Mills JD, Hadley K, Bailes JE. Dietary supplementation with the omega-3 fatty acid docosahexaenoic acid in traumatic brain injury. Neurosurgery 2011;68(2):474–81.

34. Gower-Winter SD, Levenson CW. Zinc in the central nervous system: from molecules to behavior. Biofactors 2012;38:186–93.

35. Suh SW, Won SJ, Hamby AM, et al. Decreased brain zinc availability reduces hippocampal neurogenesis in mice and rats. J Cereb Blood Flow Metab 2009;29:1579–86.

36. Cho E, Hwang JJ, Han SH, et al. Endogenous zinc mediates apoptotic programmed cell death in the developing brain. Neurotox Res 2010;17:156–66.

37. Morris DR, Levenson CW. Zinc in traumatic brain injury: from neuroprotection to neurotoxicity. Curr Opin Clin Nutr Metab Care 2013;16:708–11.

38. Choi BY, Kim JH, Kim HJ, et al. Zinc chelation reduces traumatic brain injury-induced neurogenesis in the subgranular zone of the hippocampal dentate gyrus. J Trace Elem Med Biol 2014;28(4):474–81.

39. Jamall OA, Feeney C, Zaw-Linn J, et al. Prevalence and correlates of vitamin D deficiency in adults after traumatic brain injury. Clin Endocrinol (oxf) 2016;85(4):636–44.

40. Aminmansour B, Nikbakht H, Ghorbani A, et al. Comparison of the administration of progesterone versus progesterone and vitamin D in improvement of outcomes in patients with traumatic brain injury: a randomized clinical trial with placebo group. Adv Biomed Res 2012;1:58.

41. Maiese K, Chong ZZ, Hou J, et al. The vitamin nicotinamide: translating nutrition into clinical care. Molecules 2009;14(9):3446–85.
42. Hoane MR, Gilbert DR, Holland MA, et al. Nicotinamide reduces acute cortical neuronal death and edema in the traumatically injured brain. Neurosci Lett 2006; 408:35–9.
43. Hoane MR, Kaplan SA, Ellis AL. The effects of nicotinamide on apoptosis and blood-brain barrier breakdown following traumatic brain injury. Brain Res 2006;1125:185–93.
44. Holland MA, Tan AA, Smith DC, et al. Nicotinamide treatment provides acute neuroprotection and GFAP regulation following fluid percussion injury. J Neurotrauma 2008;25(2):140–52.
45. Vonder Haar C, Peterson TC, Martens KM, et al. Vitamins and nutrients as primary treatments in experimental brain injury: clinical implications for nutraceutical therapies. Brain Res 2016;1640:114–29.
46. Hoane MR, Pierce JL, Holland MA, et al. Nicotinamide treatment induces behavioral recovery when administered up to 4 hours following cortical contusion injury in the rat. Neuroscience 2008;154(3):861–8.
47. Swan AA, Chandrashekar R, Beare J, et al. Preclinical efficacy testing in middle-aged rats: nicotinamide, a novel neuroprotectant, demonstrates diminished preclinical efficacy after controlled cortical impact. J Neurotrauma 2011;28(3): 431–40.
48. Shear DA, Dixon CE, Bramlett HM, et al. Nicotinamide treatment in traumatic brain injury: operation brain trauma therapy. J Neurotrauma 2016;33(6):523–37.
49. Wu A, Ying Z, Gomez-Pinilla F. Vitamin E protects against oxidative damage and learning disability after mild traumatic brain injury in rats. Neurorehabil Neural Repair 2010;24(3):290–8.
50. Ishaq GM, Saidu Y, Bilbis LS, et al. Effects of a-tocopherol and ascorbic acid in the severity and management of traumatic brain injury in albino rats. J Neurosci Rural Pract 2013;4(3):292–7.
51. Razmkon A, Sadidi A, Sherafat-Kazemzadeh E, et al. Administration of vitamin C and vitamin E in severe head injury: a randomized double-blind controlled trial. Clin Neurosurg 2011;58:133–7.
52. Adhihetty P, Beal M. Creatine and its potential therapeutic value for targeting cellular energy impairment in neurodegenerative diseases. Neuromolecular Med 2008;10(4):275–90.
53. Braissant O. Creatine and guanidinoacetate transport at blood-brain and blood-cerebrospinal fluid barriers. J Inherit Metab Dis 2012;35(4):655–64.
54. Beal MF. Neuroprotective effects of creatine. Amino Acids 2011;40(5):1305–13.
55. Andres RH, Ducray AD, Schlattner U, et al. Functions and effects of creatine in the central nervous system. Brain Res Bull 2008;76:329–43.
56. Wallimann T, Wyss M, Brdiczka D, et al. Intracellular compartmentation, structure and function of creatine kinase isoenzymes in tissues with high and fluctuating energy demands: the 'phosphocreatine circuit' for cellular energy homeostasis. Biochem 1992;281:21–40.
57. Sullivan P, Geiger J, Mattson M, et al. Dietary supplement creatine protects against traumatic brain injury. Ann Neurol 2000;48(5):723–9.
58. Dolder M, Walzel B, Speer O, et al. Inhibition of the mitochondrial permeability transition by creatine kinase substrates: requirement for microcompartmentation. J Biol Chem 2003;278:17760–6.
59. Sestili P, Martinelli C, Colombo E, et al. Creatine as an antioxidant. Amino Acids 2011;40:1385–96.

60. Mazzeo A, Beat A, Singh A, et al. The role of mitochondrial transition pore, and its modulation, in traumatic brain injury and delayed neurodegeneration after TBI. Exp Neurol 2009;218(2):363–70.

61. Meyer LE, Machado LB, Santiago AP, et al. Mitochondrial creatine kinase activity prevents reactive oxygen species generation: antioxidant role of mitochondrial kinase-dependent ADP re-cycling activity. J Biol Chem 2006;281(49): 37361–71.

62. Braissant O, Henry H, Beard E, et al. Creatine deficiency syndromes and the importance of creatine synthesis in the brain. Amino Acids 2011;40:1315–24.

63. Watanabe A, Kato N, Kato T. Effects of creatine on mental fatigue and cerebral hemoglobin oxygenation. NeuroScience Res 2002;42:279–85.

64. McMorris T, Harris R, Swain J, et al. Effect of creatine supplementation and sleep deprivation, with mild exercise, on cognitive and psychomotor performance, mood state, and plasma concentrations of catecholamines and cortisol. Psychopharmacology (Berl) 2006;185(1):93–103.

65. Rae C, Digney AL, McEwan SR, et al. Oral creatine monohydrate supplementation improves brain performance: a double-blind, placebo-controlled, crossover trial. Proc R Soc Lond B 2003;270(1529):2147–50.

66. Ling J, Kritikos M, Tiplady B. Cognitive effects of creatine ethyl ester supplementation. Pharmacology 2009;20(8):673–9.

67. Signoretti S, Di Pietro V, Vagnozzi R, et al. Transient alterations of creatine, creatine phosphate, N-acetylaspartate and high-energy phosphates after mild traumatic brain injury in the rat. Mol Cell Biochem 2010;333(1–2):269–77.

68. Yang MS, DeWitt DS, Becker DP, et al. Regional brain metabolite levels following mild experimental head injury in the cat. J Neurosurg 1985;63(4):617–21.

69. Scheff S, Dhillon H. Creatine-enhanced diet alters levels of lactate and free fatty acids after experimental brain injury. Neurochem Res 2004;29(2):469–79.

70. Saraiva AL, Ferreira AP, Silva LF, et al. Creatine reduces oxidative stress markers but does not protect against seizure susceptibility after severe traumatic brain injury. Brain Res Bull 2012;87(2–3):180–6.

71. Skellaris G, Kotsiou D, Tamiolak M, et al. Prevention of complications related to traumatic brain injury in children and adolescents with creatine administration: an open label randomized pilot study. J Trauma 2006;61(2):322–9.

72. Skellaris G, Nasis G, Kotsiou M, et al. Prevention of traumatic headache, dizziness, and fatigue with creatine administration. A pilot study. Acta Paediatr 2008; 97(1):31–4.

73. Zhu H, Bian C, Yuan J, et al. Curcumin attenuates acute inflammatory injury by inhibiting the TLR4/MyD88/NF-kB signaling pathway in experimental traumatic brain injury. J Neuroinflammation 2014;11:59.

74. Sharma S, Zhuang Y, Ying Z, et al. Dietary curcumin supplementation counteracts reduction in levels of molecules involved in energy homeostasis after brain trauma. Neuroscience 2009;161(4):1037–44.

75. Wu A, Ying Z, Schubert D, et al. Brain and spinal cord interaction: a dietary curcumin derivative counteracts locomotor and cognitive deficits after brain trauma. Neurorehabil Neural Repair 2011;25(4):332–42.

76. Yu L, Fan Y, Ye G, et al. Curcumin inhibits apoptosis and brain edema induced by hypoxia-hypercapnia brain damage in rat models. Am J Med Sci 2015; 349(6):521–5.

77. Wang CW, Chan CLW, Ho RTH, et al. The effect of qigong on depressive and anxiety symptoms: a systematic review and meta-analysis of randomized controlled trials. Evid Based Complement Alternat Med 2013;2013:716094.

78. Oh B, Butow P, Mullan B, et al. Impact of medical qigong on quality of life, fatigue, mood and inflammation in cancer patients: a randomized controlled trial. Ann Oncol 2010;21:608–14.
79. Lynch M, Sawynok J, Kiew C, et al. A randomized controlled trial of qigong for fibromyalgia. Arth Res Ther 2012;14:R178.
80. Lauch R, Cramer H, Hauser W, et al. A systematic review and meta-analysis of qigong for fibromyalgia syndrome. Evid Based Complement Alternat Med 2013; 2013:635182.
81. Li F, Harmer P, Fitzgerald K, et al. Tai chi and postural stability in patients with Parkinson's disease. N Engl J Med 2012;366(6):511–9.
82. Tsang WW. Tai chi training is effective in reducing balance impairments and falls in patients with Parkinson's disease. J Physiother 2013;59(1):55.
83. Gao Q, Leung A, Yang Y, et al. Effects of tai chi on balance and fall prevention in Parkinson's disease: a randomized controlled trial. Clin Rehabil 2014;28(8): 748–53.
84. Mańko G, Ziolkowski A, Mirski A, et al. The effectiveness of selected tai chi exercise in a program of strategic rehabilitation aimed at improving the self-care skills of patients aroused from prolonged coma after severe TBI. Med Sci Moni 2013;19:767–72.
85. Wei GX, Xu T, Fan FM, et al. Can tia chi reshape the brain? A brain morphometry study. PLoS One 2013;8(4):e61038.
86. Jahnke R, Larkey L, Rogers C, et al. A comprehensive review of health benefits of qigong and tai chi. Am J Health Promot 2010;24(6):e1–25.
87. Wang C. Tai chi and rheumatic diseases. Rheum Dis Clin North Am 2011;37(1): 19–32.
88. Available at: http://www.dailycupofyoga.com/2012/06/09/5-different-types-of-yoga-which-one-suits-you-the-best/. Accessed June 18, 2016.
89. Tiedemann A, O'Rourke S, Sesto R, et al. 12 week Iyengar yoga program improved balance and mobility in older community-dwelling people: a pilot randomized controlled trial. J Gerontol A Biol Sci Med Sci 2013;68(9):1068–75.
90. Telles S, Raghavendra BR, Naveen KV, et al. Changes in autonomic variables following two meditative states described in yoga texts. J Altern Complement Med 2013;19(1):35–42.
91. Silverthorne C, Khalsa SB, Gueth R, et al. Respiratory, physical, and psychological benefits of breath-focused yoga for adults with severe traumatic brain injury (TBI): a brief pilot study report. Int J Yoga Therap 2012;22:47–51.
92. Chan W, Immink MA, Hillier S. Yoga and exercise for symptoms of depression and anxiety in people with post-stroke disability: a randomized, controlled pilot trial. Altern Ther Health Med 2012;18(3):34–43.
93. Kabat-Zinn J. Chronic pain patients based on the practice of mindfulness meditation: theoretical consideration and preliminary results. Gen Hosp Psychiatry 1982;4:33–47.
94. Zeidan F, Martucci KT, Kraft RA, et al. Brain mechanisms supporting the modulation of pain by mindfulness meditation. J Neurosci 2011;31(14):5540–8.
95. Azulay J, Smart CM, Mott T, et al. A pilot study examining the effect of mindfulness-based stress reduction on symptoms of chronic mild traumatic brain injury/post-concussive syndrome. J Head Trauma Rehabil 2013;28(4): 323–31.
96. Bedard M, Felteau M, Mazmanian D, et al. Pilot evaluation of a mindfulness-based intervention to improve quality of life among individuals who sustained traumatic brain injuries. Disabil Rehabil 2003;25(13):722–31.

97. Hanna-Pladdy B, Berry ZM, Bennett T, et al. Stress as a diagnostic challenge for postconcussive symptoms: sequelae of mild traumatic brain injury or physiological stress response. Clin Neuropsychol 2001;15(3):289–304.

98. Stephenson KR, Simpson TL, Martinez ME, et al. Changes in mindfulness and posttraumatic stress disorder symptoms among veterans enrolled in mindfulness-based stress reduction. J Clin Psychol 2017;73(3):201–17.

99. Bormann JE, Thorp SR, Wetherell JL, et al. Meditation-based mantram intervention for the veterans with posttraumatic stress disorder: a randomized trial. Psychol Trauma 2013;5(3):259–67.

100. Bormann JE, Gifford AL, Shively M, et al. Effects of spiritual mantram repetition on HIV outcomes: a randomized controlled trial. J Behav Med 2006;29(4): 359–76.

101. Oman D, Bormann JE. Mantram repetition fosters self- efficacy in veterans for managing PTSD: a randomized trial. Psychol Relig Spirituality 2015;7(1):34.

102. Bormann J, Liu L, Thorp S, et al. Spiritual wellbeing mediates PTSD change in veterans with military-related PTSD. Int J Behav Med 2012;19(4):496–502.

103. Bormann JE, Thorp S, Wetherell JL, et al. Meditation-based mantram intervention for veterans with posttraumatic stress disorder: a randomized trial. Psychol Trauma 2013;5(3):259.

Medicolegal Issues in Traumatic Brain Injury

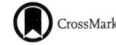

Nathan D. Zasler, MD, FAAPM&R, FACRM, BIM-C, FIAIME, DAIPM, CBIST[a,b,c,d,e,]*, Erin Bigler, PhD[f]

KEYWORDS

- Physical medicine and rehabilitation • Physiatry • Independent medical evaluation
- Neuropsychology • Neuroimaging • Medicolegal

KEY POINTS

- Medicolegal expert testimony in cases involving TBI requires a different skill base than clinical practice.
- Physiatrists involved in medicolegal work involving TBI cases must understand the ethical, legal, and business caveats that come with such undertakings and their disparities from standard clinical practice.
- The standards for assessment and diagnostic formulation in medicolegal work involving persons with TBI must meet current standards of community practice and opinion and medicolegal testimony (ie, Daubert standards).
- Physiatric examiners must understand and appropriately use medicolegal terminology.
- When providing expert testimony in cases involving TBI, the physiatric examiner must understand how to incorporate preinjury, injury, and postinjury information, the latter including but not limited to neurodiagnostics and neuropsychological testing, into their diagnostic formulations and opinions regarding apportionment and causality.

INTRODUCTION

Physiatrists involved in the medicolegal assessment of persons with traumatic brain injury (TBI) have many challenges facing them including but not limited to (1) how to fully assess the causality, apportionment, and impact of the myriad impairments that may occur after such injuries, direct and indirect; (2) how to ensure that the examinee provides optimal effort and valid performance; (3) how to formulate opinions to

Disclosure Statement: Both authors are engaged in medicolegal consultation as part of their overall professional practice and receive monies for same.
[a] Concussion Care Centre of Virginia, Ltd, 3721 Westerre Parkway, Suite B, Richmond, VA 23233, USA; [b] Tree of Life Services, Inc, Richmond, VA, USA; [c] Department of Physical Medicine and Rehabilitation, Virginia Commonwealth University, Richmond, VA, USA; [d] Department of Physical Medicine and Rehabilitation, University of Virginia, Charlottesville, VA, USA; [e] IBIA; [f] Brigham Young University, 1001 Kimball Tower, Provo, UT 84602, USA
* Corresponding author. C/O Concussion Care Centre of Virginia, 3721 Westerre Parkway, Suite B, Richmond, VA 23233.
E-mail address: nzasler@cccv-ltd.com

Phys Med Rehabil Clin N Am 28 (2017) 379–391
http://dx.doi.org/10.1016/j.pmr.2016.12.012
1047-9651/17/© 2016 Elsevier Inc. All rights reserved.

pmr.theclinics.com

provide the necessary assistance that the triers of fact in the case require; (4) how to strive to maintain neutrality and ethical practice in an adversarial environment ripe with nonobjective influences and potential for bias; and (5) how to provide a holistic bio-psychosocial analysis of the case while acknowledging any limitations, as they may exist, in the data, analysis, and/or conclusions.

The formal medicolegal evaluation or so-called independent medical evaluation (IME) provides an opportunity for a nontreating physiatrist to perform an assessment of an individual for purposes of opining on a potential wide range of issues emanating from a claimed TBI. Within that context the physician must know how to take a thorough and relevant history, perform a relevant hands-on evaluation, review all neurodiagnostics (including neuropsychological and neuroimaging evaluations), and generate a report that addresses the claimed TBI related consequences (discussed later).

CONTROVERSIES AND CAVEATS

Traditional IME training, regardless of the specialty organization responsible for said training, holds that there is no physician-patient relationship in the context of an IME.[1] In this context, the physician becomes the examiner and the person being assessed, the examinee. It should also be noted that an examiner-examinee relationship in the absence of a treating relationship would dictate that the examiner not share opinions regarding their examination findings and/or conclusions. The party who retained the examiner to conduct the IME should be the only person or persons receiving such information. Traditional training also dictates an absence of confidentiality in such a setting (ie, if the examinee tells you they murdered someone then you have the legal and ethical responsibility to report what was conveyed).[1] It is also important to remember that the IME document is privileged and should only be released to the requesting agency unless otherwise appropriately subpoenaed.

Some organizations' IME ethical guidelines run contrary to the espoused traditional practices.[2] For example, the American Medical Association (AMA) has stipulated that there is a limited patient-physician relationship in the context of an IME.[3] Additionally, the AMA code further edified that one had to maintain patient confidentiality as outlined in Opinion 5.09 dealing with IMEs, which specifically stipulates that confidentiality is to be maintained as with any other "patient" except as "required by law."[4] The AMA ethics code further directs physicians involved in IMEs to "disclose fully potential or perceived conflicts of interest," noting: "The physician should inform the patient about the terms of the agreement between himself or herself and the third party, as well as the fact that he or she is acting as an agent of that entity." The authors have concerns about stipulating that one is an agent for the retaining party given the implications of advocacy for said party when one's role by definition should be neutral as a nonadvocate for any side involved in the litigation.

Physiatrists are often challenged to apply general clinical ethics to unfamiliar medicolegal situations. Many organizations offer their own versions of board certification. The criteria for attainment of these certifications vary from merely paying a fee, to a requirement for formal training, practical experience, and written and/or oral examination. Board certification and at a minimum board eligibility should serve as the foundation for providing any medicolegal testimony. Further subspecialty certifications, such as the American Board of Physical Medicine and Rehabilitation Brain Injury Medicine Certification can further bolster one's credentials if testifying on TBI-related cases. Other organizational certifications may be of value in the context of learning IME practice nuances but one should carefully investigate the organization's reputation and scope of training, and membership and certification requirements. Experience, training, and additional credentials including publication and speaking record can serve an expert well in terms of knowledge base and ultimately being accepted by the court to meet "expert" criteria.

The potential liability that an examiner may have for opinions expressed in the context of the examination and/or for any real or claimed psychological or physical injury that the examinee may have sustained in the examination process is rarely considered by medical practitioners. Clinicians are not immune to legal action for work performed in the context of such evaluations and should ensure that their medical malpractice insurance specifically covers all dimensions of their medicolegal practice. Practitioners must also realize that IMEs are generally viewed by State Medical Boards as constituting the practice of medicine; therefore, performing IMEs or testifying in states where one is not licensed puts one at risk for being charged and even convicted of practicing medicine without a license.

THE MEDICOLEGAL EXAMINATION: AN OVERVIEW

The general requirement for ensuring ethical conduct in any form of medicolegal evaluation is rendered even more imperative when confronted by the complex, often subtle range of impairments and associated disability that may occur after TBI, particularly when more mild. The evaluator must be cognizant of the relative attribution of postinjury impairment to the TBI itself versus comorbid conditions including but not limited to posttraumatic psychological, musculoskeletal, and/or peripheral neurologic disorders. It should be understood that in most cases the IME occurs as a one-time event, thereby necessitating as complete an assessment as feasible in the context of the time permitted, which often is limited by opposing counsel and/or the court. Setting the assessment standards high by adhering to ethical conduct while using evidence-based assessment methodologies that meet current consensus practice standards should be every expert physiatrist's goal.[5]

Evaluators are expected to provide equal measures of respect to the examinee including courtesy, dignity, and fairness and spend adequate time in the assessment process. Certain forms of assessment may need to be provocative, either psychologically or physically, to evoke symptoms and/or signs relevant to making diagnostic formulations in a case. In this context, testing should always be performed for symptom and sign validity, performance validity, effort, and response bias to ensure that the presentation and testing results accurately reflect the examinee's condition. Experts should keep in mind that depending on the evaluation circumstances examinees may overreport, underreport, and accurately report their symptoms and some may do a combination of the aforementioned, consciously and/or unconsciously.

In common with the judiciary, the duty of impartiality is owed equally to all litigating parties. It is the evaluator's task to conduct the evaluation in a fair manner and to present the results fully and objectively without advocacy for any party involved. The expert, first and foremost, remains a physician and should follow the Hippocratic Oath at all times.

MEDICOLEGAL TERMINOLOGY

Several terms and phrases are unique to the world of clinicolegal practice that should be familiar to anyone who serves as an expert witness.[6]

- Aggravation: a permanent worsening of a pre-existing impairment/condition.
- Apportionment: the act of assigning responsibility of a particular event or injury to a certain proportion or percentage of an examinee's particular impairment.

- Causality: the act of relating a particular consequence, such as an impairment, to a specific event or set of events in time.
- Exacerbation: a temporary worsening of a pre-existing impairment/condition.
- Maximum medical improvement: therapy phraseology that emanates from Worker's Compensation literature in the AMA Guides to Evaluation of Permanent Impairment, the meaning of which has evolved over time and remains consensus as opposed to evidence based.[7] In the sixth edition of the Guides to Evaluation of Permanent Impairment, it is conceptualized as "a date from which further recovery or deterioration is not anticipated, although over time (beyond 12 months) there may be some expected change." It is important to note if there is potential for future improvement and/or decline depending on the nature of the specific injury and impairments (ie, poorly controlled epilepsy).
- Medical probability: the statistical likelihood that the medical event in question is more likely than not (greater than 50%) going to occur or occurred because of a particular event, which is different from the traditional levels of "significance" used in hypothesis testing (ie, .01 level of significance).

ETHICAL CAVEATS

The American Academy of Physical Medicine and Rehabilitation published a white paper with recommendations for expert witness testimony.[8] There has been no updated version of this document published since its initial release. This document indicates that the expert witness should serve to educate the court as a whole, rather than representing one side or the other, independent of which side retained the expert. The ultimate test for accuracy and impartiality is whether reports or testimony could be presented without alteration for use by either the plaintiff or the defendant.

Three additional recommendations are emphasized: (1) identification of opinions that are personal and not necessarily held by other physicians, (2) making a clear distinction between medical malpractice and medical maloccurrence when analyzing case evidence, and (3) willingness to submit transcripts of depositions and/or courtroom testimony for peer review.

The role of the evaluator should be passive in relationship to the evaluee and his/her family. The evaluator neither seeks nor accepts any duty of care, and must explicitly, firmly, and unambiguously discourage any expectation of or request for care. Avoiding conflicts between differing professional roles is equally important given the potential for compromising objectivity and credibility.[9]

The main ethical caveats in the context of providing testimony on cases involving TBI should include the following:

- Substantive experience in the area in which one is to testify
- Limitation of testimony to one's sphere of medical expertise
- Professional conduct, including language, at all times
- Maintaining a nonadvocacy position
- Provision of findings that are favorable and unfavorable with regards to the case in question
- Avoidance of mixing expert roles
- Avoidance of adversarial posturing
- Address the science behind the opinions and not those persons providing the opinions (ie, avoid denigration of fellow professionals)
- Avoid scenarios with potential conflict of interest (by perception or in reality)
- Remain objective and unbiased at all times

- Charge for your time as an expert not for the activity you are engaged in
- Save all notes and testing generated during the IME

REVIEW OF EXPERT ROLES IN MEDICOLEGAL CASES

Relevant to physicians and other professionals, Blau[10] identified three different and conflicting roles for professionals working in medicolegal settings: (1) treating doctor, (2) expert witness, and (3) trial consultant. Great caution should be taken to avoid engaging in more than one of these roles in a particular case; however, treating doctors are often asked by lawyers to serve as experts to save on expenses. Each role has a unique set of responsibilities that, because of conflicting expectancies and pressures, increases risk of compromising objectivity. Every effort should be made to avoid placing the practitioner in a conflictual relationship with their patient and with their own practice ethics because one must be an advocate for their patient and cannot therefore be "neutral" as a treater/expert.

A further role existing in some circumstances is that of "peer or case reviewer." This professional is retained to review the case evidence without direct assessment of the evaluee (evidentiary review), and/or to critically evaluate the opinions in the case. Not all clinicians are comfortable with performing a strictly evidentiary review and offering expert opinions about a claimant or a peer based solely on documentation without interview or direct evaluation. Some practitioners stipulate that their peer review work product should be used only for internal review purposes and not proffered for medicolegal purposes.

INDEPENDENT MEDICAL EVALUATION TIPS FOR TRAUMATIC BRAIN INJURY CASES

- Always obtain a retention letter and a signed retention/consultative agreement.
- Always make sure you request clear documentation as to why you are being retained and what specifically you are being asked to do.
- Establish ground rules with all sides before the examination/evaluation.
- Have the examinee sign a consent for evaluation, photography, and videography, as relevant, and a document stipulating the expectancies from them as the examinee (ie, be honest, cooperative, and put forth full effort).
- Strive to use standardized, objective, normed, and generally accepted evaluation tools/examinations in the context of the evaluation including tests of effort; response bias; and sign, symptom, and performance validity.
- Always request an opportunity to talk with corroboratory sources.
- Avoid third-party observers given their potential to denigrate examinee performance and when not possible acknowledge the potential negatives of same in the IME report.[11,12]
- Avoid pejorative language in the context of direct assessment and/or in the report itself.

THE INDEPENDENT MEDICAL EVALUATION EXAMINATION

Every effort should be made to optimize examinee performance during an IME. These evaluations can be anxiety provoking particularly when seen by an expert physician retained by opposing counsel. It is therefore of utmost importance to make sure the examinee knows that the examiner is there to advocate for the truth and not for any party involved in the litigation process. Making sure that there is consent given for the evaluation by the examinee or their guardian and that the examinee and/or guardian fully understand what is involved in the evaluation process should be a priority from the first moments of the encounter. Examinees should be educated to ask questions if they are unclear on any directions during the examination and to inform the examiner if they require a break, need to take medications, or are having discomfort because of an examination procedure.

The examiner should make every effort to obtain as complete a history as possible from the person being assessed and corroboratory sources. The latter is often not permitted by opposing counsel when conducting defense examinations but remains no less critical in that context. The history taken must include preinjury, injury, and postinjury information. It is equally imperative to clarify all potentially relevant comorbidities, especially social/situational stressors that may or may not be injury related, nonrestorative sleep, pain issues, over-the-counter and prescription medication prescription history, drug treatment response history and side effects, and any substance use/abuse, among other historically relevant points. The examinee and appropriate corroboratory sources should be interviewed to determine what the claimed impairments are deemed to be by them that are consequential to the TBI being litigated. As much information as possible should be obtained about the initial injury and details regarding same, timing of symptom and sign onset, changes over time, response to treatment, compliance with said treatment, and current status and functional limitations. Information regarding functional limitations with activities of daily living (basic and higher level), mobility, communication, psychosocial function, sexuality, cognition, behavior/personality, avocational pursuits, and work should all be explored.[1,13,14]

A complete elemental neurologic examination should be performed including standardized and normed measures of cognitive and behavioral function. Any medicolegal assessment should consider for effort, response biases, and sign and symptom validity.[1,15,16] Examiners should also use relevant assessment tools that address functional abilities germane to the examinee's level of neurologic impairment, such as the Functional Independence Measure, Disability Rating Scale, Coma Recovery Scale Revised. For cases involving mild TBI, the expert should be aware of current forensic neuropsychiatric issues germane to this group of patients.[17,18] The examiner should review all questionnaires and tests to make sure they are fully completed.

THE INDEPENDENT MEDICAL EVALUATION REPORT

The report should be presented in an organized and systematic fashion including the referring source, nature of evaluation, all records reviewed, complete delineation of testing performed, and results from same (for complete transparency some examiners even include their handwritten notes).[19] **Box 1** provides the suggested areas to be included in any IME report.

EXPERT WITNESS TESTIMONY: PREPARATION AND PERFORMANCE

There are several rules that experts should adhere to with regard to providing testimony when serving as an expert witness.[20,21] These rules include the following:

- Always be prepared; review relevant documentation as needed including your notes and report before providing any testimony.
- Always expect the unexpected question (just because a question is asked does not mean you need to answer it if it is not relevant to your testimony; ie, you can refuse to answer or take the fifth).
- Be honest and if you do not know something acknowledge so.
- Be a teacher (that is educate the triers of fact on the matters of relevance in the case).

Box 1
IME content in a TBI case

Demographic details including name, address, birth date, age, sex, handedness, and social security number/license number

Referral source: name, position, company, address, telephone, fax, and email

Party responsible for payment; may be different than party that retained

Type of report (ie, IME, peer review, consultant report)

Documents requested and reviewed

Documents requested but not received at time of report issuance

History of present illness (per records and per examinee and corroboratory sources)

Past medical and mental health history

Family medical history

Psychosocial history including any history of abuse, substance use/abuse, marital history, counseling, and hobbies among other areas of inquiry

Educational history including any history of learning disability, school problems (eg, being held back, behavioral issues, failing grades)

Vocational history including current and prior jobs, physical requirements of same, and duration of employment

Military service history including duration, status of discharge, and rank achieved

Legal history, including civil and criminal, as applicable

Review of systems

Assessment including physical examination (neurologic, musculoskeletal, and related relevant systems based on injury history) and cognitive behavioral testing with inclusion of positive and negative findings and response bias, effort, and symptom, sign, and performance validity assessment results

Diagnostic impressions with identification of which are injury related, not injury related, versus possibly injury related

Maximum medical improvement status

Impairment ratings as requested (generally based on AMA Guides to Evaluation of Permanent Impairment)

Prognostic opinions regarding general status as related to TBI and as necessary broken down into specific impairment-related prognoses and return to work prognosis

Causality and apportionment opinions

Risk and restrictions as related to the injury/TBI in question

Life expectancy or median survival time opinions as requested/relevant

Recommendations for treatment or further diagnostic studies

Edification clauses focusing on caveats regarding the report content, implications, liability, and potential for altering opinions if additional information is provided

Relevant appendices

- Always ask to read your deposition, whether discovery or de bene esse.
- Always dress and present professionally for any legal proceeding.
- Avoid head nods, always speak clearly, use proper grammar, project your voice, and avoid being monotone.

- If you do not understand the question say so and/or ask for it to be rephrased.
- If you misspeak, correct yourself and remember your answer is not being timed, so think before you speak.
- Only answer the question asked, no more, no less unless you believe you are being set-up by opposing counsel, then elaborate only to clarify (if the other attorney needs you to say more they will ask you).
- Avoid becoming argumentative or confrontational with opposing counsel.
- Only testify on the basis of medical probability unless otherwise asked.
- Decline answering hypotheticals if you believe your answer will be used to confound your expert opinion.
- Always be prepared to provide a rationale and scientific explanation that meets general consensus standards in your field for each and every expert opinion you have provided.

NEUROPSYCHOLOGICAL ASSESSMENT: A PHYSIATRIC PRIMER

Cognitive and behavioral functioning may be altered in a variety of ways following a significant TBI. As outlined in Jason R. Soble and colleagues' article, "Neuropsychological Evaluation in TBI," in this issue, neuropsychology has developed and standardized methods to measure the neurobehavioral and neurocognitive sequelae associated with TBI. For the physiatrist needing to render a medicolegal opinion, it is important to know how to extract the most meaningful and objective information from a neuropsychological evaluation to render opinions regarding cognitive-behavioral impairment and implied disability.

Neuropsychology is built on the foundation comparing standardized test performance of the individual with a large normative sample.[22] Typically, an examinee's test score is referenced to a bell curve distribution as shown in **Fig. 1**. By plotting this information, the clinician can visualize how a particular cognitive score or behavioral measure compared with other individuals. As shown in **Fig. 1**, neuropsychological test scores typically are referenced as standard (mean = 100; standard deviation [SD] = 15), scaled (mean = 10; SD = 3), T- (mean = 50; SD = 10), and/or percentile scores.[22] There are several approaches to interpreting a low score:

- Deficit model: considers low scores that fall below the average or "normal" range (at or below 1 SD) as potentially reflecting impairment.

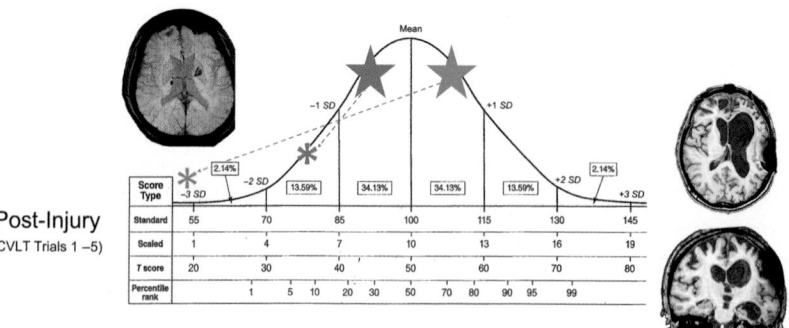

Fig. 1. Bell curve and the interpretation of neuropsychological test results. Red, severe TBI; blue, mild TBI; asterisk, actual postinjury memory score; star, baseline estimate memory; SD, standard deviation.

- Discrepancy model: considers low scores to reflect impairment if they substantially deviate from inferred premorbid ability based on educational testing and records, employment history, and anecdotal information.
- Deficit pattern model: assumes the clustering of where maximum performance occurs on various tests, or using the best performance scores permits estimating a general level of premorbid functioning and where deficits reside.

Most neuropsychologists use a combination of these approaches and other methods, but all have limitations.[22,23]

Limitations of Neuropsychological Test Findings in a Medicolegal Setting

Regardless of the approach used a major limitation of neuropsychological assessment is that currently it is not done in a naturalistic setting, which hampers the so-called ecological validity of neuropsychological test results.[24–28] For neuropsychological tests to be standardized they always have to be administered in the exact same manner, using the same questions, prompts, and queries for each test item. Given this artificiality and limits of the assessment setting, it becomes immediately apparent that some neuropsychological measures may inadequately tap real-world questions and ability to function. This is where reliable work-place information and/or input from family and colleagues who knew the person before and after injury may be instrumental.

Additionally, there is the issue of whether a patient is exhibiting maximum effort in performing the task. Underperforming on a mental measure could be interpreted as a deficit, when in fact there is not an impairment. Unfortunately, this is a complicated issue with no universal solution. In the context of a medicolegal case involving TBI measures of symptom validity testing (SVT) and performance validity testing (PVT) should be administered and specifically commented on within the neuropsychological report because whenever litigation is present the specter of secondary gain is always present. The Institute of Medicine has provided overview on this topic (http://nationalacademies.org/hmd/Activities/SelectPops/TestingSSADisability.aspx). A major interpretative challenge associated with SVT and PVT measures is that brain injury alone may alter neurologic function associated with task engagement, motivation, and task performance such that neurologically impaired patients may "fail" these measures because of the brain injury and not because of overreporting and/or underperforming as an attempt to manipulate the assessment.[29]

Possibly the biggest problem forensically in neuropsychology is that there is no agreed on neuropsychological test battery uniformly used.[30] Often, this merely provides legal fodder for active debate on which tests were used and their appropriateness for assessing the inferred impairment, if present. Legal debates like this become confusing to the triers of fact as to how different neuropsychologists can examine the same patient, ostensibly using the same or similar neuropsychological assessment instruments, yet have diametrically opposite viewpoints. Legal debates about these limitations of neuropsychological test findings can turn into endless legal tit-for-tat arguments (eg, just as they can with medical expert opinions on such issues as prognosis and life expectancy).

How can greater objectivity within a medicolegal setting be brought to the trier of fact? Fortunately, given twenty-first century neuroimaging technology, neuropsychological test findings are integrated with neuroimaging and other elements of the overall medical assessment, thereby lessening the ambiguity of clinical correlation between brain injury and outcome. Because neurocognitive and neurobehavioral sequelae may occur as a consequence of multifaceted factors, it is the author's recommendation that the best use of neuropsychological findings is integrated with a physiatric approach and contemporary neuroimaging findings. Indeed, it is our recommendation that no conclusions can be made from neuropsychological test findings without this kind of integration.

NEUROIMAGING AND NEUROPSYCHOLOGY: MEDICOLEGAL IMPLICATIONS FOR THE PHYSIATRIST

Computed tomography is most commonly performed acutely with MRI more commonly performed as a follow-up procedure.

Because frontotemporal and deep white matter neuropathologic changes associated with TBI are the most likely abnormalities to be identified by neuroimaging studies, abnormalities within these regions tend to relate to slowed processing speed, altered attention/concentration including working memory, along with impairments in episodic memory and/or executive functioning.[22] Damage to these regions may also alter emotional regulation without associated cognitive impairment. Given these relationships, in the TBI patient with positive neuroimaging identified by accepted and objective standards and impairments in one or all of those domains, clinical correlation can be established.

Unfortunately, a noncomplicated mild TBI case with negative imaging including MRI at follow-up constitutes the most challenging type of case. Neither neuroimaging or neuropsychological assessment as stand-alone procedures can diagnosis this condition. Furthermore, changes in mood, sleep disorder, chronic pain, and related medical conditions including posttraumatic stress disorder and depression may produce cognitive and neurobehavioral changes similar to what occurs after TBI, particularly when mild. As such, test findings from a neuropsychological assessment alone without other information cannot diagnosis mild TBI. The history and circumstances of the event that injures the individual, their initial signs and symptoms, and the post-injury course are the factors that define whether a TBI occurred, not some test score on a neuropsychological measure. Additionally, headache, lethargy and fatigue, apathy, and related symptoms have no specific neuropsychological assessment method for evaluation but may occur in the patient with TBI.

The physiatrist evaluating the patient after mild TBI should expect that the neuropsychological test results will generally be either subtle or nondescript and unremarkable. When it is clear that significant trauma has occurred, neurologic signs and/or symptoms have ensued consistent with a concussive brain injury, and SVT/PVT assessments are all passed, yet, the patient persists in having neurosymptoms, they may be part of the ill-defined group of patients with persistent postconcussion symptomatology (see Blessen C. Eapen and colleagues' article, "Disorders of Consciousness"; and Rebecca N. Tapia and Blessen C. Eapen's article, "Rehabilitation of Persistent Symptoms After Concussion," in this issue).

THE FUTURE OF NEUROPSYCHOLOGY AND NEUROIMAGING IN PHYSIATRIC EXPERT TESTIMONY

In the presence of traditionally identified pathology, these techniques can provide more descriptive quantitative information about the pathology.[31] However, it takes time for these techniques to be more routinely incorporated into diagnostic decision making. As outlined by a position statement from the American Society for Neuroradiology, there are emerging guidelines on how these advanced neuroimaging methods can be used in the medicolegal setting.[32] As these techniques evolve they hold promise to provide the physiatrist with additional biomarker information about the injury to the brain and how it relates to medical prognosis and outcome in TBI.

PRACTICAL RECOMMENDATIONS

Interpreting psychological test results has long been criticized as speculative when it comes to explaining behavior. Major university and medical center–based training programs in clinical neuropsychology emphasize objective and concise report writing with conclusions summarized in a few pages. Although there may be a considerable amount to discuss about a case, in TBI the questions are straightforward. Did this patient sustain a TBI? Are there neuroimaging findings consistent with having sustained a TBI? Can the neuropsychological findings be interpreted within the context of what neuroimaging and the medical history reflect? Are there residual deficits that can be reliably demonstrated in the test findings that interfere with the patient's activities of daily living? Answers to these questions can be accomplished with brevity in report writing.

Stuss[33] offered the following six principles in the neuropsychological interpretation of the TBI patient, paraphrased as follows:

- Everything must make sense
- The severity of TBI must be defined by the acute injury characteristics
- Symptoms gradually improve
- Rules of logic must always apply
- Decisions should be based on "competent, multidisciplinary, longitudinal research"
- The evaluation be conducted knowledgeably with appropriate assessment metrics

Following these guidelines should lead to appropriate interpretation of test findings.

SUMMARY

Medicolegal expert work is rife with challenges across several spheres including legal, ethical, and medicolegal. The physiatrist who engages in such work must take the time to ensure an intimate knowledge of these various areas to not only conduct quality work but also to ensure provision of unbiased opinions that will truly assist the triers of fact in advocating for appropriate and fair settlement. In that context, physiatrists must also understand that they have potential liability on several different levels in the context of conducting this type of work including having the potential to be sued or charged with practicing medicine without a license. Profitable as such work may often be, clinicians need to be prepared to be put "under the microscope." The process, by its nature, is often adversarial, stressful, and time consuming. Medicolegal expert work requires a high level of sophistication in terms of methodology, assessment techniques, diagnostic formulation skills, and written and oratory skills that is different from those required in daily clinical practice.

ACKNOWLEDGMENTS

The authors thank Ms Lori Kramer for assistance with proofing and Dr Sara Etheredge DPT for assistance with article preparation.

REFERENCES

1. Ameis A, Zasler ND, Martelli MF, et al. Clinicolegal issues. In: Zasler N, Katz D, Zafonte R, editors. Brain injury medicine: principles and practice. 2nd edition. New York: Demos Publishers; 2013. p. 1391–414.
2. American Medical Association, Council on Ethical and Judicial Affairs. Code of medical ethics: current opinions with annotations. Washington, DC: AMA; 1996.

3. American Medical Association Policy. E-10.03 patient-physician relationship in the context of work-related and independent medical examinations. Chicago (IL): American Medical Association; 2005. Available at: www.ama-assn.org. Accessed June 8, 2016.
4. American Medical Association Policy. E-5.09 confidentiality industry-employed physicians and independent medical examiners. Chicago (IL): American Medical Association; 2005. Available at: www.ama-assn.org. Accessed June 8, 2016.
5. Daubert v Merrell Dow Pharmaceuticals, Inc. 509 US 579, 113 S. Ct. 2786, 125 L. Ed. 2d 469, (1993 US).
6. Department of Consumer & Business Services. Community Worker's Compensation. Guide to providing independent medical exams. (OR): 2015. Available at: http://www.cbs.state.or.us/wcd/communications/publications/4913.pdf. Accessed June 8, 2016.
7. Rhondinelli RD, Genovese E, Katz RT, et al. Guides to the evaluation of permanent impairment. 6th edition. Chicago: American Medical Association; 2008.
8. American Academy of Physical Medicine and Rehabilitation. Expert witness testimony (white paper). Washington, DC: AAPMR; 1992.
9. Acting as an expert in medico-legal proceedings. Canadian Medical Protective Association Website. 2009. Available at: https://www.cmpa-acpm.ca/-/acting-as-an-expert-in-medico-legal-proceedings. Accessed June 10, 2016.
10. Blau T. The psychologist as expert witness. New York: John Wiley & Sons; 1984.
11. Constantinou M, McCaffrey RJ. The effects of 3rd party observation: when the observer is a video camera. Arch Clin Neuropsychol 2002;18(7):788–9.
12. Howe LLS, McCaffrey RJ. Third party observation during neuropsychological evaluation: an update on the literature, practical advice for practitioners, and future directions. Clin Neuropsychol 2010;24:518–37.
13. Granacher R. Traumatic brain injury: methods for clinical and forensic neuropsychiatric assessment. 3rd edition. New York: CRC Press; 2015.
14. Zasler ND, Ameis A, Martelli MF. Medicolegal issues associated with motor vehicle collisions: medical perspective. In: Duckworth MP, Iezzi T, O'Donohue WT, editors. Motor vehicle collisions: medical, psychosocial, and legal consequences. Oxford (United Kingdom): Elsevier; 2008. p. 467–502.
15. Martelli MF, Nicholson K, Zasler ND. Assessment of response bias. In: Zasler N, Katz D, Zafonte R, editors. Brain injury medicine: principles and practice. 2nd edition. New York: Demos Publishers; 2013. p. 1415–36.
16. Zasler ND. Validity assessment and the neurological physical exam. NeuroRehabilitation 2015;36(4):401–13.
17. Wortzel HS, Arciniegas DB. The DSM-5 approach to the evaluation of traumatic brain injury and its neuropsychiatric sequelae. NeuroRehabilitation 2014;34(4):613–23.
18. Wortzel HS, Granacher RP. Mild traumatic brain injury update: forensic neuropsychiatric implications. J Am Acad Psychiatry Law 2015;43(4):499–505.
19. CMPA General Counsel. Preparing medico-legal reports: suggestions for physicians - duties and responsibilities. Ottawa (Canada): Canadian Medical Protective Association; 2008. Available at: https://www.cmpa-acpm.ca/-/preparing-medico-legal-reports-suggestions-for-physicians. Accessed June 8, 2016.
20. Brodsky SL. Testifying in court: guidelines and maxims for the expert witness. Washington, DC: American Psychological Association; 1991.
21. Sullivan JD. The medico-legal expertise: solid medicine, sufficient legal and a measure of common sense. Mcgill J Med 2008;9(2):147–51.

22. Lezak MD, Howieson DB, Bigler ED, et al. Neuropsychological assessment. New York: Oxford University Press; 2012.
23. Mortensen EL, Gade A, Reinisch JM. A critical note on Lezak's 'best performance method' in clinical neuropsychology. J Clin Exp Neuropsychol 1991;13(2): 361–71.
24. Gioia GA, Isquith PK. Ecological assessment of executive function in traumatic brain injury. Dev Neuropsychol 2004;25(1–2):135–58.
25. Parsons TD. Virtual reality for enhanced ecological validity and experimental control in the clinical, affective and social neurosciences. Front Hum Neurosci 2015; 9:660.
26. Spooner DM, Pachana NA. Ecological validity in neuropsychological assessment: a case for greater consideration in research with neurologically intact populations. Arch Clin Neuropsychol 2006;21(4):327–37.
27. Sbordone RJ. The hazards of strict reliance on neuropsychological tests. Appl Neuropsychol Adult 2014;21(2):98–107.
28. Sbordone RJ, Purisch AD. Hazards of blind analysis of neuropsychological test data in assessing cognitive disability: the role of confounding factors. Neuro-Rehabilitation 1996;7(1):15–26.
29. Bigler ED. Effort, symptom validity testing, performance validity testing and traumatic brain injury. Brain Inj 2014;28(13–14):1623–38.
30. Silverberg ND, Crane PK, Dams-O'Connor K, et al. Developing a cognition endpoint for traumatic brain injury clinical trials. J Neurotrauma 2017;34(2): 363–71.
31. Wilde EA, Hunter JV, Bigler ED. A primer of neuroimaging analysis in neurorehabilitation outcome research. NeuroRehabilitation 2012;31(3):227–42.
32. Meltzer CC, Sze G, Rommelfanger KS, et al. Guidelines for the ethical use of neuroimages in medical testimony: report of a multidisciplinary consensus conference. AJNR Am J Neuroradiol 2014;35(4):632–7.
33. Stuss DT. A sensible approach to mild traumatic brain injury. Neurology 1995; 45(7):1251–2.

Toward a Postmodern Pragmatic Discourse Semioethics for Brain Injury Care

Empirically Driven Group Inquiry as a Dialogical Practice in Pursuit of the Peircean Aesthetic Ideal of 'Reasonableness'

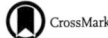

Gary Goldberg, BASc, MD

KEYWORDS

- Ethics • Semiotics • Semioethics • Brain injury • Pragmatism
- Postmodern philosophy • Biosemiotics

KEY POINTS

- A study of ethics requires the ability to examine and understand the nature of the experience of the subject and recognize the foundational status of dynamic process and relationality.
- A new postmodern philosophic framework that recognizes the fundamental importance of relational functions is required to address the complex ethical dilemmas encountered in brain injury care adequately.
- Brain injury is best understood as 'an assault on the personal' played out in the context of the subjectivity of the injured person.
- Using an approach informed by 'semioethics,' the exceptionality of the injured person is fully honored and respected.
- 'Semioethics' can provide a framework for navigating the consensus-seeking dialogical inquiry that strives for a response to an ethical dilemma.

Disclosure Statement: The author has no financial conflicts to disclose.
Hunter Holmes McGuire VA Medical Center, Physical Medicine and Rehabilitation Service (117A), 1201 Broad Rock Boulevard, Richmond, VA 23249, USA
E-mail addresses: gary.goldberg@va.gov; gary.goldberg.md@gmail.com

Phys Med Rehabil Clin N Am 28 (2017) 393–411
http://dx.doi.org/10.1016/j.pmr.2016.12.013
1047-9651/17/Published by Elsevier Inc.

pmr.theclinics.com

It's life, Jim, but not as we know it.
—*Lyric from Star Trekkin' by John O'Connor, Grahame Lister, and Rory Kehoe*

Ethics simply would not exist in the absence of real relationships that either reduce or increase real suffering in others. Therefore, we need to understand both the nature of experience and our connections to others.
—*Arthur Zajonc[1(p10)]*

In an effort to understand everything in terms of matter and mechanism, I believe that we have indeed made a tragic error in discounting the qualitative experience of life. Subjective experience is all we have, and science itself is built upon it. Instead of fearing the subjective, we need to befriend it . . . the world is pregnant with lived experience, and it is time to turn to that experience and to the essentially subjective character of reality, to accept the infant child some would deny.
—*Arthur Zajonc[1(p13)]*

INTRODUCTION

"Doing the right thing"—realizing the course of conduct that *ought* to be taken—in the process of enacting ethical decision making when it comes to the challenges posed by acquired brain injury (ABI) presents a broad variety of provocative difficulties and vexations. Furthermore, the process for how to best arrive at a satisfactory solution to an ethical dilemma presented in the context of ABI care is not defined definitively. This paper argues that one of the main reasons that this is so is because we are in critical need of a transformation in the fundamental philosophic paradigm for understanding brain injury and its consequences, particularly when faced with axiological concerns that revolve around subjective meaning and value as distinct from 'fact,' in the context of the personal—that is, the experiential—which are central issues for ethical decision making. The physicist, author, and educator, Arthur Zajonc, whose research concerns a reorientation of science toward human life and ethics, asks "Where do mind and morality meet?", and that is precisely the crux of the matter. Mind and morality meet in the context of subjectivity, a subjectivity that 'never disappears (but) . . . is our friend, not the enemy science has made it out to be'[1(p13)]—science in the dominant paradigm of mechanistic 'scientism,' that is. A study of ethics requires the ability to examine and understand the nature of the experience of the *subject*—the experiencing human being—and, in that context, to recognize the need to realize the foundational status of dynamic process and relationality, as opposed to the indolent mechanistic materiality attributable to the "unresolved residue of antiquated thinking from the seventeenth century that still pervades the twenty-first century treatment of the mind."[1(p10)] It could well be argued that medicine, as a moral practice,[2] including, in particular, for the purposes of this paper, ABI rehabilitation, requires the same.[3,4] To be alive is to be a dynamic processual subject—a living, experiencing being coupled to the exterior world through a myriad of different relationships, ranging from relatively simple impassive interactions with inanimate objects—like the keyboard I am typing on—to highly complex and provocative interpersonal connections and exchanges with other living beings including those of particular—although certainly not exclusive—interest, involving other human persons. To be human is to have a unique array of 'lived' experiences acquired during a 'lived' trajectory that constitute a dynamic 'life-world'[1,5] played out in the culturally propelled context of a species-specific human *Umwelt*—where the *Umwelt* is the species-specific external world as known to and understood by the subject in terms of the meaning and relevance of the various features of the surrounding environment and circumstances as self-assessed.[6-9] Ethics is all about the intersubjective encounter and the navigation of the intrapersonal and interpersonal. It centers on the relationship between persons—both living human and nonhuman subjects—and how to effectively and properly engage with and become engaged in provocative relational situations and value-laden contexts. To be able to do ethics involves the extraction of meaning from experience and the assignment of value to the relational.

In this paper, it will be argued that the dominant 'modern' philosophic paradigm in which the Western world is so deeply saturated and on which the Newtonian scientific paradigm, since the beginning of the 'Age of Enlightenment,' has been grounded—its dualism, nominalism, depersonalization, and the intentional deletion and bracketing out of the subjective being—the experience of the observer—along with bracketing out of each and every nonhuman organism populating the planet, and its inability to address the crucial and foundational nature of *relationality* and *communication*—including cultural influences—in the quest to understand conscious experience and, with it, the nature of personhood—makes it very difficult, if not impossible, to recognize and fully understand the deep nature of the 'personal'—that is, *subjective being*—in the context of fully nuanced human existence. In the context of modern nominalistic philosophy wherein relation is considered an illusory imposed invention of the mind, real ethics is effectively precluded. Ethics cannot be performed adequately without an understanding that emanates from the personal, an understanding that begins with subjectivity—with the direct experience of the subject—and necessarily incorporates the relational. Ethics is not possible in an impersonal world of encasketed and effectively sequestered and insular 'thinking machines'—the scenario laid out by Cartesian nominalism that denies the reality of the relational, including the influence of the cultural—assuming that the mind 'makes it all up' and imposes its own relational structure—and places an impenetrable wall separating the subjective mind-dependent realm generated inside the head ('*ens rationis*') from the objective mind-independent world outside ('*ens reale*'), the true existence of which can only be inferred in the context of the modern worldview. For the modern philosophic paradigm, the world seems to be organized because it is the human mind that is endowed with the ability to generate the organizing structure, the overlaid logical order that it imposes on reality. But what if it really works the other way around? What if the human mind is logically ordered the way it is because it is a product of the discoverable logic of the reality of the natural world—the mind that pervades nature—from whence it emerged over eons through an expansive and long-enduring evolutionary process? That really would change everything. We now have clues from relativity and quantum mechanics indicating that the logic of the Newtonian paradigm—the logic of hard-core scientific materialism—with its effective elimination of the subjective observer from the system studied, leads to a false objectivism. Instead, what the 'new physics' of relativity and quantum mechanics indicates is that the presence of the subject matters—"subjectivity is real, and real at every level of analysis"[1(p13)]—and that it is a necessary and integral element of the scientific worldview whose presence and participation cannot be discounted or eliminated. In the new physics, observations are subject to the subject.

A new postmodern framework, indeed, an emerging 'new age' of human understanding[10,11] is entailed—a 'postmodern' framework that recognizes and incorporates the fundamental importance of communication, sociality, and intersubjective collaboration throughout the natural world—but particularly for the self-reflecting human species for which ethics, as the capacity to perceive what is happening, imagine what could be, and then reflect on what *ought* to be done, is not only a possibility, but an *obligation*—a new nonnominalistic view that recognizes that relations, although invisible and essentially incapable of being detected directly by the senses, are nevertheless very *real* existents discoverable through inquiry. Furthermore, relations operate at a suprasubjective level,[12] over and above the entities linked together by the relation, making possible a context-dependent flexible interaction between the mind-dependent—that is, what cannot be without the participation of mind—and the mind-independent—that is, the 'things' that constitute the real world regardless of whether or not they are 'objectified'—that is, 'known' to a finite mind. In this new postmodern worldview, these two fundamental realms can interpenetrate freely and openly in accordance with relational context.[13]

To be a human person is directly and intimately connected to the process through which the human brain and nervous system, in the context of its embodiment as situated in the further context of our immediate and larger environment with all its complexity (populated with 'objects'—that is, known entities—many of whom—certainly the living organisms including fellow humans—are also themselves subjects) and affordances for agency, gives rise to and makes possible subjective experience. Therefore, recovering the subjective and having a philosophic framework that honors and allows for the full understanding and appreciation of the subjective, of the phenomena that occur in the experience of the human person, is a necessary prerequisite for engaging in the quest for acceptable ethical decision making in the context of caring for the brain-injured human person.

It will be argued that the process of extracting meaning from subjective experience in the personal context—the ability to understand and infer what is 'significant' or meaningful—ultimately involves 'semiosis'—the 'action of signs'—that makes possible the flexible context-dependent interaction between *ens rationis* and *ens reale* spanning past, future, and the here-and-now in such an interpretation, and makes experience, itself, possible.[14-18] Furthermore, the scientific foundation of the emerging field of biosemiotics[18-24]—the study of semiosis as the process through which meaning is extracted from subjective experience in the context of living organisms viewed as complex purposive systems with intentionality[25] that function in the embedded framework of their environmental context—offers a scientific theory of meaning based on the interaction between living things and their inner and outer worlds—the *Innenwelt* and the *Umwelt*—meaning that is mediated through semiosis. If what really matters in the ethical context is the axiological—the determination and understanding of value and meaning—then biosemiotics can be viewed as a scientific enterprise capable of grounding a theory of moral valuation, thus providing a philosophic foundation for an ethics capable of bridging the gap between fact and value, the natural and the cultural, reconciling science and morality and enabling progress of our societal ethic.[26] Cobley[27] has recently provided a detailed and cogent 3-fold argument for precisely how the possibility of an ontology of ethics is linked to biosemiotics in the context of the species-specific features—including linguistic capacity—of the human *Umwelt*:

1. Through the capacity of language to displace, in both time and space, through semiosis, events in other times and places, events that have not yet occurred (ie, as 'fictions'), as well as in the anticipation of how things *could become*, referenced to how they currently are (ie, conditions can get better—or get worse).
2. Through the aspects of the *Umwelt* that actively contribute to affective experience, from suffering to satisfaction to joy.
3. Through the specific experience of 'otherness' or 'alterity' distinguished from but referenced to the experience of 'self' that develops in the context of the human *Umwelt*.

Cobley maintains that ethics, as opposed to being "the idea of . . . a moral system" that arose from the "sound moral judgment of a rational, unified consciousness," is the result of the circumstances of the species-specific human *Umwelt* that emphasize the difference in "kind and degree" between the functionality and disposition of the human versus other natural organisms, as well as what specifically characterizes the human being as a "natural subject."[27(p61)]

Brain injury, because the human brain effectively is the bodily organ most intimately involved with subjective human experience, self-identity, and awareness, and the extraction of generalizable meaning from experience, is "an assault on the personal,"[28(p34)] a fundamental transformation of the central functions of the subject with ABI both in terms of how they experience themselves and how they experience their world, as well as how they function as a conscious agent within the context of their life-world. ABI can have a powerful influence on self-identity[29–32] and the process of recovery can entail a complex process of phenomenologically oriented personal narrative reconstruction.[32,33] Correspondingly, we need to have a new postmodern philosophic paradigm that helps us to recover a deep understanding of what it truly means "to be a person"[34]—to understand what constitutes a human person—an approach that allows us to engage in ordered and systematic scientific discourse regarding pragmatic ethical concerns with regard to such "persons,"[35] especially under the significantly transfiguring circumstances of ABI and its life-altering impact on the subjectivity and selfhood—that is, self-awareness and agency—of the person affected.

Not only does brain injury deeply affect the subjectivity of the person injured—that is, their existence as a human person—because of the potentially significant aspects of personhood impacted (eg, personality, self-identity, capacity to communicate, emote, perceive, act, empathize, and function as a moral agent, to identify only a few of the myriad ways that ABI can alter subjective being), it can also produce significant problematic impairment of self-awareness.[36,37] In addition, the injured human person can initiate self-protective adaptive strategies "in attempts of the organism to come to terms with"[38(p245)] the effects of the injury as self-perceived and understood, schemes that may unintentionally exacerbate the impairment of functionality and precipitate an existential emotional decompensation that Kurt Goldstein termed a "catastrophic reaction."[38,39] Because subjectivity is defined through its relations to objects and other subjects—including other human persons—that constitute the *Umwelt* of the injured person, it also affects all those other human persons who are engaged relationally with the injured person (ie, all those human others who find themselves entangled in the injured person's 'semiotic web')—their family, their employer, their friends, and everyone else in their relational network. In addition, in the context of treatment, everyone involved in their medical care becomes a part of this intersubjective relational network in which the injured individual is embedded. In the process of addressing the challenges of ethical decision making, members of an ethics committee who may be specially consulted to assist with this process are further added into this intricate extended network. This group rapidly becomes a very complex web of dynamic communication and ongoing relational interaction, through which information as well as affective coloration can pulse—involving channels that are both linguistic and extralinguistic.

This article presents a brief sketch of a recommended approach to ethical decision making in the context of ABI care with all of these considerations in mind. Various reasons why ABI poses significant ethical challenges have been briefly touched on here and a limited sample of the sources of these challenges are itemized in **Box 1**.

AS McGrath HAS POINTED OUT

The treatment and rehabilitation of people with acquired brain injury is a potent and distinctive source of ethical dilemmas because it involves profound novelty,

Box 1
Limited sample of sources of ethical challenge encountered in acquired brain injury care

Impact of level of consciousness and inferred sentience in minimally conscious states

Determination and significance of brain viability versus brain death

Appropriate versus unrealistic expectations

Communicating unfavorable information in an appropriate and empathic manner

Decision making in the face of uncertainty regarding ultimate outcomes

Influence of premorbid affective health and personality

What to do when the patient is incapacitated and no family or friends are available

Questions of level of volitional control, agency, and capacity to predict consequences of actions taken

Accountability for actions and responsibility for consequences pursuant to actions taken by patient

Impact on perception and treatment of the patient as a moral agent

Impact of alterations in physical appearance and physical movement

Impact of alterations in ability to perform basic self-care functions

Impact of impairment of instrumental activities of daily living (eg, cooking, shopping, finances, etc)

Impact of alterations in judgment and insight

Impact of alterations in agency and executive function (eg, planning, time management, etc)

Impact of alterations in the ability to engage in abstraction

Impact of behavioral disinhibition and agitated behavior

Impact of alterations in various forms of memory function

Impact of various neuropsychiatric complications of acquired brain injury (eg, mood disorders, seizures, psychosis)

Overall impact on other persons (eg, family caregivers) in the patient's relational network

Impact on spirituality and faith in the context of the struggle to adjust to altered identity

Limitations on the ability to communicate accurately and intelligibly

Impact of alteration in emotional regulation and contextual expression

Impact of impaired self-awareness and the ability to make appropriate adjustments to change in self-identity

Impact of maladaptive compensatory strategies (eg, depression, anxiety, catastrophic reaction, etc)

Impact of various other forms of cognitive impairment (eg, regulation of attention, perception, anosognosia, apraxia, etc)

Impact on capacity for effective decision making

Impact of impairment in interpretation of nonverbal cues from others

Impact of impairment in the ability to empathize and on various aspects of emotional intelligence

Impact of inability to generate an income (ie, vocational disability)

Impact of inability to drive a vehicle

Impact of inability to independently navigate home community

Need to identify an appropriate safe discharge environment; obligations to train those who will assume responsibility

Availability of and access to outpatient follow-up care after discharge from inpatient treatment *great complexity, only partial information, and a coming together of several different value systems and assumptive worlds.*[40(p12)]

The exclusive application of the so-called principlist approach to the performance of analytical decision making in the context of these ethical challenges will be critiqued and an alternative approach founded in semioethics will be proposed. An argument will be made for developing an alternative empirically driven person-centered approach to ethical decision making that operates by cycling between case-specific empirical data gathering and ethical review and group inquiry performed as a dialogical practice involving multiple stakeholders.[35,41,42]

The 'architectonic' organizational chart of the sciences developed by the great American philosopher, Charles Sanders Peirce, is introduced briefly as the systematic source of the philosophic foundation of the herein proposed approach to ethics in ABI, noting particularly where ethics fits into this system, as well as touching briefly on the triadic structure of the sign relation as conceived by Peirce in the context of his semiotic proposal for the manner in which semiosis, the process of sign action, serves to allow organisms to interpret experience in the world so as to extract meaningful and generalizable knowledge from it. We then look at implications of Peirce's postmodern philosophic framework for the practice of ethics and the shared scientific process of searching for consensus through discourse guided by ethical ideals.

In appreciating and coming to understand the ubiquitous and fundamental importance of semiosis as a crucial process that infuses the cosmos, the human species, having the capacity not only *to use* semiosis in communication and valuation—as does every other living organism—but also *to know and reflect on* the fact that there *are* sign relations and to develop an understanding of what such signs do and are all about, is the unique 'semiotic animal' on the planet quite distinct from the concept of the rational animal—the animal capable of reasoning—that 'thinks itself into existence'—the *res cogitans* so famously branded by René Descartes.[43,44] The semiotic animal has the capacity to elevate itself, through its response to the semiotically mediated experience of alterity—of 'otherness,' from an animal capable of mere self-justifying rationalization into an animal capable of discerning what is *reasonable—what is the right thing to do*—in the context of the encounter with alterity.[45] As Deely writes:

The rationality of the rational animal may be abstractly considered as closed unto itself, but experientially it is bound up with and inseparable from otherness; and this same rationality, as the capacity for being reasonable, appears against the horizon of otherness not abstractly and closed off but rather as—precisely—the ability to grasp the reason of things presented within objectivity.[45(p720)]

As such, the human being is subject to an expanded and semiotically informed concept of semioethics,[45–47] a species-specific ethical obligation to preserve and safeguard the welfare of the 'Earthbound' other—all the semiotically enmeshed living inhabitants of Gaia, each creature presenting itself as other to the self—that emerges directly from the recognition and understanding of the human person as the one and only known semiotic animal.[45,48]

AS PETRILLI STATES

[S]emioethics offers the broadest view possible on existence available today to the so-called 'semiotic animal'—or human being, who is also the cosmically responsible agent. Therefore, not only must we do justice to the human capacity for semioethics on a theoretical level, but we must also evidence our vital,

inexorable need for this semioethical capacity . . . not just for the sake of safe-guarding human life but all of life generally over the entire planet . . . indeed, today more than ever . . . not only must we explain and understand this capacity (for semioethics), but we must stress our inescapable need for it, our need to cultivate our semioethical propension in the most conscientious, imaginative and responsible manner possible for the health of semiosis at large and therefore for identity itself. Otherness requires nothing less.[45]

THE 'PRINCIPLIST PARADIGM' IS INADEQUATE

The predominant paradigm that dominates conventional bioethics is principlist in its approach[49] and is based on the moral theory of key guiding normative principles presumed to be universally applicable, such as those set out by Beauchamp and Childress.[50] This paradigm is based on the 4 major principles of autonomy, beneficence, nonmaleficence, and justice (**Box 2** for selected ethical issues organized in accordance with such principles) that then become the reference points for all of the moral obligations that arise in a clinical context. The problem, as demonstrated by Fiester[49] among others, is that this approach can be readily compromised and reduced into a simplified and mindless 'principlist paradigm checklist' so that a purely normative assessment is made with prescriptive recommendations generated based entirely on a limited and reductive set of ethical concerns that do not come close to addressing the full range of moral obligations that arise in complex clinical situations and recognizing the context-dependent and culturally influenced nuances that characterize the special circumstances of each individual case.[49] This is 'cookbook' bioethics and it is just not adequate in identifying and adequately addressing all of the significant and varied moral issues that arise in complex clinical cases. As Fiester notes in her critique of the principlist paradigm:

> The effect of the principlist paradigm is a narrowing of the moral lens through which clinical ethics cases are viewed at the cost of missing important moral issues and the moral obligations they generate.[49(p685)]

The principlist paradigm also, as Fiester points out, leads to an inadequate identification of moral obligations because it separates obligations regarding *communication* with patients and caregivers from the recommendations drawn from application of the principle-based 'ethics,' per se. Although important for the moral issues that it does manage to identify, the fateful fault with the principlist approach is that this separation of communication from ethics is a 'false dichotomy' because "ineffective communication causes patients harm, and thus good, effective communication is an ethical obligation."[49(p689)] In the context of the thesis of this paper, this sundering of communication from the detached theory-based analytical paradigm can be understood as the difference between, on the one hand, an ethics that is derived from the perspective of modernism wherein the process of 'doing ethics' involves identifying and applying a set of 'principles' as universally pertinent 'ideas' used to prescribe a course of action that discounts the subjectivity of its human participants, from, on the other hand, a semiotically informed 'semioethics' that fully and holistically recognizes the subjectivity of all those human persons participating in the process and underlines the need to ensure that adequate contact and detailed, respectful, and sufficient communication occurs every step of the way, including full recognition of the powerful cross-cultural influences that the presumptive universality of core principles disregards,[51] and that all *reasonable* moral obligations, especially those lying outside the scope of the 'principles,' are recognized and addressed. What distinguishes the process

---

Box 2
Some bioethics principles and related concerns that may apply in acquired brain injury care

Nonmaleficence

a. Do no harm.

b. What is considered 'harmful'?

Beneficence

a. Facilitate recovery.

b. Weighing risks versus benefits.

c. Improve functionality.

d. Relieve and, where possible, prevent suffering.

e. Making sure that communication of all relevant information is clear and appropriate.

f. Respecting cultural differences

g. What is considered 'beneficial'? What is in the best interest of the patient?

Autonomy

a. Fundamental right to self-determination and independent agency.

b. Does patient have the current capacity to exercise decision making freedom?
   i. Ability to communicate choices clearly.
   ii. Ability to understand provided information.
   iii. Ability to reason and make correct inferences.
   iv. Ability to recognize circumstances and project consequences and their impact.

c. Is there a surrogate decision maker identified in case one is needed? How have they been designated?

d. Has the patient made their desires known clearly? Can they now? Have they in the past?

e. If there is an advance directive, are circumstances such that it should or should not be invoked?

f. Balancing autonomy with assessed risk of self-harm or harm to others.

g. When is the authority to limit autonomy indicated and justified?

h. Has the brain injury significantly altered self-awareness such that judgment and insight are impaired to the point where the risks of significant harm to self or others are judged to be significant?

Justice

a. Recognizing the roles and rights of all stakeholders in the process.

b. Recognizing the roles and rights of the injured person and how they could be affected by the injury.

c. Resource management.

d. Access to care.

e. Justification of resource use based on medical necessity.

f. Is there sufficient scientific evidence to justify clinical decision making?

---

of implementing semioethics, as opposed to conventional modernist ethics, is the manner in which all key information is gathered, shared, and communicated in a relational context, all relevant empirical data necessary to fully appreciate the unique circumstances of the case are obtained, the manner in which there is open-mindedness and sensitivity to plurality and diversity conveyed through context, disavowal of the temptation to avoid the affect involved in difficult communicative encounters, and the manner in which all the moral obligations evident through the semiotically expanded moral lens, including those that emerge in the context of the intersubjective relational encounter with the subjectivity of the other person(s) involved,[27,45,52,53] are taken into account and acted upon. In this manner, the exceptionality of the person as a natural subject operating holistically in the relational context of his or her culturally conditioned species-specific *Umwelt*—in the context of subjective experience through which meaning and value relative to the subject emerges—is fully honored and respected.[24]

PHILOSOPHIC FOUNDATIONS IN PEIRCEAN SEMIOTICS AND THE PROCESS OF SEMIOSIS

It will not be possible in the limited space here to do justice to or to properly recognize the foundational nature of the 'architectonic' philosophic system worked out by Charles Sanders Peirce—who Alfred North Whitehead, in a 1936 letter to Charles Hartshorne, referred to as the "American Aristotle"—in bringing human subjectivity and the experiential (ie, the phenomenological) back into the realm of scientific inquiry with the resultant revival of a cogent form of experientially founded realism based on an ontology of relations linked to the pervasive presence of semiosis (ie, the 'action of signs') permeating nature and the cosmos.[12,15] Signs are indications of relational being. Anything can be a sign, not as itself, but in relation to another—its 'object'—for 'an other'—its 'interpretant.' Suffice it to say that it is the irreducibly triadic logic—the tripartite sign relation between the 3 relata of which it is constituted: the 'sign vehicle' or 'representamen' (that which signifies or 'represents'), the 'object' (that to which the sign vehicle obtains), and the interpretant (that for which—or for whom—the relational association between the sign-vehicle and the object is provoked)—of the Peircean semiotic that offers the prospect of constructive 'repair' of the instigating and often infuriating binary oppositions—the dichotomous impasses—that heavily populate the modern landscape.

In a brief summary of the Peircean triadic sign concept, Hoffmeyer states the following:

> [T]he sign unites tokens of three fundamental categories, the categories of First-ness ('feeling'), Secondness ('resistance') and Thirdness ('mediation'), usually expressed by the terms subject or representamen (Firstness), object (Second-ness) and interpretant (Thirdness) . . . the central point that is so easily overlooked here is that the sign doesn't exist materially, it happens. The sign is an event . . . It was one of Peirce's major insights that since all thought takes time, all thought takes the form of sign processes ('semiosis'). Logic is therefore based on the tri-adicity of the sign relation. And so, biosemiotics claims, is cognition not only in humans, but in all other organisms as well.[54(pp244–245)]

The process of Peircean semiosis, the sign relation, and the action of signs are illustrated in **Figs. 1** and **2**.

Anything that serves the purpose of *mediation* or *lawful interconnection* that makes experience intelligible, or what Peirce called 'thirdness' in the context of his phenomenological list of categories (and in the context of his process metaphysics, 'evolutionary' or 'creative' love), underwrites the possibility of a creative and stochastic but still continuously interconnected (ie, 'synechistic') evolutionary process emergent through the so-mediated balanced interplay between the source of creative

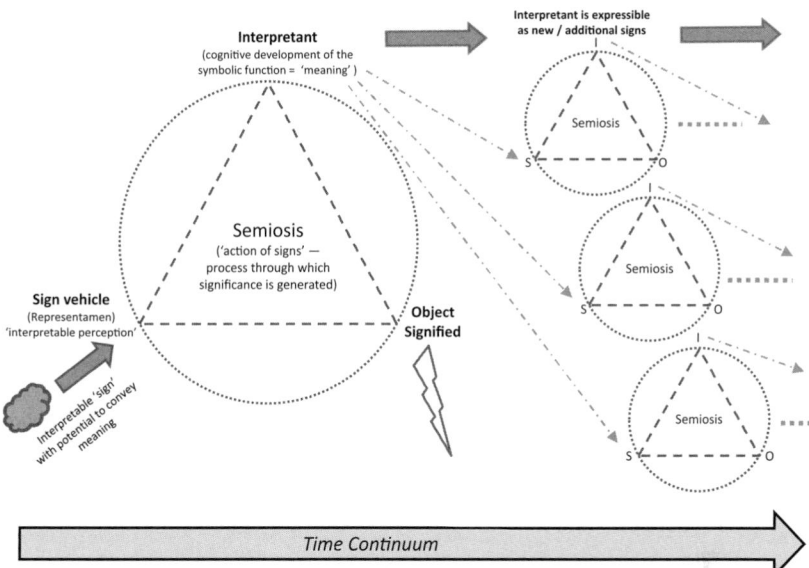

Fig. 1. The process of infinite semiosis. A schematic portrayal of how the process of semiosis unfolds to form the semiotic 'web' of experientially mediated meaning making and communication that takes place in the sign-perfused 'semiosphere'—a 'sphere of sign processes and elements of meaning that constitute a frame of understanding within which biology must work.'[20] The perceptible 'sign vehicle' or 'representamen'—in this case 'storm clouds'—is connected to the 'object'—a 'lightning strike,' the anticipation of which—the 'interpretant,' which is the meaning extracted from the relation of the sign vehicle to the object signified—in turn, becomes a sign linking to further possible meaningful inferences and decisions regarding, for example, action to be taken to avoid being struck by lightning. (*Courtesy of* Martin J. Irvine, MD, Founding Director of the Communication, Culture and Technology Program at Georgetown University, Washington, DC; with permission.)

possibility, pure chance ('firstness'), and the source of stability, 'brute-force' actuality (the world of rigidly conjoined dyadic oppositions—ie, 'secondness').[55–58]

A summary outline of Peirce's architectonic system is provided in **Box 3**, showing how and where ethics fits into the overall picture, and how ethics emerges from Peirce's philosophic system.[57] Peirce viewed ethics as one of the normative sciences, superordinate to 'logic' as semiotic, and subordinate to aesthetics. As opposed to individual pleasure (hedonism) or the general greater good of society (utilitarianism), Peirce identified the ultimate good or *summum bonum,* in the context of his metaphysical view of the evolutionary process through which mind actualizes, as the "growth of concrete reasonableness."[59] As Petrilli states:

> The most advanced developments in reason and knowledge are achieved through the creative power of reasonableness and are fired by the power of love, agapasm: 'the impulse projecting creations into independency and drawing them into harmony' (CP 6.288).[59(p239)]

Peirce, who was a Harvard-trained chemist and made his living as a scientist, viewed his philosophic system as providing a basis for seeking truth through the process of scientific inquiry where the raw data are empirical data accessed through experience, the scientific examination of which Peirce called 'phaneroscopy'—what is more commonly referred to in philosophic circles as 'phenomenology.' Peirce

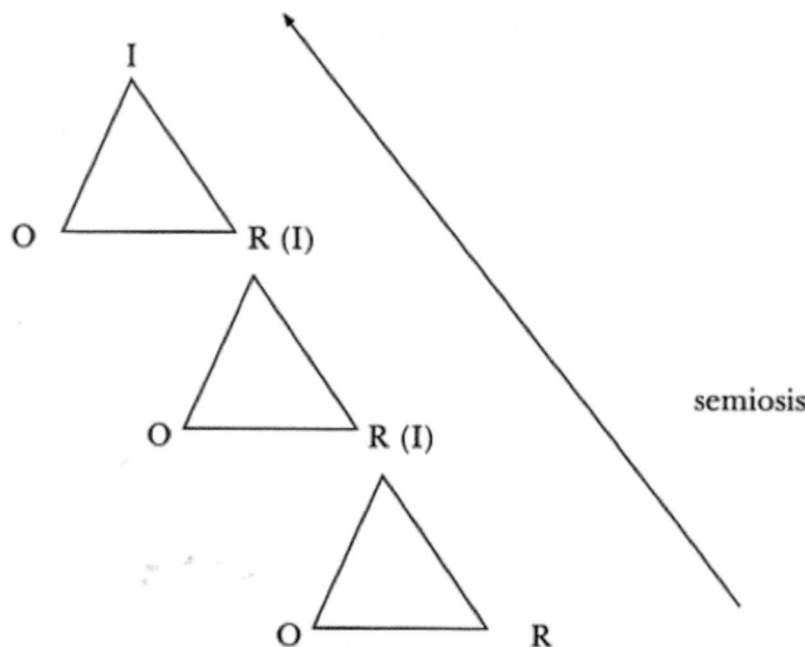

Fig. 2. The unfolding of 'infinite semiosis' through an interpretive process network whereby the interpretant (I) becomes the representamen (R) related to the signified object (O) for the next interpretive event in the semiotic sequence.

begins with the fundamental assumption that nothing is beyond the reach of inquiry, that the truth emerges through an open process of inquiry carried out by a semiotically enmeshed community of like-minded inquirers using logically based investigational methods to seek deeper insights into the lawful structure of reality. The basis of truth-seeking inquiry is the systematic registration of the empirical, those phenomena available to the inquirer through direct experience of the world, to which the linked logical elements of abduction (ie, the creative process of intuiting a reasonable explanatory conjecture in the form of a testable hypothesis), deduction (ie, those experientially accessible empirical observations logically predicted by the hypothesis), and induction (ie, the ordered search for the presence of a finite set of such observations from which the likelihood of the hypothesis being true can be inferred) are recurrently applied in the ongoing search for the lawful structure of reality.

Peirce thus considered ethics to be a normative science along with aesthetics and logic with the goal of defining norms for what is to be considered admirable and desired, how one is to conduct oneself accordingly in a deliberate and self-controlled manner and with the correct 'attitude,' and what methods (ie, the application of semiotics as logic) can be used to seek out and identify the estimable. As noted, Peirce defines the ultimate aesthetic ideal as what he called the 'growth of concrete reasonableness'—a manifestation of mind in nature—that permits an increase in the shared communal understanding of and reasoned insight into the true lawful nature of reality.[60(p130)] Nubiola reviewed how Peirce understood this overarching aesthetic ideal as basically the mediational lawfulness of the evolving universe and that Peirce repeatedly testifies to "reasonableness being essentially the same in its operation in

Box 3
The organizational relationship between the sciences according to the architectonic classification scheme of C.S. Peirce

1. Sciences of discovery ('heuretic' sciences)
   a. Mathematics (science that draws necessary conclusions about hypothetical objects)
   b. Positive sciences (sciences that seek positive assertions of fact)
      i. Philosophy ('cenoscopy'—science of universally available positive phenomena accessible to anyone in normal daily experience)
         1. Phenomenology ('phaneroscopy'—science of what appears in everyday experience)
            a. Theory of cenopythagorean categories or 'predicaments'; modes of being
               i. Firstness (Quality of 'feeling'; pure 'being' without assertion; potentiality; chance; reference to a pure abstract form or 'ground'; 'beginning'; monadic)
               ii. Secondness (haecceity; alterity; an 'other' different from all the rest; encounter ('second' with a 'first'); resistance; reaction; 'brute force'; actuality; reference from relate to correlate; 'end'; dyadic)
               iii. Thirdness (mediation; habit; law; intelligibility; significance; purpose; displacement; generality; continuity; reference to an interpretant; 'between'; triadic)
         2. Normative sciences (science seeking to discover good ways of achieving recognized objectives)
            a. Esthetics ('growth of concrete reasonableness'—ultimate ideal of human life—that is, achievement of a state of higher understanding of nature)
            b. Ethics (defines life's purpose: conduct as self-control that commits to the ultimate ideal as that which sanctions action—that is, the 'growth of concrete reasonableness')
            c. General logic ('semeiotic'—determining concrete reasonableness as the locus of Peirce's truth theory and fallibilism)
               i. Speculative grammar ('analytical'–including the classification of the triadic sign relation)
               ii. Critic (structure and form of the process of argument; the modes of inference)
                  1. Abduction (generate the hypothesis)
                  2. Deduction (determine the necessary consequences)
                  3. Induction (Are these consequences detected in samples?)
               iii. Methodeutic (how to properly conduct scientific inquiry)
                  1. Pragmaticism as a regulative principle of inquiry: the whole meaning of a hypothesis is in its conceivable practical effects (ie, via 'impact on experience').
                  2. Scientific method
         3. Metaphysics (science of the ultimate reality behind appearances)
            a. General/ontological (locus of Peirce's form of 'scholastic realism')
            b. Theological/psychic
            c. Physical evolutionary process
               i. Modes of evolutionary process
                  1. Tychasm (chance)
                  2. Anancasm (mechanical actuality)
                  3. Agapasm (creative love)
               ii. Synechism/continuity of space–time and law/everything is continuously connected
      ii. Special sciences ('idioscopy'—science of new positive phenomena only accessible through use of specialized equipment and/or application of a specialized form of experiment)
         1. Physical sciences
         2. Psychic sciences
2. Sciences of review (classification schemes; taxonomy; synthetic systematics)
3. Practical sciences (technological 'applied' science)

the universe, in nature and in the human mind."[60(p130)] Nubiola went on to say that "this element of Thirdness and of law is essentially irreducible to a dyadic analysis as the scientistic materialism of Peirce's times tried to do, and as contemporary naturalism tries to do today as well."[60] In Peirce's own words, "Under this conception, the ideal of conduct will be to execute our little function in the operation of the creation by giving a hand toward rendering the world more reasonable whenever, as the slang is, it is 'up to us' to do so."[61] For Peirce, then, ethics involves doing what is determined to be most likely to produce an outcome that increases the reasonableness of the situation under consideration given the specific empirical observations.

Thus, ethics becomes a question of seeking human conduct that facilitates the growth of practical wisdom conceived of as insightful pragmatic common sense accessed through logical inquiry aimed at the growth of concrete reasonableness, via the discovery of lawful mediation that addresses the situation. Ethical conduct is viewed as a deliberate pursuit of action informed by such wisdom, a pursuit of "reason fired by love,"[59] that serves to make the world a more reasonable and better understood place, not only through individual conduct, although that is where it starts, but also through exemplary behavior that engenders and encourages similar behavior in others, via a collective social process. The goal of growing concrete reasonableness in the world then requires becoming a social catalyst for such growth in a community of similar inquirers through consistent and sustained ethical action that facilitates the shared collective pursuit of ethical ideals. In a paper seeking to define what Peirce sought as the ideals that define the 'good life,' Aydin[62] notes that, in the pursuit of ethical conduct, Peirce applies the same principles of seeking truth and elucidating logical lawfulness—a process of successive approximation through an empirical search guided by logical procedure and carried out by a closely knit community of inquirers, in this case with respect to the ideals in accordance with which to conduct our actions, through the process of generalization:

> According to Peirce, we should not concern ourselves too much with questions about what we as individual moral actors should or should not do. We should rather consider our thinking and acting as part of a broader development with a common history and common future. What is important is not what I think but what eventually should be thought. From that perspective, the very first command is that we ought to acknowledge that there is a higher business than our own.[62(p439)]

Thus, the search for the ethical ideal of increased reasonableness is something that can only take place in the context of an empirical process carried on by a community of similarly minded inquirers. In comparing and contrasting Peirce's postmodern semiotic approach to the a priori rationalism of the prototypical modern philosopher, Immanuel Kant, Aydin goes on:

> The ultimate aim that ought to govern our conduct does not coincide with our actual rational nature, but is something to be attained in the future by an unlimited community (of inquirers)...the basis of Peirce's ethics cannot lie in (already) knowing what the good is, for the function of ethics consists precisely in the search for what the good could be.[62(p439)]

For Peirce, the good is not accessible in a set of a priori principles, but "something that is the object of a common quest."[62(p450)] In his view, the ethical process does not involve applying a set of given principles received as products of rational thought. The process involves an inherently social collaborative pursuit carried out as an empirical process by a group of inquirers with a common purpose—a concerted quest for shared ideals. In the end, the performance of ethics involves a process through which we search "beyond our active individual lives and become part of a cosmic process that transcends us; only by overcoming our disconnected and fragmented human individuality, can we become genuine persons"[62(p450)] engaged in this process. This might possibly allow Peirce to be seen as a 'postliberal' humanist, so that Peirce-inspired semioethics entails what Petrilli[48,59] and Petrilli and Ponzio,[53] following Levinas,[52] have termed a *humanism of alterity*, leading to the notion that Peirce, rather than at first glance seeming to be antihumanist or posthumanist, may actually be acknowledged as "a humanist in a different and even better sense."[62(p450)]

SUMMARY

Subsequent experience of life has taught me that the only thing that is really desirable without a reason for being so, is to render ideas and things reasonable. One cannot well demand a reason for reasonableness itself. Logical analysis shows that reasonableness consists in association, assimilation, generalization, the bringing of items together into an organic whole —which are so many ways of regarding what is essentially the same thing. In the emotional sphere this tendency toward union appears as Love; so that the Law of Love and the Law of Reason are quite as one.

—Charles Sanders Peirce[63(p332)]

Here in the early years of the twenty-first century, a majority of philosophers and scientists are naturalists. But in the public sphere . . . on questions of morality and meaning, religion and spirituality are given a preeminent place. Our values have not yet caught up with our best ontology. They had better start catching up.

—Sean Carroll[64(p418)]

What, then, are the implications of these various philosophic considerations for how ethical decision making should be carried out as they arise in ABI care? Clearly, the process should be guided by the recognition and appreciation of the subjective being of the patient as a suffering other human person experiencing a very difficult process, recognizing that an empathic understanding and response to their experience in dealing with their challenges is crucial and, in fact, obligatory in the process of caring. The need for empathic understanding extends to those individuals in the semiotic network of the patient who are also directly and significantly affected by the varied consequences and implications of the injury. Effective communication among all parties involved is an ongoing critical concern that must be monitored and addressed whenever inadvertent miscommunication occurs. An empirical person-centered approach[65] that emphasizes the careful gathering together and assembly of the data specific to the circumstances of the individual case is preferred to the insensitive and unrefined application of normative principles independent of detailed specific context. Widdershoven and colleagues[42] describe an empirical approach based on "hermeneutic ethics and responsive evaluation" that "regards experience as the concrete source of moral wisdom" and this approach may also connect the ethical process to the crucial context-sensitive issues that arise in each individual case.[41] Facilitation of open dialogue and guided consensus formation through ongoing discourse between clinicians, the patient, and key stakeholders can permit the process to address pragmatic issues through a coordinated discourse-intensive group inquiry.[35] As Cooke maintains in proposing a "pragmatic discourse ethics," "the process of inquiry contains its own normative structure as it aims to discover norms."[35(p653)] In the frame of Peirce's philosophy, this implies an empirical process of inquiry directed to the joint discovery and implementation of ethical ideals that guide decision making so as to maximize the likelihood of the most reasonable outcome given the constraints imposed by often dire circumstances.

Finally, it is suggested that recognition of the pervasive presence of the process of semiosis as the 'action of signs' that anchors subjectivity—through which the import of relationality becomes evident and pragmatic meaning emerges from subjective experience—can provide an important nondualistic, nonnominalistic, postmodern philosophic framework in which to seek out, through communitarian inquiry, *reasonable* responses to difficult, value-laden, ethical challenges that suffuse the practice of brain injury care. Facts alone are not enough when "meaning matters."[26] The problem of knowledge necessarily assumes preceding problems of an axiological nature.[66]

The emerging concept of a biosemiotically informed ethics—semioethics—can be seen to provide a general framework for navigating the challenging and provocative consensus-seeking dialogical process involved in striving to hit upon a response to each and every unique situation that presents itself in the forum of bioethics—a response around which all those involved in the process can come to a consensus regarding how best to facilitate the continued growth of concrete reasonableness in the face of the significant challenges imposed by the injury.[66]

There are several recent references to which the interested reader is referred that specifically address the overall approach to ethics in brain injury care in more detail than can be considered here.[67–69] This author has found the monograph by McGrath[69] to be of particular value thanks to several illustrative case presentations and the pragmatic applicability of her discussion and presentation of the issues to the clinical treatment setting.

Also of significant note is a recent monograph authored by a nationally prominent neuroethicist directed to the lay public.[70] Fins depicts some of the most difficult and provocative emerging ethical concerns in brain injury care, including challenging controversies surrounding the assessment and care of patients with severe injuries who are in minimally conscious states, having survived catastrophic injuries owing to the impressive advancements that have occurred over the past few decades in acute trauma care. Broadly acceptable realistic solutions to such ethical challenges that maximize the growth of concrete reasonableness are likely to be elusive. Simultaneously meeting the potentially competing conditions of both rationality *and* relationality, ensuring that there is balanced and just opportunity for input from all relevant stakeholders, will require a demanding discursive process of consensus building across broad swaths of society.

REFERENCES

1. Zajonc A. Mind and morality: where do they meet? Minding Nature 2015;8(2): 10–15. Available at: www.arthurzajonc.org/publications/mind-and-morality-where-do-they-meet/. Accessed February 7, 2017.
2. Pellegrino E. Toward a reconstruction of medical morality. Am J Bioeth 2006;6: 65–71.
3. Baron RJ. An introduction to medical phenomenology: I can't hear you while I'm listening. Ann Intern Med 1985;103:606–11.
4. Goldberg G. Medical phenomenology and stroke rehabilitation. An introduction. Top Stroke Rehabil 2011;18:1–5.
5. Zahavi D. Subjectivity and selfhood. Investigating the first-person perspective. Cambridge (MA): MIT Press; 2005.
6. Kull K. Umwelt. In: Cobley P, editor. The Routledge companion to semiotics. London: Routledge; 2010. p. 348–9.

7. Sagan D. Introduction: Umwelt after Uexküll. In: Uexküll J, von Uexküll M, O'Neil JD, editors. A foray into the worlds of animals and humans: with a theory of meaning. (Joseph D O'Neil translation of 1940 ed.). Minneapolis (MN): University of Minnesota Press; 2010. p. 3.

8. Kull K. On semiosis, ümwelt, and semiosphere. Semiotica 1998;120:299–310.

9. Deely J. Semiotic entanglement: the concepts of environment, Umwelt, and Lebenswelt in semiotic perspective. Semiotica 2014;199:7–42.

10. Deely J. The four ages of understanding. The first postmodern survey of philosophy from ancient times to the turn of the twenty-first century. Toronto: University of Toronto Press; 2001.

11. Deely J. Postmodernity as the unmasking of objectivity: identifying the positive essence of postmodernity as a distinct new era in the history of philosophy. Semiotica 2011;183:31–57.

12. Deely J. Objective reality and the physical world: relation as key to understanding semiosis. Green Lett 2015;19:267–79. Available at: http://www.tandfonline.com/loi/rgrl20. Accessed February 7, 2017.

13. Deely J. Semiosis and human understanding. In: Pelkey J, Matthews SW, Sbrocchi LG, editors. Semiotics 2014: the semiotics of paradox. Ottawa (ON): Legas Publishing; 2015. p. 643–82.

14. Deely J. Introducing semiotic. Its history and doctrine. Bloomington (IN): Indiana University Press; 1982.

15. Bains P. The primacy of semiosis. An ontology of relations. Toronto: University of Toronto Press; 2014.

16. Deely J. Basics of semiotics. Bloomington (IN): Indiana University Press; 1990.

17. Sebeok TA. Signs. An introduction to semiotics. Toronto (Canada): University of Toronto Press; 1994.

18. Hoffmeyer J. Signs of meaning in the universe. Translated by BJ Haveland. Bloomington (IN): Indiana University Press; 1996.

19. Barbieri M. Introduction to biosemiotics: the new biological synthesis. Berlin: Springer; 2007.

20. Hoffmeyer J. Biosemiotics. An examination into the signs of life and the life of signs. Scranton (PA): University of Scranton Press; 2008.

21. Kull K, Deacon T, Emmeche C, et al. Theses on biosemiotics. Prolegomena to a theoretical biology. Biol Theor 2009;4:167–73. Available at: http://link.springer.com/journal/13752. Accessed February 7, 2017.

22. Favareau D, editor. Essential readings in biosemiotics. Anthology and commentary. Berlin: Springer; 2009.

23. Emmeche C, Kull K, editors. Towards a semiotic biology. Life is the action of signs. London: Imperial College Press; 2011.

24. Favareau D. Why this now? The conceptual and historical rationale behind the development of biosemiotics. Green Lett 2015;19:227–42.

25. Deely J. Intentionality and semiotics. A story of mutual fecundation. Scranton (PA): University of Scranton Press; 2007.

26. Beever J. Meaning matters: the biosemiotic basis of bioethics. Biosemiotics 2012;5:181–91.

27. Cobley P. Ethics cannot be voluntary. In: Colbley P, editor. Cultural implications of biosemiotics. Berlin: Springer; 2016. p. 61–73.

28. McGrath JC. The person at the centre of rehabilitation. In: McGrath JC, editor. Ethical practice in brain injury rehabilitation. Oxford (United Kingdom): Oxford University Press; 2007. p. 34–51.

29. Muenchberger H, Kendall E, Neal R. Identity transition following traumatic brain injury: a dynamic process of contraction, expansion and tentative balance. Brain Inj 2008;22:979–92.

30. Levack WMM, Boland P, Taylor WJ, et al. Establishing a person-centered framework of self-identity after traumatic brain injury: a grounded theory study to inform measure development. BMJ Open 2014;4:e004630.

31. Walsh RS, Muldoon OT, Gallagher S, et al. Affiliative and 'self-as-doer' identities: Relationships between social identity, social support, and emotional status amongst survivors of acquired brain injury (ABI). Neuropsychol Rehabil 2015;25:555–73.

32. Morris SD. Rebuilding identity through narrative following traumatic brain injury. J Cogn Rehabil 2004;22:15–21. Available at: http://www.jofcr.com/jcrarchives/vol22/V22I2Morris.pdf. Accessed February 7, 2017.

33. Fraas MR, Calvert M. The use of narratives to identify characteristics leading to a productive life following acquired brain injury. Am J Speech Lang Pathol 2009;18: 315–28.

34. Deely J. Toward a postmodern recovery of 'person'. Espíritu LXI 2012;143:147–65.

35. Cooke EF. On the possibility of a pragmatic discourse bioethics. Putnam, Habermas, and the normative logic of bioethical inquiry. J Med Philos 2003;28:635–53.

36. Lou HC, Changeux JP, Rosenstand A. Towards a cognitive neuroscience of self-awareness. Neurosci Biobehav Rev 2016. http://dx.doi.org/10.1016/j.neubiorev.2016.04.004.

37. Ham TE, Bonnelle V, Hellyer P, et al. The neural basis of impaired self-awareness after traumatic brain injury. Brain 2014;137:586–97.

38. Goldstein K. The effect of brain damage on the personality. Psychiatry 1952;15: 245–60.

39. Prigatano GP. Personality disturbances associated with traumatic brain injury. J Consult Clin Psychol 1992;60:360–8.

40. McGrath JC. The ethical challenge posed by acquired brain injury. Adv Clin Neurosci Rehabil 2008;8:12.

41. Musschenga AW. Empirical ethics, context-sensitivity, and contextualism. J Med Philos 2005;30:467–90.

42. Widdershoven G, Tineke A, Molewijk B. Empirical ethics as dialogical practice. Bioethics 2009;23:236–48.

43. Deely J. Defining the semiotic animal. A postmodern definition of the human being superseding the modern definition "Res Cogitans". Am Catholic Philosophical Q 2005;79:461–81.

44. Deely J. Semiotic animal. A postmodern definition of 'Human Being' transcending patriarchy and feminism. South Bend (IN): St. Augustine's Press; 2010.

45. Petrilli S. Semioethics, subjectivity and communication. For the humanism of otherness. Semiotica 2004;148:69–92.

46. Deely J. Why the semiotic animal needs to develop a semioethics. In: Deely J, Sbrocchi LG, editors. Semiotics 2008: specialization, semiosis, semiotics. Ottawa (ON): Legas Publishing; 2009. p. 716–28.

47. Deely J. From semiotics to semioethics. Or how does responsibility arise in semiosis? In: Monahan S, Smith B, Prewitt TJ, editors. Semiotics 2004/2005. Ottawa (ON): Legas Publishing; 2007. p. 242–61.

48. Petrilli S. The self as a sign, the world, and the other: living semiotics. London: Transaction Publishers; 2013.

49. Fiester A. Viewpoint: why the clinical ethics we teach fails patients. Acad Med 2007;82:684–9.

50. Beauchamp T, Childress J. The principles of biomedical ethics. 5th edition. New York: Oxford University Press; 2001.
51. Traphagan JW. Rethinking autonomy. A critique of principlism in biomedical ethics. Albany (NY): SUNY Press; 2013.
52. Levinas E. Humanism of the other. Translated by N Poller. Champaign (IL): University of Illinois Press; 2006.
53. Petrilli S, Ponzio A. Semiotics unbounded. Interpretive routes through the open network of signs. Toronto (Canada): University of Toronto Press; 2005.
54. Hoffmeyer J. Semiotic scaffolding: a unitary principle gluing life and culture together. Green Lett 2015;19:243–54.
55. de Waal C. Peirce. A guide for the perplexed. New York: Bloomsbury Academic Press; 2013.
56. Colapietro V. C.S. Peirce, 1839-1914. In: Marsoobian A, Ryder J, editors. The Blackwell guide to American philosophy. Malden (MA): Blackwell Publishing; 2003. p. 75–100.
57. Atkin A. Peirce. New York: Routledge; 2016.
58. Ochs P. Charles Sanders Peirce. In: Griffin DR, editor. Founders of constructive postmodern philosophy. Peirce, James, Bergson, Whitehead and Hartshorne. Albany (NY): SUNY Press; 1993. p. 43–89.
59. Petrilli S. Neglected aspects of Peirce's writings: contributions to ethics and humanism. Southern Semiotic Review 2013;2:235–52.
60. Nubiola J. What reasonableness really is. Transactions of the Charles S Peirce Society 2009;45:125–34.
61. Hartshorne CH, Weiss P, editors. Collected papers of C.S. Peirce, vol. 1. Cambridge (MA): Harvard University Press; 1958. p. 1931–5, 615.
62. Aydin C. On the significance of ideals. Charles S. Peirce and the good life. Transactions of the Charles S Peirce Society 2009;45:422–43.
63. Peirce CS. Clark University, 1889–1899: Decennial celebration. In: Wiener PP, editor. Charles S. Peirce: selected writings. (Values in a universe of chance). New York: Dover Publications; 1958. p. 331–5.
64. Carroll S. The big picture. On the origins of life, meaning, and the universe itself. New York: Penguin Random House; 2016.
65. Stewart M, Brown JB, Weston WW, et al. Patient-centered medicine. Transforming the clinical method. 2nd edition. Oxfordshire (United Kingdom): Radcliffe Medical Press; 2003.
66. Petrilli S. Identity today and the critical task of semioethics. Am J Semiot 2015;31: 55–116.
67. Savage TA. Ethical considerations. In: Zollman FS, editor. Manual of traumatic brain injury rehabilitation. Assessment and management. New York: Demos Medical; 2016. p. 499–506.
68. Banja JD, Fins JJ. Ethics in brain injury medicine. In: Zasler ND, Katz DJ, Zafonte RD, editors. Brain injury medicine. 2nd edition. New York: Demos Medical; 2013. p. 1374–90.
69. McGrath JC. Ethical practice in brain injury rehabilitation. Oxford (United Kingdom): Oxford University Press; 2007.
70. Fins JJ. Rights come to mind. Brain injury, ethics, and the struggle for consciousness. New York: Cambridge University Press; 2015.

Research Frontiers in Traumatic Brain Injury
Defining the Injury

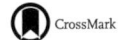

Andrew J. Gardner, PhD[a],*, Shirley L. Shih, MD, MS[b],
Elizabeth V. Adamov, DO[b], Ross D. Zafonte, DO[b,c]

KEYWORDS

- Research • Neuroimaging • Serum biomarkers • Blood biomarkers • Genetics
- Physiology • Phenotypes

KEY POINTS

- Traumatic brain injury (TBI) is a dynamic field of research that has benefited from continued advancement in technology and ongoing developments across various scientific fields.
- TBI assessment, management, and prognosis has been improved through neuroimaging, biomarkers, genetics, and physiology studies.
- TBI premorbid risk, pathophysiology, and clinical phenotype are important considerations that influence clinical outcomes.

INTRODUCTION

Traumatic brain injury (TBI) is a dynamic field of research that has exploded in the past decade. This increasing research interest has largely been associated with the continued advancement in technology (eg, neuroimaging) and ongoing developments across various scientific fields (eg, serum and blood biomarkers, genetics, and physiology), but also largely driven by the fact that TBI is a significant public health concern. It remains one of the leading causes of death among young adults and

Disclosure: See last page of article.
[a] Sports Concussion Program, Hunter New England Local Health District, Centre for Stroke and Brain Injury, School of Medicine and Public Health, University of Newcastle, University Drive, Callaghan, New South Wales 2308, Australia; [b] Department of Physical Medicine and Rehabilitation, Spaulding Rehabilitation Hospital, Harvard Medical School, 300 1st Avenue, Boston, MA 02129, USA; [c] Massachusetts General Hospital Home Base Program, Brigham and Women's Hospital, Massachusetts General Hospital, Red Sox Foundation, Boston, MA 02129, USA
* Corresponding author. Sports Concussion Program, Calvary Mater Hospital, Hunter New England Local Health District, Level 5 McAuley Building, Waratah, New South Wales 2298, Australia.
E-mail address: Andrew.Gardner@neurogard.com.au

Phys Med Rehabil Clin N Am 28 (2017) 413–431
http://dx.doi.org/10.1016/j.pmr.2016.12.014
1047-9651/17/© 2016 Elsevier Inc. All rights reserved.

pmr.theclinics.com

accounts for approximately one-half of all trauma-related fatalities globally.[1] The World Health Organization estimates that between 150 and 300 individuals per 100,000 are affected by TBI worldwide, of which around 10 million TBI-related hospitalizations or deaths occur annually.[1] In the United States alone, it is estimated that approximately 1.5 to 2 million Americans sustain a TBI annually. TBIs account for around 1.4 million emergency room visits, 275,000 hospital admissions, and 52,000 deaths in the United States each year. They contribute to approximately 30% of all deaths in the United States, annually.[2] TBI also has an enormous social and financial cost, with estimates of the annual financial burden associated with TBI ranging between $9 and $10 billion. TBI often results in residual symptoms that affect an individual's cognition, movement, sensation, and/or emotional functioning. Recovery and rehabilitation from TBI may require considerable resources and may take years.

Multidisciplinary approaches to TBI research have provided considerable insights into this injury, and epidemiologic studies have exposed the public health impact of TBI in relation to age, gender, and socioeconomic variables to incidence, prognosis, and outcome. In this special issue of *Physical Medicine and Rehabilitation Clinics of North America* on TBI, other articles have discussed fundamental issues such as the mechanism of injury, the biomechanics, pathophysiology, diagnosis, management, assessment/investigation(s), various postinjury sequelae, and potential long-term consequences. Therefore, the aim of this review is to provide an overview of the various new research approaches ("frontiers") that have been adopted around the world examining TBI, to discuss advancements in clinical trials, and to provide an overview of possible directions for future research. This discussion includes an overview of a range of TBI research, from sports concussion to severe TBI, from acute and subacute injury to long-term and chronic outcomes, from assessment and management to prognosis, specifically examining recent neuroimaging, biomarkers, genetics, and physiologic studies. The current review is less focused on discussing the underpinnings and background of the various technologies discussed (see other articles in this special issue for specific details) and more focused on the research findings and advancements in the TBI field. We also do not review potential novel treatment paradigms.

NEUROIMAGING

Neuroimaging has been explored elsewhere in greater detail in this special issue (see Elisabeth Wilde 'Neuroimaging'). The increasing sophistication of advanced neuroimaging techniques has provided researchers (and clinicians) with an incredible insight, not only into the structure of the brain, but also into various aspects of its function (eg, connectivity, metabolism, blood flow, perfusion, magnetization transfer effect, and local field inhomogeneities).[3] Neuroimaging now has an increasingly important role in the clinical diagnosis and management of TBI. A number of advanced neuroimaging techniques that go beyond the capabilities of computed tomography (CT) and structural MRI have been increasingly used in TBI research. There are many variables that may affect the quality of data (the image resolution) that these techniques can acquire (ie, the magnetic field strength, the head coil specifications, improved filling of k-space), but also the processing of the data after acquisition. These processing techniques can sometimes rely on the manufacturer's automated software, but others are operator dependent, which means that the data can vary depending on the expertise of the operator. A number of these techniques and their capabilities have been outlined in a previous review.[3]

NEUROIMAGING RESEARCH
Diffusion Tensor Imaging Traumatic Brain Injury Literature Summary

Diffusion tensor imaging (DTI) has become a frequently used technique in TBI research. There are 3 main approaches for DTI analysis (**Table 1**).

Significant differences in the various DTI metrics (fractional anisotropy, mean diffusivity, and apparent diffusion coefficient) have been observed across all levels of TBI severity, in adults and children. The reported DTI changes have revealed a correlation with injury severity,[4–8] functional outcome,[9–11] neurologic function,[12] and cognitive function.[9,13] A recent systematic review of the DTI literature in sports concussion suggested that DTI may have potential for early identification of athletes with unresolved concussions who are at high risk for a poor outcome, which may assist in more specific and effective clinical management; however, consistency across methodology within the field would improve interpretation of the data across studies.[14]

MR Spectroscopy Traumatic Brain Injury Literature Summary

MR spectroscopy MRS is an MR technique that calculates the biochemistry or neurometabolite alteration by observing the structure, dynamics, reaction state, and chemical environment of molecules. MRS has been used increasingly to investigate the presence of metabolite alteration after TBI, especially in tissue with no or little visible injury on conventional imaging. The various neurometabolites seen on MRS at 3T have been previously summarized elsewhere.[15]

MRS has been touted as a reliable technique for providing early prognostic information in relation to clinical outcome in some patient groups.[16,17] A recent systematic review of the MRS literature in sports concussion suggested that MRS may have potential as a tool for identifying altered neurophysiology and monitoring recovery in adult athletes, even beyond the resolution of postconcussive symptoms and other investigation techniques returning to normative levels.[15]

Functional MRI Traumatic Brain Injury Literature Summary

Functional MRI (fMRI) has been used to examine functional activation in all levels of TBI severity in both adults[18,19] and children.[20–22] fMRI has demonstrated a dissociation between TBI and comparison groups in their allocation of cortical resources to the encoding, maintenance, and retrieval phases of working memory. In adolescent moderate to severe TBI, increased activation during encoding and retrieval of letters of a memory task was observed using event-related fMRI, whereas the healthy matched control group displayed increased activation during maintenance relative to encoding

Table 1	
Three common DTI analysis approaches	
Technique	**Capabilities**
ROI	Predetermined regions in the brain are examined and the DTI metrics are calculated for these regions. This approach is appropriate where specific regions are expected to have been affected.
Tractography	Fiber tractography uses the collection of water molecules around fiber tracts to reconstruct the tracts.
VBA or TBSS	Enables a holistic approach without designating a specific anatomic location for analysis.

Abbreviations: DTI, diffusion tensor imaging; ROI, region of interest; TBSS, tract-based spatial statistics; VBA, voxel-based analysis.

and retrieval.[23] fMRI has also been effective in understanding and tracking recovery of mild TBI (mTBI),[24–26] in addition to the effects of rehabilitation in more severe TBI,[27–29] including understanding disorders of consciousness and arousal.[30–32]

Resting State Functional MRI Traumatic Brain Injury Literature Summary

Examining what the brain does at rest (ie, resting state fMRI) has revealed altered activation patterns in veterans of the wars in Iraq and Afghanistan who had sustained 1 or more mTBIs, compared with veterans who had not been exposed to blasts and had not sustained a TBI during deployment.[33]

Susceptibility Weighted Imaging Traumatic Brain Injury Literature Summary

The extent of hemorrhage as observed on susceptibility weighted imaging has been shown to correlate with injury severity as measured by the Glasgow Coma Scale, coma duration, and long-term outcome in children.[34] The exact role of minor hemorrhage and its influence on prognosis is unclear.

Arterial Spin Labeling Traumatic Brain Injury Literature Summary

Arterial spin labeling has shown promise in characterizing regional brain function in more severe TBI where task-evoked responses are difficult to obtain, determining the relation between changes in regional cerebral blood flow and cognitive deficits for identification of potential pharmacologic or therapeutic targets, and as a biomarker for pharmaceutical trials.[35] Perfusion parameters can be of interest both in acute mTBI as well as during the subacute and later phases of recovery from more moderate to severe TBI, to chronicle both transient and persistent TBI-related changes in cerebral perfusion.

Magnetoencephalography Traumatic Brain Injury Literature Summary

Magnetoencephalography possesses considerable potential for use in mTBI where traditional MR investigation is unrevealing.[36–39] Magnetoencephalography seems to be sensitive to abnormal neuronal signals resulting from axonal injury, signified by focal or multifocal low-frequency neuronal magnetic signal (delta-band 1–4 Hz, or theta-band 5–7 Hz) that can be measured directly and localized. Such work may help to define preexisting patterns (ie, attention deficit hyperactivity disorder [ADHD] and those with TBI).

SERUM AND BLOOD BIOMARKERS

Discovering biomarkers or biological signals for specific diseases and/or injuries has become and increasing focus of many researchers and clinicians across a number of fields of study, including TBI. At present, the discovery of an accurate biochemical assessment for identifying objectively the extent of damage after TBI remains elusive. Four decades ago, a seminal paper on the evaluation of cerebrospinal fluid (CSF) levels of cyclic AMP as a potential biomarker of depth of coma was published.[40] An increase in Glasgow Coma Scale score was associated with increased cyclic AMP in the CSF of individuals with severe TBI. Subsequently, the interest in elucidating and characterizing novel and selective TBI biomarkers has increased exponentially. Advancements in neuroproteomics have resulted in a number of candidates for serum and blood biomarkers of TBI. Indeed, some serum and blood TBI biomarker candidates have been studied for a number of years in this context. The various serum and blood biomarkers that have been investigated in the context of TBI are summarized in **Table 2**.

Table 2
Serum and blood biomarkers

Biomarkers	Description and Function
S-100B	A calcium-binding peptide produced mainly by astrocytes that exert paracrine and autocrine effects on neurons and glia. It is thought to be involved in the regulation of a number of cellular processes such as cell cycle progression and differentiation.
Tau	Proteins that stabilize microtubules. They are produced through alternative splicing of a single gene called *MAPT* (microtubule-associated protein tau). When tau proteins become defective and fail to adequately stabilize microtubules, pathologies of the nervous system can develop.
NSE	A specific serum marker for neuronal damage. It is a 78 kD gamma-homodimer and represents the dominant enolase-isoenzyme found in neuronal and neuroendocrine tissues.
GFAP	An intermediate-filament protein that is highly specific for cells of astroglial lineage. It is an intermediate filament protein that is expressed by numerous cell types of the CNS, including astrocytes, and ependymal cells.
UCH-L1	A deubiquitinating enzyme found in nerve cells throughout the brain. It is thought to be involved in cell machinery that degrades extraneous proteins.
IL-1B	A proinflammatory cytokine thought to contribute to the development of posttraumatic astrogliosis.

Abbreviations: CNS, central nervous system; GFAP, glial fibrillary acidic protein; IL-1B, interleukin-1β; NSE, neuron-specific enolase; S100B, S100 calcium-binding protein B; UCH-L1, ubiquitin carboxy-terminal hydrolase L1.

S-100B Traumatic Brain Injury Literature Summary

- CSF and serum S-100B concentrations have been reported to be higher in TBI patients compared with subarachnoid hemorrhage.[41]
- S-100B concentrations in CSF and serum were significantly higher in patients with an unfavorable outcome compared with patients with a good outcome.[41]
- Serum S-100B concentrations on admission to hospital, and at 24 hours after injury, had among the greatest predictive value for poor status at 72 hours.[42]
- Significant correlations in serum S-100B and Glasgow Outcome Scale score at 6 months.[41]
- High initial S-100B levels (>0.7 μg/dL) in serum are associated with 100% mortality.[41]
- Patients with intracerebral lesions on brain CT scan or with bad clinical evolution were identified using S-100B serum concentrations with a sensitivity of 100% and a specificity of 30%.[43]
- In severe TBI, S-100B concentrations were significantly higher in patients who died compared with survivors.[44]
- S-100B samples at 24, 48, 72, and 96 hours have been found to be useful tools for predicting mortality, with 72 hours providing the best prediction.[44]

Tau Traumatic Brain Injury Literature Summary

- Microtubule-associated protein tau was increased at days 0, 30, and 90 in TBI cases compared with controls. Maximum tau levels were recorded at 24 hours.[45]
- Day 0 tau was excellent at discriminating complicated mTBI from controls.[45,46]

Neuron-Specific Enolase Traumatic Brain Injury Literature Summary
- In severe TBI patients, only the 48-hour neuron-specific enolase samples collected were found to be useful tools for predicting mortality, with neuron-specific enolase samples at 24, 72, and 96 hours not found to be predictive.[44]
- Neuron-specific enolase has demonstrated a potential for determining outcomes at 6 months.[47]

Glial Fibrillary Acidic Protein Traumatic Brain Injury Literature Summary
- Plasma glial fibrillary acidic protein (GFAP) was increased at days 0, 30, and 90 in TBI cases compared with controls. Maximum GFAP levels were recorded at 24 hours.[45] Day 0 GFAP was excellent at discriminating complicated mTBI from controls.[45] GFAP concentration was found to strongly predict outcome after pediatric TBI, and has been recommended as a candidate biomarker for pediatric TBI.[48] Day 7 GFAP levels predicted a poorer Glasgow Outcome Scale score (1–3) at 1 year.[49]

Ubiquitin Carboxy-Terminal Hydrolase L1 Traumatic Brain Injury Literature Summary
- The ubiquitin carboxy-terminal hydrolase L1 (UCH-L1) concentration was found to strongly predict outcome after pediatric TBI, and has been recommended as a candidate biomarker for pediatric TBI.[48] Higher serum levels of UCH-L1 were observed in brain-injured children compared with controls.[48] A stepwise increase in UCH-L1 concentrations over the continuum of mild to severe TBI was observed.[48] UCH-L1 holds the potential to detect acute intracranial lesions as assessed by CT.[48] Serum UCH-L1 concentrations strongly predicted a poor outcome in this study.[48] However, another study of UCH-L1 in pediatric mTBI did not find significant differences between pediatric mTBI compared with orthopedic injury controls, and UCH-L1 concentrations did not predict postconcussion symptom scale scores over the first month after injury.[50]

Interleukin-1B Traumatic Brain Injury Literature Summary
- There is a paucity of studies that have examined circulating interleukin (IL)-1 changes after TBI, which may be a reflection of the challenges associated with measuring this protein in human TBI.[51] Serum levels of IL-1B collected at 6 hours after severe TBI have been found to be associated with Glasgow Coma Scale,[52] whereas increased serum IL-6 has been shown to be useful for the differential diagnosis of increased intracranial pressure after TBI.[53] A favorable Glasgow Outcome Scale score (4–5) at 1 year was predicted by higher admission IL-6.[49] Nonsurvivors at 1 year had day 7 IL-6 serum levels of greater than 71.26 pg/mL.[49]

GENETICS

There are currently a number of genes that are associated with TBI outcome that can be quite variable and unpredictable. The variability in post-TBI presentation of individuals with similar injury severity and preinjury intellect and educational background suggests that factors other than injury severity also have an important impact on TBI outcome. One such factor may be an individual's genotype. Genetics influence the response to and recovery from TBI. It is a dynamic area and, as such, providing an exhaustive list of potential candidate genes and alleles here is not possible owing to space limitations. So, much like in the neuroimaging section, this section provides a brief overview of research in this field. An array of genetic responses are triggered by TBI both in the acute and subacute stages after injury.[54]

Apolipoprotein E (ApoE) has historically been the most commonly studied gene, and it has been found to influence rehabilitation outcome, coma recovery, and risk of posttraumatic seizures, as well as cognitive and behavioral functions after injury. Other genes have been investigated to a lesser extent, such as catechol-o-methyltransferase (COMT) and DRD2, which may influence the degree of executive dysfunction by altering dopaminergic system function. IL genes have a role in post-TBI neuronal inflammation, and polymorphisms of the p53 gene may modulate post-TBI apoptosis. The angiotensin-converting enzyme gene may affect TBI outcome via mechanisms of cerebral blood flow and/or autoregulation, and the calcium channel, voltage-dependent, P/Q type, alpha-1A (CACNA1A) gene may exert influence via the calcium channel and its effect on delayed cerebral edema (**Table 3**).[55]

Apolipoprotein E Traumatic Brain Injury Literature Summary
- The ε4 allele is associated with poor outcomes after TBI.[56–58]
- It is unlikely that ApoE genotype influences cognitive function in the initial recovery period after TBI, regardless of injury severity.[59]

Table 3
TBI and genetics

Gene	Description and Function
ApoE	A complex glycolipoprotein that facilitates the uptake, transport, and distribution of lipids. A 4-exon gene codes for ApoE on chromosome 19 in humans. There are 3 major alleles: ε2, ε3, and ε4.
ACE	Plays a central role in regulation of blood pressure through the conversion of angiotensin I to angiotensin II. The ACE gene is located n chromosome 17 and has a common insertion/deletion mutation in intron 16.
CACNA$_1$A	The CACNA$_1$A gene codes for the α-1 subunit (pore-forming component) of the neuronal calcium channel. The functional polymorphisms in this gene might therefore alter the downstream effects of the influx of calcium into the neuron that is triggered at the time of TBI.
COMT	An enzyme that metabolizes catecholamine neurotransmitters (ie, dopamine, epinephrine, and norepinephrine).
BDNF	Initially manufactured as a precursor protein and then cleaved to BDNF and stored in and released from secretory vesicles in response to neural activity. It facilitates both early and late long-term potentiation, a process critical to the formation and maintenance of episodic and working memory.
NGB	A protein found in neurons of both the peripheral and central nervous system that appears to convey some resilience to hypoxic/ischemic insult, perhaps by facilitating oxygen transport across the blood–brain barrier or enhancing availability of oxygen to mitochondria.
DRD$_2$	Located on chromosome 11, there are more than a dozen polymorphisms described for this gene, 3 that result in amino acid substitutions and 2 that reduce the expression of DRD$_2$ receptors.
IL	The IL-1 family consists of 2 proinflammatory interleukins (α and β) and an IL receptor antagonist (IL-1RA). IL-6 is a proinflammatory cytokine that has been associated with hippocampal neurogenesis.
TP53	Considered a facilitator in orchestrating both cell growth arrest and the onset of apoptosis.

Abbreviations: ACE, angiotensin-converting enzyme; ApoE, apolipoprotein E; BDNF, brain-derived neurotrophic factor; CACNA$_1$A, calcium channel, voltage-dependent, P/Q type, alpha-1A; COMT, catechol-o-methyltransferase; DRD$_2$, dopamine D$_2$ receptor; IL, interleukin; NGB, neuroglobin gene.

- The influence of ApoE ε4 allele on neuropsychological testing, functional outcome, and in pediatric populations has been found to be variable and complex, although a review found that the ApoE ε4 allele adversely influences recovery after TBI, particularly with respect to dementia-related outcomes and outcomes after severe TBI.[60]
- A recent metaanalysis concluded that ApoEε4 allele is associated with the long-term functional outcome of patients with TBI.[61]
- Another recent metaanalysis concluded that ApoEε4 allele does not have a detrimental effect on cognition after TBI.[62]
- A further metaanalysis and metaregression concluded that the ApoEε4 allele is important to the prognosis of pediatric TBI, but not for adult TBI; this effect may be time dependent.[63]

Angiotensin-Converting Enzyme Traumatic Brain Injury Literature Summary
- Significant effects on TBI outcome were found for 3 neighboring tag single nucleotide polymorphisms in the codominant (genotypic) model of inheritance.
- Genetic variations in a specific region of the angiotensin-converting enzyme gene possibly influences outcomes of TBI patients.[64]
- The presence of 1 or more D alleles was associated with a mortality of 36.4% compared with 7.1% for 2 alleles.[65]
- D allele carrier patients (insertion/deletion) performed worse than those with 1 allele homozygous (I/I) polymorphism on tests involving attention and processing speed.[66]

Calcium Channel, Voltage-Dependent, P/Q Type, Alpha-1A Traumatic Brain Injury Literature Summary
- The CACNA1A gene may exert an influence via the calcium channel and its effect on delayed cerebral edema.[55]

Catechol-o-Methyltransferase Traumatic Brain Injury Literature Summary
- The COMT Met (158) allele was associated with higher nonverbal processing speed compared with Val (158)/Val (158) homozygotes after controlling for demographics and injury severity.[67]
- The COMT Val (158) Met polymorphism did not associate with mental flexibility or with verbal learning.[67] The COMT genotypes have been suggested to play a role of in the long-term recovery of executive function after pediatric TBI.[68] COMT polymorphism (3 COMT genotype groups; Val/Val, Val/Met, and Met/Met) did not differ in terms of neuropsychological performance or functional outcome after controlling for age, education, and severity of injury.[69]

PHYSIOLOGY OF TRAUMATIC BRAIN INJURY

In the last decade, significant growth in our understanding of the multifocal physiologic disruption that occurs after TBI has also elucidated its complexity. Macroscopic neural disruption from TBI may include edema, inflammation, ischemia, and necrosis. However, even in the absence of macroscopic neural sequelae, such as in cases of mTBI or concussion, elaborate cellular and subcellular disturbances may occur.

Minutes to Days After Brain Injury

Biomechanical forces on cerebral tissue can result in neuronal and glial cytoskeletal disruption, causing axonal, dendritic, and astrocytic damage.

- Axons, in particular, are prone to damage owing to stretching. The term traumatic axonal injury has been used to describe post-TBI microscale axonal disruptions.[70]
  - Across the spectrum of severity of TBI, cognitive impairments have recently been linked to white matter tract disruption owing to diffuse axonal injury.[71]
  - Although a disconnected axon may not necessarily cause neuronal cell death, this process hampers neuronal activity severely. The neuron may survive, but is not functional.[70] This type of microstructural neural tissue injury, although not readily apparent on CT, has been demonstrated on advanced imaging such as DTI and fractional anisotropy.[70]
  - Microtubules can also be damaged by axonal stretching, hampering axonal bidirectional transport, diminishing synaptic activity, and potentially resulting in axonal disconnection and disrupted neurotransmission.[70]

Traumatic insult also causes mechanodisruption of the cell membrane and results in ionic and neurotransmitter flux as well as increased oxidative stress.[72]

- Massive glutamate release, potassium efflux, and intracellular calcium and sodium accumulation initiate a cascade of injurious intracellular events.[72]
  - Increased intracellular calcium signals phosphorylation of axonal neurofilaments, altering their structure, and initiates proteolytic injury to other cytoskeletal components.
  - Calcium sequestration into the mitochondria via several known transporters results in mitochondrial dysfunction, oxidative stress, and free radical formation.
- Oxidative stress damages proteins, and hampers cellular protein degradation, causing toxic accumulation of defective proteins.
  - The ubiquitin–proteasome system, responsible for the controlled degradation of intracellular proteins and organelles, functions improperly in cerebral autopsy studies of humans with TBI.[73]
  - Recently, extracellular tau protein accumulation has been demonstrated after severe TBI.[74] This is a similar finding to that reported in several neurodegenerative disorders such as Alzheimer disease, tauopathies, amyotrophic lateral sclerosis, and Parkinson disease.[70,75,76]

To restore homeostasis, the injured brain requires additional energy.

- High glucose consumption is noted immediately after TBI. For unclear reasons, however, there is then a period of glucose metabolic depression, which varies in duration. At this time, cerebral glucose uptake is diminished.
- Because the cerebral blood flow volume usually does not match the metabolic demand of the injured tissue, energy demands are not met. This imbalance may also occur owing to cerebral vascular changes or glucose transport irregularity, among other theories.[70] An additional complicating factor, specifically in blast TBI, is cerebral vasospasm.[77]
- The energy crisis renders the cell vulnerable to chronic dysfunction. Cytochrome c release from mitochondria, along with activation of intracellular proteases, may then lead to cell death via apoptosis or necrosis.

This period of metabolic energy crisis may also render the neural tissue more vulnerable to repeat injury, which is of particular importance in sports-related concussion.[70]

- The risk for potentially fatal outcomes after repeat mTBI occurs with greatest incidence within the first 10 days of initial impact.[70]

- Impaired glucose metabolism lasts longer with repeat injury soon after initial impact.[70] Symptomatically, this period correlates with impaired working memory in animal studies, and lasts longer when repeat injury occurs before full metabolic recovery.[70]
- Such processes may be more pronounced in the younger brain. As the human brain continues to develop into the early 20s, cerebral glucose requirements in the pediatric population are generally higher.[78]
- The duration of this more susceptible metabolic state varies among the injured individuals, posing a clinical challenge in providing return to play recommendations.

Weeks to Months After Brain Injury

The current view of TBI is that of more of a disease process rather than single event. Pathophysiology, therefore, extends beyond the initial injury. Chronic sequelae of brain injury have been characterized by gross and microscopic pathologic findings.

- A recent study showed that chronically ongoing atrophy and cell death weeks to months after injury, specifically in the frontal and temporal lobes, is linked with chronic neurocognitive impairments at 12 months after TBI.[79]
- More recently, aggregation of tau protein in brains of patients with known repeated concussive blows, a hypothetical entity termed chronic traumatic encephalopathy, has gained attention.[80]
- A chronic upregulation of inflammatory cytokines have also been noted after TBI, suggesting that this disease process features a chronic inflammatory state.[70,81]
  - There is microglial activation and resulting inflammatory damage to brain tissue.[82]
  - Ongoing white matter atrophy in the corpus callosum months to years after TBI has been demonstrated.[71] Increased risk of Alzheimer disease and other dementias after TBI are being examined currently. Inflammation of the substantia nigra is proposed to contribute to developing Parkinson disease after TBI.[70,81] A recent study by Crane and colleagues[58] demonstrated an association between TBI with loss of consciousness and development of Parkinson disease, Lewy bodies, and microinfarcts. However, Crane's group did not find a link between TBI and Alzheimer disease.[58]

In summary, biomechanical forces to the brain with or without structural injury can initiate a neurochemical and metabolic response that is characterized by membrane potential disruption and ionic imbalances, resulting in an excitotoxic injury cascade and metabolic crisis owing to unmet energy requirements. This ionic imbalance, neurotransmitter dysfunction, and other changes in cellular function may lead to chronic cell dysfunction, neurodegeneration, and cell death. Connections are being examined between the neurophysiologic cellular processes after TBI and early and long-term clinical symptoms.

UNDERSTANDING THE PREINJURY AND POSTINJURY PHENOTYPE

Recent literature has expanded our understanding of the aggregate characteristics that may either (1) predispose an individual to sustain a TBI or (2) exacerbate the symptoms and prolong the recovery from TBI. This section summarizes the key demographic, neuropsychiatric, and behavioral attributes that typify the individual before and after TBI.

Gender

In general, males have higher rates of TBI compared with females. The rates of TBI-related visits to the emergency department, hospitalizations, and deaths in 2010 were 29% higher in men compared with women.[83] However, female athletes participating in sports with comparable rules to their male counterparts sustain more concussions and have a longer recovery.[84,85] This may be secondary to reduced dynamic stabilization of the head–neck segment in females.[86]

Prior Head Injury

A history of prior head injury increases the risk of a repeat head injury by 2 to 5.8 times.[84] In addition, athletes with a history of concussion experience more concussion-related symptoms compared with those with a first concussion.[87–89] In a case-control study of individuals diagnosed with mTBI in the emergency department, individuals with prior mTBI had increased odds (odds ratio, 18.36; 95% confidence interval, 8.60–39.17) of experiencing persistent postconcussive symptoms compared with controls matched for age, sex, and injury mechanism.[90] However, it remains unclear whether a prior concussion prolongs the recovery from subsequent concussions.[91,92]

Headache History and Symptomatology

Headache is the most frequently reported symptom after TBI, with prevalence as high as 44% for individuals with moderate to severe TBI and up to 91% for individuals with mTBI.[93] Migraine headache is the most common headache type after TBI, reported by up to 40% of individuals experiencing headache.[94] Those with migrainous symptoms experience more severe postconcussive symptoms[95] and have a protracted recovery.[91,96] Females are more likely to report a history of preinjury migraine headache and have higher rates of posttraumatic headache than males.[94] However, preinjury migraine history has not been associated with prolonged TBI recovery.[84,91]

Attention Deficit Disorder/Attention Deficit Hyperactivity Disorder

It is well-documented in the literature that individuals with attention deficit disorder (ADD)/ADHD are at greater risk for accidents and injuries.[97–99] A preinjury diagnosis of ADD/ADHD is associated with increased risk of sustaining a TBI and possibly with prolonged recovery. In a study of 139 National College Athletic Association Division I athletes, 50.4% of athletes with self-reported ADHD had experienced at least 1 concussion compared with only 14.4% of athletes without ADHD.[100] A cross-sectional study of 3993 Canadian adults with a history of self-reported TBI demonstrated increased odds of scoring positive on an ADHD screen (odds ratio, 2.49; 95% confidence interval, 1.54–4.04) and reporting a lifetime diagnosis of ADHD (odds ratio, 2.64; 95% confidence interval, 1.40–4.98) compared with those without a TBI history, controlling for sex, age, and education.[101] A metaanalysis of 5 studies on mTBI and ADHD that included 3023 mTBI patients and 9716 control subjects demonstrated a significant association between mTBI and ADHD with a relative risk of 2.0. However, the association with mTBI was weak for antecedent ADHD (relative risk, 0.98) and instead much stronger for ADHD subsequent to mTBI (relative risk, 2.2).[102] However, to shed light on the directionality of association, the same research team followed with a study demonstrating a strong association between mTBI and antecedent ADHD.[103] In individuals with mTBI, those with a history of ADHD experienced more severe postconcussive symptoms compared with those without ADHD.[103] In children with mTBI, those with ADHD had significantly higher rates of disability and lower rates of recovery than children without ADHD, even after controlling for age, sex, initial Glasgow Coma Scale score, hospital duration of stay, injury mechanism, other extracranial injuries, and duration of follow-up.[104]

Psychiatric Comorbidities: Depression, Anxiety, and Posttraumatic Stress Disorder

There is a high prevalence of psychiatric disorders in individuals with TBI, with rates of major depression and anxiety disorders ranging from 25% to 50% and 10% to 70%, respectively,[105] and rates of posttraumatic stress disorder ranging from 11% to 27%.[106,107] Up to 40% of individuals with TBI have 2 or more comorbid psychiatric disorders.[105] A history of TBI is associated with an increased odds of neurologic and psychiatric disease, including mild cognitive impairment, Alzheimer disease, Parkinson disease, depression, mixed affective disorders, and bipolar disorder.[108] A pre-injury psychiatric diagnosis is the most significant predictor of developing a psychiatric disorder after TBI, including major depressive disorder[109–111] and anxiety disorders.[110] Additionally, recent studies indicate that 22% to 45% of individuals without a premorbid psychiatric history develop a psychiatric disorder after TBI.[110,112]

Alcohol and Substance Use

There is a strong association between alcohol and/or substance use and TBI; however, the directionality of this association is unclear. Individuals with a history of pre-injury substance use are at particularly high risk of developing a substance use disorder after TBI, often resulting in poorer outcomes.

Summary

Understanding the pre-TBI "phenotype" becomes imperative as we identify potential targets for risk stratification and prevention, and comprehending the postinjury symptom constellation will identify opportunities for early clinical intervention.

FUTURE DIRECTIONS

The field of TBI is exploding with new research and fresh insight into the structural, physiologic, metabolic, and phenotypic manifestations of a traumatic insult to the brain. New and exciting arenas of TBI research include the following:

1. Translational research from laboratory and animal models to clinical paradigms of TBI.
   - Alternative substrate therapy including interventions at the mitochondrial level (eg, calcium transport blockers), targets of tau-related pathology, and special diets (eg, ketogenic diet).[78,113]
   - Pathophysiologic consequences of repeated head trauma.
2. DTI, fMRI, and fractional anisotropy to test novel neuropsychological constructs and identify associated neuroanatomical correlates.
   - Unmyelinated versus myelinated axon susceptibility and age-related implications.
   - Physiologic significance of changes measured by fMRI in the blood oxygen level-dependent signal.
   - Chronic substantia nigra atrophy with loss of dopaminergic neurons as a result of TBI.
   - Blood, urine, and CSF biomarkers of TBI to detect injury and/or determine prognosis.
     - Immature brain: heme oxygenase-1, heat shock protein 60, myelin basic protein, and s100b.[78]

○ Mature brain: alpha II spectrin, bcl-2, glial fibrillary acidic protein, heat shock protein 70, spectrin breakdown products, and tau protein.[78]

3. Genetic epidemiology and genome-wide association studies to identify genetic variants that introduce differential susceptibility to TBI. This process includes the creation and use of large biological data repositories (biobanks) for population-based studies.

   • Ion channelopathies associated with malignant edema of second impact syndrome.
   • Polymorphic alleles in genes such as APOE, BDNF, DRD2/ANKK1, and COMT.

As we delve deeper into the complex processes that underlie the injured brain, identifying the mechanistic links becomes the new frontier in TBI research. By understanding the relationship between premorbid risk, pathology, and the presenting phenotype, we can develop targeted therapies to improve outcomes.

SUMMARY

Technological advancements and scientific breakthroughs across a number of other medical and scientific fields have been the catalyst for progress in understanding TBI of all severities. This has provided TBI researchers and clinical trial investigators with constant opportunities to investigate innovative and novel methods to better understand this important disorder. This paper focused on research frontiers in TBI, from neuroimaging, serum and blood biomarkers, genetics, physiology, and finally to clinical trials. Although presented separately, the most effective studies incorporate a multifocal, multidisciplinary approach to advancing our understanding of TBI.

DISCLOSURE STATEMENT

A.J. Gardner has a clinical practice in neuropsychology involving individuals who have sustained sport-related concussion (including current and former athletes). He serves, in a voluntary capacity, as a member of the Australian Rugby Union (ARU) concussion advisory group. He has also served as a consultant to the ARU in a remunerated role from July 2016. He has received travel funding from the Australian Football League (AFL) to present at the Concussion in Football Conference in 2013. Previous grant funding includes the NSW Sporting Injuries Committee, the Brain Foundation and the Hunter Medical Research Institute (HMRI), supported by Jennie Thomas. He is currently receiving research funding through the HMRI, supported by Anne Greaves. S.L. Shih, E.V. Adamov, and R.D. Zafonte have nothing to disclose.

REFERENCES

1. Basso A, Previgliano I, Servadei F. Traumatic brain injuries. In: Aarli JA, editor. Neurol. Disord. Public Heal. Challenges. Geneva (Switzerland): World Health Organization; 2006. p. 164–76.
2. Faul M, Xu L, Wald MM, et al. Traumatic brain injury in the United States: emergency department visits, US Department of Health and Human Services, Centers for Disease Control & Prevention, hospitalizations, and deaths. Atlanta (GA): 2010.
3. Shenton ME, Hamoda HM, Schneiderman JS, et al. A review of magnetic resonance imaging and diffusion tensor imaging findings in mild traumatic brain injury. Brain Imaging Behav 2012;6:137–92.
4. Arfanakis K, Haughton VM, Carew JD, et al. Diffusion tensor MR imaging in diffuse axonal injury. AJNR Am J Neuroradiol 2002;23:794–802.

5. Benson RR, Meda SA, Vasudevan S, et al. Global white matter analysis of diffusion tensor images is predictive of injury severity in traumatic brain injury. J Neurotrauma 2007;24:446–59.
6. Betz J, Zhuo J, Roy A, et al. Prognostic value of diffusion tensor imaging parameters in severe traumatic brain injury. J Neurotrauma 2012;29:1292–305.
7. Wilde EA, Debakey ME, Ramos MA, et al. Diffusion tensor imaging of the cingulum bundle in children after traumatic brain injury. Dev Neuropsychol 2010;35:333–51.
8. Yuan W, Holland S, Schmithorst V, et al. Diffusion tensor MR imaging reveals persistent white matter alteration after traumatic brain injury experienced during early childhood. AJNR Am J Neuroradiol 2007;28:1919–25.
9. Levin HS, Wilde EA, Chu Z, et al. Diffusion tensor imaging in relation to cognitive and functional outcome of traumatic brain injury in children. J Head Trauma Rehabil 2008;23:197–208.
10. Huisman TAGM, Schwamm LH, Schaefer PW, et al. Diffusion tensor imaging as potential biomarker of white matter injury in diffuse axonal injury. Am J Neuroradiol 2004;25:370–6.
11. Wozniak JR, Krach L, Ward E, et al. Neurocognitive and neuroimaging correlates of pediatric traumatic brain injury: a diffusion tensor imaging (DTI) study. Arch Clin Neuropsychol 2007;22:555–68.
12. Caeyenberghs K, Leemans A, Geurts M, et al. Brain-behavior relationships in young traumatic brain injury patients: DTI metrics are highly correlated with postural control. Hum Brain Mapp 2010;31:992–1002.
13. Kumar R, Husain M, Gupta RK, et al. Serial changes in the white matter diffusion tensor imaging metrics in moderate traumatic brain injury and correlation with neuro-cognitive function. J Neurotrauma 2009;26:481–95.
14. Gardner A, Kay-Lambkin F, Stanwell P, et al. A systematic review of diffusion tensor imaging findings in sports-related concussion. J Neurotrauma 2012;29:2521–38.
15. Gardner A, Iverson GL, Stanwell P. A systematic review of proton magnetic resonance spectroscopy findings in sport-related concussion. J Neurotrauma 2014;31:1–18.
16. Brenner T, Freier MC, Holshouser BA, et al. Predicting neuropsychologic outcome after traumatic brain injury in children. Pediatr Neurol 2003;28:104–14.
17. Yeo RA, Phillips JP, Jung RE, et al. Magnetic resonance spectroscopy detects brain injury and predicts cognitive functioning in children with brain injuries. J Neurotrauma 2006;23:1427–35.
18. Cazalis F, Feydy A, Valabrègue R, et al. fMRI study of problem-solving after severe traumatic brain injury. Brain Inj 2006;20:1019–28.
19. Maruishi M, Miyatani M, Nakao T, et al. Compensatory cortical activation during performance of an attention task by patients with diffuse axonal injury: a functional magnetic resonance imaging study. J Neurol Neurosurg Psychiatry 2007;78:168–73.
20. Lovell MR, Pardini JE, Welling J, et al. Functional brain abnormalities are related to clinical recovery and time to return-to-play in athletes. Neurosurgery 2007;61:352–60.
21. Scheibel RS, Pearson DA, Faria LP, et al. An fMRI study of executive functioning after severe diffuse TBI. Brain Inj 2003;17:919–30.
22. Scheibel RS, Newsome MR, Steinberg JL, et al. Altered brain activation during cognitive control in patients with moderate to severe traumatic brain injury. Neurorehabil Neural Repair 2007;21:36–45.

23. Newsome MR, Scheibel RS, Hanten G, et al. Brain activation while thinking about the self from another person's perspective after traumatic brain injury in adolescents. Neuropsychology 2010;24:139–47.

24. Chen J-K, Johnston KM, Collie A, et al. A validation of the post concussion symptom scale in the assessment of complex concussion using cognitive testing and functional MRI. J Neurol Neurosurg Psychiatry 2007;78:1231–8.

25. Chen J-K, Johnston KM, Frey S, et al. Functional abnormalities in symptomatic concussed athletes: an fMRI study. Neuroimage 2004;22:68–82.

26. Jantzen KJ, Anderson B, Steinberg FL, et al. A prospective functional MR imaging study of mild traumatic brain injury in college football players. AJNR Am J Neuroradiol 2004;25:738–45.

27. Kim Y-H, Yoo W-K, Ko M-H, et al. Plasticity of the attentional network after brain injury and cognitive rehabilitation. Neurorehabil Neural Repair 2009;23:468–77.

28. Strangman G, O'Neil-Pirozzi TM, Burke D, et al. Functional neuroimaging and cognitive rehabilitation for people with traumatic brain injury. Am J Phys Med Rehabil 2005;84:62–75.

29. Strangman GE, O'Neil-Pirozzi TM, Goldstein R, et al. Prediction of memory rehabilitation outcomes in traumatic brain injury by using functional magnetic resonance imaging. Arch Phys Med Rehabil 2008;89:974–81.

30. Gosseries O, Pistoia F, Charland-Verville V, et al. The role of neuroimaging techniques in establishing diagnosis, prognosis and therapy in disorders of consciousness. Open Neuroimag J 2016;10:52–68.

31. Soddu A, Gomez F, Heine L, et al. Correlation between resting state fMRI total neuronal activity and PET metabolism in healthy controls and patients with disorders of consciousness. Brain Behav 2016;6:e00424.

32. Laureys S, Schiff ND. Coma and consciousness: paradigms (re)framed by neuroimaging. Neuroimage 2012;61:478–91.

33. Wilde EA, Bouix S, Tate DF, et al. Advanced neuroimaging applied to veterans and service personnel with traumatic brain injury: state of the art and potential benefits. Brain Imaging Behav 2015;9:367–402.

34. Trainor TP, Fitts JP, Grolimund D, et al. Grazing-incidence XAFS studies of aqueous Zn(II) on sapphire single crystals. J Synchrotron Radiat 1999;6: 618–20.

35. Van Boven RW, Harrington GS, Hackney DB, et al. Advances in neuroimaging of traumatic brain injury and posttraumatic stress disorder. J Rehabil Res Dev 2009;46:717–57.

36. Cairns NJ, Bigio EH, Mackenzie IRA, et al. Neuropathologic diagnostic and nosologic criteria for frontotemporal lobar degeneration: consensus of the Consortium for Frontotemporal Lobar Degeneration. Acta Neuropathol 2007;114: 5–22.

37. Huang M-X, Nichols S, Baker DG, et al. Single-subject-based whole-brain MEG slow-wave imaging approach for detecting abnormality in patients with mild traumatic brain injury. Neuroimage Clin 2014;5:109–19.

38. Huang M, Risling M, Baker DG. The role of biomarkers and MEG-based imaging markers in the diagnosis of post-traumatic stress disorder and blast-induced mild traumatic brain injury. Psychoneuroendocrinology 2016;63:398–409.

39. Robb Swan A, Nichols S, Drake A, et al. Magnetoencephalography slow-wave detection in patients with mild traumatic brain injury and ongoing symptoms correlated with long-term neuropsychological outcome. J Neurotrauma 2015; 32:1510–21.

40. Rudman D, Fleischer A, Kutner MH. Concentration of 3', 5' cyclic adenosine monophosphate in ventricular cerebrospinal fluid of patients with prolonged coma after head trauma or intracranial hemorrhage. N Engl J Med 1976;295: 635–8.

41. Kellermann I, Kleindienst A, Hore N, et al. Early CSF and serum S100B concentrations for outcome prediction in traumatic brain injury and subarachnoid hemorrhage. Clin Neurol Neurosurg 2016;145:79–83.

42. DeFazio MV, Rammo RA, Robles JR, et al. The potential utility of blood-derived biochemical markers as indicators of early clinical trends following severe traumatic brain injury. World Neurosurg 2014;81:151–8.

43. Bouvier D. Interest of S100B protein blood level determination in severe or moderate head injury. Ann Biol Clin (Paris) 2013;71:145–50.

44. Rodriguez-Rodriguez A, Egea-Guerrero JJ, Gordillo-Escobar E, et al. S100B and neuron-specific enolase as mortality predictors in patients with severe traumatic brain injury. Neurol Res 2016;38:130–7.

45. Bogoslovsky T, Wilson D, Chen Y, et al. Increases of plasma levels of glial fibrillary acidic protein, tau, and amyloid beta up to 90 days after traumatic brain injury. J Neurotrauma 2017;34(1):66–73.

46. Shahim P, Tegner Y, Wilson DH, et al. Blood biomarkers for brain injury in concussed professional ice hockey players. JAMA Neurol 2014;71:684–92.

47. Gao J, Zheng Z. Development of prognostic models for patients with traumatic brain injury: a systematic Review. Int J Clin Exp Med 2015;8:19881–5.

48. Mondello S, Kobeissy F, Vestri A, et al. Serum concentrations of ubiquitin C-terminal hydrolase-L1 and glial fibrillary acidic protein after pediatric traumatic brain injury. Sci Rep 2016;6:28203.

49. Raheja A, Sinha S, Samson N, et al. Serum biomarkers as predictors of long-term outcome in severe traumatic brain injury: analysis from a randomized placebo-controlled Phase II clinical trial. J Neurosurg 2016;1:1–11.

50. Rhine T, Babcock L, Zhang N, et al. Are UCH-L1 and GFAP promising biomarkers for children with mild traumatic brain injury? Brain Inj 2016;30(10): 1231–8.

51. Kossmann T, Hans V, Imhof HG, et al. Interleukin-6 released in human cerebrospinal fluid following traumatic brain injury may trigger nerve growth factor production in astrocytes. Brain Res 1996;713:143–52.

52. Tasci A, Okay O, Gezici AR, et al. Prognostic value of interleukin-1 beta levels after acute brain injury. Neurol Res 2003;25:871–4.

53. Jeter CB, Hergenroeder GW, Hylin MJ, et al. Biomarkers for the diagnosis and prognosis of mild traumatic brain injury/concussion. J Neurotrauma 2013;30: 657–70.

54. Dutcher SA, Michael DB. Gene expression in neurotrauma. Neurol Res 2001;23: 203–6.

55. Jordan BD. Genetic influences on outcome following traumatic brain injury. Neurochem Res 2007;32:905–15.

56. Jordan D, Relkin NR, Ravdin LD, et al. Apolipoprotein E epsilon4 associated with chronic traumatic brain injury in boxing. JAMA 1997;279:136–40.

57. Chen XH, Johnson VE, Uryu K, et al. A lack of amyloid beta plaques despite persistent accumulation of amyloid beta in axons of long-term survivors of traumatic brain injury. Brain Pathol 2009;19:214–23.

58. Crane PK, Gibbons LE, Dams-O'Connor K, et al. Association of traumatic brain injury with late-life neurodegenerative conditions and neuropathologic findings. JAMA Neurol 2016;73(9):1062–9.

59. Padgett CR, Summers MJ, Vickers JC, et al. Exploring the effect of the apolipoprotein E (APOE) gene on executive function, working memory, and processing speed during the early recovery period following traumatic brain injury. J Clin Exp Neuropsychol 2016;38:551–60.

60. Lawrence DW, Comper P, Hutchison MG, et al. The role of apolipoprotein E epsilon (epsilon)-4 allele on outcome following traumatic brain injury: a systematic review. Brain Inj 2015;29:1018–31.

61. Li L, Bao Y, He S, et al. The association between apolipoprotein e and functional outcome after traumatic brain injury: a meta-analysis. Medicine (Baltimore) 2015;94:e2028.

62. Padgett CR, Summers MJ, Skilbeck CE. Is APOE epsilon4 associated with poorer cognitive outcome following traumatic brain injury? A meta-analysis. Neuropsychology 2016;30(7):775–90.

63. Kassam I, Gagnon F, Cusimano MD. Association of the APOE-epsilon4 allele with outcome of traumatic brain injury in children and youth: a meta-analysis and meta-regression. J Neurol Neurosurg Psychiatry 2016;87:433–40.

64. Dardiotis E, Fountas KN, Dardioti M, et al. Genetic association studies in patients with traumatic brain injury. Neurosurg Focus 2010;28:E9.

65. Kehoe AD, Eleftheriou KI, Heron M, et al. Angiotensin-converting enzyme genotype may predict survival following major trauma. Emerg Med J 2008;25:759–61.

66. Ariza M, Matarin M, Del Junqué C, et al. Influence of Angiotensin-converting enzyme polymorphism on neuropsychological subacute performance in moderate and severe traumatic brain injury. J Neuropsychiatry Clin Neurosci 2006;18:39–44.

67. Winkler EA, Yue JK, McAlister TW, et al. COMT Val 158 Met polymorphism is associated with nonverbal cognition following mild traumatic brain injury. Neurogenetics 2016;17:31–41.

68. Kurowski BG, Backeljauw B, Zang H, et al. Influence of catechol-o-methyltransferase on executive functioning longitudinally after early childhood traumatic brain injury: preliminary findings. J Head Trauma Rehabil 2016;31:E1–9.

69. Willmott C, Withiel T, Ponsford J, et al. COMT Val158Met and cognitive and functional outcomes after traumatic brain injury. J Neurotrauma 2014;31:1507–14.

70. Giza CC, Hovda DA. The new neurometabolic cascade of concussion. Neurosurgery 2014;75:S24–33.

71. Johnson VE, Stewart W, Smith DH. Axonal pathology in traumatic brain injury. Exp Neurol 2013;246:35–43.

72. MacFarlane MP, Glenn TC. Neurochemical cascade of concussion. Brain Inj 2015;29:139–53.

73. Sakai K, Fukuda T, Iwadate K. Immunohistochemical analysis of the ubiquitin proteasome system and autophagy lysosome system induced after traumatic intracranial injury: association with time between the injury and death. Am J Forensic Med Pathol 2014;35:38–44.

74. Rubenstein R, Chang B, Davies P, et al. A novel, ultrasensitive assay for tau: potential for assessing traumatic brain injury in tissues and biofluids. J Neurotrauma 2015;32:342–52.

75. Scott G, Ramlackhansingh AF, Edison P, et al. Amyloid pathology and axonal injury after brain trauma. Neurology 2016;32:342–52.

76. Magnoni S, Esparza TJ, Conte V, et al. Tau elevations in the brain extracellular space correlate with reduced amyloid-β levels and predict adverse clinical outcomes after severe traumatic brain injury. Brain 2012;135:1268–80.

77. Alford PW, Dabiri BE, Goss JA, et al. Blast-induced phenotypic switching in cerebral vasospasm. Proc Natl Acad Sci U S A 2011;108:12705–10.

78. Giza CC, Mink RB, Madikians A. Pediatric traumatic brain injury: not just little adults. Curr Opin Crit Care 2007;13:143–52.

79. Wright MJ, McArthur DL, Alger JR, et al. Early metabolic crisis-related brain atrophy and cognition in traumatic brain injury. Brain Imaging Behav 2013;7: 307–15.

80. McKee AC, Stern RA, Nowinski CJ, et al. The spectrum of disease in chronic traumatic encephalopathy. Brain 2013;136:43–64.

81. Smith C, Gentleman SM, Leclercq PD, et al. The neuroinflammatory response in humans after traumatic brain injury. Neuropathol Appl Neurobiol 2013;39: 654–66.

82. Johnson VE, Stewart JE, Begbie FD, et al. Inflammation and white matter degeneration persist for years after a single traumatic brain injury. Brain 2013;136: 28–42.

83. Centers for Disease Control and Prevention National Center for Injury Prevention and Control. Rates of TBI-related deaths by age group—United States, 2001-2010. Injury prevention and control: traumatic brain injury and concussion. Centers for Disease Control and Prevention. Available at: http://www.cdc.gov/traumaticbraininjury/data/rates_bysex.html. Accessed July 21, 2016.

84. Harmon KG, Drezner JA, Gammons M, et al. American Medical Society for Sports Medicine position statement concussion in sport. Br J Sports Med 2013;47:15–26.

85. Marar M, McIlvain NM, Fields SK, et al. Epidemiology of concussions among United States high school athletes in 20 sports. Am J Sports Med 2012;40: 747–55.

86. Tierney RT, Sitler MR, Swanik CB, et al. Gender differences in head-neck segment dynamic stabilization during head acceleration. Med Sci Sports Exerc 2005;37:272–9.

87. Schatz P, Moser RS, Covassin T, et al. Early indicators of enduring symptoms in high school athletes with multiple previous concussions. Neurosurgery 2011;68: 1562–7 [discussion: 1567].

88. Bruce JM, Echemendia RJ. Concussion history predicts self-reported symptoms before and following a concussive event. Neurology 2004;63:1516–8.

89. Iverson GL, Gaetz M, Lovell MR, et al. Cumulative effects of concussion in amateur athletes. Brain Inj 2004;18:433–43.

90. Wojcik SM. Predicting mild traumatic brain injury patients at risk of persistent symptoms in the Emergency Department. Brain Inj 2014;28:422–30.

91. Lau B, Lovell MR, Collins MW, et al. Neurocognitive and symptom predictors of recovery in high school athletes. Clin J Sport Med 2009;15203:216–21.

92. Slobounov S, Slobounov E, Sebastianelli W, et al. Differential rate of recovery in athletes after first and second concussion episodes. Neurosurgery 2007;61: 338–44 [discussion: 344].

93. Lucas S. Posttraumatic headache: clinical characterization and management. Curr Pain Headache Rep 2015;19:48.

94. Lucas S, Hoffman JM, Bell KR, et al. Characterization of headache after traumatic brain injury. Cephalalgia 2012;32:600–6.

95. Mihalik JP, Register-Mihalik J, Kerr ZY, et al. Recovery of posttraumatic migraine characteristics in patients after mild traumatic brain injury. Am J Sports Med 2013;41:1490–6.

96. Kontos AP, Elbin RJ, Lau B, et al. Posttraumatic migraine as a predictor of recovery and cognitive impairment after sport-related concussion. Am J Sports Med 2013;41:1497–504.

97. Pastor P, Reuben C. Identified attention-deficit/hyperactivity disorder and medically attended, nonfatal injuries: US school-age children, 1997-2002. Ambul Pediatr 2006;6:38–44.

98. Lam LT. Attention deficit disorder and hospitalization due to injury among older adolescents in New South Wales, Australia. J Atten Disord 2002;6:77–82.

99. Swensen A, Birnbaum HG, Ben Hamadi R, et al. Incidence and costs of accidents among attention-deficit/hyperactivity disorder patients. J Adolesc Heal 2004;35:346.e1–9.

100. Alosco ML, Fedor AF, Gunstad J. Attention deficit hyperactivity disorder as a risk factor for concussions in NCAA division-I athletes. Brain Inj 2014;28:472–4.

101. Ilie G, Vingilis ER, Mann RE, et al. The association between traumatic brain injury and ADHD in a Canadian adult sample. J Psychiatr Res 2015;69:174–9.

102. Adeyemo BO, Biederman J, Zafonte R, et al. Mild traumatic brain injury and ADHD: a systematic review of the literature and meta-analysis. J Atten Disord 2014;18:576–84.

103. Biederman J, Feinberg L, Chan J, et al. Mild traumatic brain injury and attention-deficit hyperactivity disorder in young student athletes. J Nerv Ment Dis 2015; 203:813–9.

104. Bonfield CM, Lam S, Lin Y, et al. The impact of attention deficit hyperactivity disorder on recovery from mild traumatic brain injury. J Neurosurg Pediatr 2013;12: 97–102.

105. Vaishnavi S, Rao V, Fann JR. Neuropsychiatric problems after traumatic brain injury: unraveling the silent epidemic. Psychosomatics 2009;50:198–205.

106. Bombardier CH, Fann JR, Temkin N, et al. Posttraumatic stress disorder symptoms during the first six months after traumatic brain injury. J Neuropsychiatry Clin Neurosci 2006;18:501–8.

107. Bryant RA, Marosszeky JE, Crooks J, et al. Posttraumatic stress disorder after severe traumatic brain injury. Am J Psychiatry 2000;157:629–31.

108. Perry DC, Sturm VE, Peterson MJ, et al. Association of traumatic brain injury with subsequent neurological and psychiatric disease: a meta-analysis. J Neurosurg 2016;124:511–26.

109. Rapoport MJ. Depression following traumatic brain injury: epidemiology, risk factors and management. CNS Drugs 2012;26:111–21.

110. Gould KR, Ponsford JL, Johnston L, et al. The nature, frequency and course of psychiatric disorders in the first year after traumatic brain injury: a prospective study. Psychol Med 2011;41:2099–109.

111. Bombardier CH, Fann JR, Temkin NR, et al. Rates of major depressive disorder and clinical outcomes following traumatic brain injury. JAMA 2010;303:1938–45.

112. Bryant RA, O'Donnell ML, Creamer M, et al. The psychiatric sequelae of traumatic injury. Am J Psychiatry 2010;167:312–20.

113. White H, Venkatesh B. Clinical review: ketones and brain injury. Crit Care 2011; 15:219.

Index

Note: Page numbers of article titles are in **boldface** type.

Phys Med Rehabil Clin N Am 28 (2017) 433–447
http://dx.doi.org/10.1016/S1047-9651(17)30013-X
1047-9651/17

Moving?

Make sure your subscription moves with you!

To notify us of your new address, find your **Clinics Account Number** (located on your mailing label above your name), and contact customer service at:

Email: **journalscustomerservice-usa@elsevier.com**

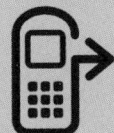

800-654-2452 (subscribers in the U.S. & Canada)
314-447-8871 (subscribers outside of the U.S. & Canada)

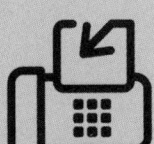

Fax number: 314-447-8029

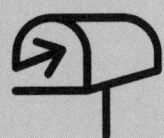

Elsevier Health Sciences Division
Subscription Customer Service
3251 Riverport Lane
Maryland Heights, MO 63043

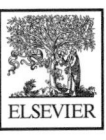
ELSEVIER

*To ensure uninterrupted delivery of your subscription, please notify us at least 4 weeks in advance of move.